THE RESEARCH BASIS FOR
AUTISM INTERVENTION

THE RESEARCH BASIS FOR AUTISM INTERVENTION

Edited by

Eric Schopler

University of North Carolina School of Medicine
Chapel Hill, North Carolina

Nurit Yirmiya and
Cory Shulman

The Hebrew University of Jerusalem
Jerusalem, Israel

and

Lee M. Marcus

University of North Carolina School of Medicine
Chapel Hill, North Carolina

KLUWER ACADEMIC/PLENUM PUBLISHERS
New York, Boston, Dordrecht, London, Moscow

Library of Congress Cataloging-in-Publication Data

The research basis for autism intervention/edited by Eric Schopler ... [et al.].
    p.   cm.
   Includes bibliographical references and index.
   ISBN 0-306-46585-X
     1. Autism—Treatment.   2. Autism—Research.   3. Autistic children—Treatment.   I.
Schopler, Eric.

   RC553.A88 R47 2001
   616.89′82—dc21

                2001025357

ISBN: 0-306-46585-X

© 2001 Kluwer Academic/Plenum Publishers, New York
233 Spring Street, New York, New York 10013

http://www.wkap.nl/

10 9 8 7 6 5 4 3 2 1

Printed in the United States of America

In memory of Lea Rabin (1928–2000 [5688–5761, Hebrew Calendar])
who inspired collaboration
at many levels

Contributors

SHOSHANA ARBELLE, Ben-Gurion University Soroka Medical Center, Beer-Sheva, 84777 Israel

DONALD B. BAILEY, JR., Frank Porter Graham Child Development Center, University of North Carolina at Chapter Hill, Chapel Hill, North Carolina 27599-8180 .

NIRIT BAUMINGER, Department of Special Education, School of Education, Bar-Ilan University, Ramat-Gan, 52900 Israel

ITEZHAK Z. BEN-ZION, Department of Child and Adolescent Psychiatry, Ben-Gurion University Soroka Medical Center, Beer-Sheva, 84777 Israel

YORAM BILU, Department of Psychology and Department of Sociology and Anthropology, The Hebrew University of Jerusalem, Mount Scopus, Jerusalem, 91905 Israel

DERMOT BOWLER, Department of Psychology, City University, London, EC1V 0HB United Kingdom

ODETTE BUKAI, Department of Psychology, The Hebrew University of Jerusalem, Mount Scopus, Jerusalem, 91905 Israel

JACOB A. BURACK, McGill University, Montreal, Quebec, H3A 1Y2, Canada

RICHARD P. EBSTEIN, S. Herzog Memorial Hospital, Jerusalem, 91351 Israel

OSNAT EREL, Department of Psychology and School of Education, The Hebrew University of Jerusalem, Mount Scopus, Jerusalem, 91905 Israel

TEMIRA FEINSILVER, S. Herzog Memorial Hospital, Jerusalem, 91351 Israel

IRIS FRIED, Ben-Gurion University Soroka Medical Center, Beer-Sheva, 84777 Israel

ANN GARFINKLE, Department of Special Education, Peabody College, Vanderbilt University, Nashville, Tennessee 37203

JOHN R. GILBERT, Department of Medicine and Center for Human Genetics, Duke University, Durham, North Carolina 27710

DAVID GLICK, Department of Biological Chemistry, Institute of Life Sciences, The Hebrew University of Jerusalem, Jerusalem, 91904 Israel

YEHUDA GOODMAN, Van Leer Institute, Jerusalem, 93114 Israel

DEBORAH D. HATTON, Frank Porter Graham Child Development Center, University of North Carolina at Chapel Hill, Chapel Hill, North Carolina 27599-8180

GRACE IAROCCI, Simon Fraser University, Burnaby, British Columbia, V5A IS6 Canada

CONNIE KASARI, Graduate School of Education and Information Studies, University of California·at Los Angeles, Los Angeles, California 90095

LEE M. MARCUS, Division TEACCH, School of Medicine, University of North Carolina at Chapel Hill, Chapel Hill, North Carolina 27599-6305

LAURENT MOTTRON, Hôpital Rivière des Prairies, Montreal, Quebec, H1E 1A4 Canada

EDNA MISHORI, Yachdav School, Tel Aviv, Israel

LUBOV NEMANOV, S. Herzog Memorial Hospital, Jerusalem, 91351 Israel

LUIGI PASTÒ, Defence and Civil Institute of Environmental Medicine, North York, Ontario, M3M 3A9 Canada

TAMMY PILOWSKY, Department of Psychology, The Hebrew University of Jerusalem, Mount Scopus, Jerusalem, 91905 Israel

MAFALDA PORPORINO, McGill University, Montreal, Quebec H3A 1Y2 Canada

LEA RABIN†, Neve Avivim, Tel Aviv, 69395 Israel

NANCY C. REICHLE, Division TEACCH, School of Medicine, University of North Carolina at Chapel Hill, Chapel Hill, North Carolina 27599-7180

ERIC SCHOPLER, Division TEACCH, School of Medicine, University of North Carolina at Chapel Hill, Chapel Hill, North Carolina 27599-6305

MICHAL SHAKED, Department of Psychology and School of Education, The Hebrew University of Jerusalem, Mount Scopus, Jerusalem, 91905 Israel

MICHAEL SHAPIRA, Department of Biological Chemistry, Institute of Life Sciences, The Hebrew University of Jerusalem, Mount Scopus, Jerusalem, 91904 Israel

CORY SHULMAN, School of Social Work and School of Education, The Hebrew University of Jerusalem, Mount Scopus, Jerusalem, 91905 Israel

LINMARIE SIKICH, Division TEACCH, School of Medicine, University of North Carolina at Chapel Hill, Chapel Hill, North Carolina 27599-7160

HERMONA SOREQ, Department of Biological Chemistry, Institute of Life Sciences, The Hebrew University of Jerusalem, Mount Scopus, Jerusalem, 91904 Israel

SIGAL TIDHAR, Department of Psychology, The Hebrew University of Jerusalem, Mount Scopus, Jerusalem, 91905 Israel

MARY E. VAN BOURGONDIEN, Division TEACCH, School of Medicine, University of North Carolina at Chapel Hill, Chapel Hill, North Carolina 27599-7180

LINDA R. WATSON, Division of Speech and Hearing, University of North Carolina at Chapel Hill, Chapel Hill, North Carolina 27599-7190

MARK WOLERY, Frank Porter Graham Child Development Center, University of North Carolina at Chapel Hill, Chapel Hill, North Carolina 27499-8180

NURIT YIRMIYA, Department of Psychology and School of Education, The Hebrew University of Jerusalem, Mount Scopus, Jerusalem, 91905 Israel

ROBERT ZIMIN, Child and Adolescent Psychiatry Unit, Sheba Medical Center, Tel Hashomer, Israel

†Deceased.

Foreword

As the past President of the Israel Society for Autism, it gives me great pleasure to congratulate Professor Schopler and his colleagues on the publication of their new book concerning the relationship between scientific research and treatment.

When we in Israel began our specifically structured education program for young children with autism, our work was based on slim to scarce know-how and information, and with no experience whatsoever. Whatever information we could gather was mostly from psychological educational centers in the U.S. One of the most important and significant connections was established between the TEACCH program of North Carolina, led and conducted by the two important scholars, Professor Eric Schopler and Professor Lee Marcus, and our Israel Society for Autism.

During our many encounters, seminars, and conferences, we profited enormously from all their accumulated expertise and scientific research, while perhaps it was also an important experience for them to see how a young society with very limited means was eventually shaping its educational program and arriving at some excellent results.

We, of course, have the highest esteem for Governor Hunt who has been following this program with so much attention and support, and we still remember his visit to Israel with distinguished representatives of the TEACCH Program.

I wish the new book every success. I know it will be an enormous contribution to all those who must cope with a difficult and painful issue—autism—for whom there is no end to the need for research and continuously improving methods of care and education.

Lea Rabin[†]

Tel Aviv
March 2000

[†]Deceased.

Preface

The relationship between North Carolina and Israel in the area of autism began in 1979 at an international conference on mental retardation in Jerusalem at which Drs. Eric Schopler and Lee Marcus gave presentations on autism and the TEACCH program. Since that visit, for the past two decades, there has been a close relationship between North Carolina and Israel in the area of autism, which has involved professionals, especially practitioners, from a variety of disciplines such as psychology, psychiatry, social work, and education. With the establishment of the North Carolina–Israel Scientific Research Program, initiated by the North Carolina–Israel Partnership, new opportunities for research collaborations were opened and a cooperative scientific workshop entitled "Research Frontiers in Autism: Genetics, Behavior and Intervention" was held in Jerusalem from June 28 to June 30, 1999. During the workshop, a group of professionals from North Carolina and from Israel presented their current research interests and projects in an attempt to find mutual areas of interest and to establish possible future collaborative projects. Other professionals working in the field of autism from the Israeli community were invited to attend. Professor Schopler delivered the keynote address at the Hebrew University of Jerusalem.

This volume is one of the many products of the workshop, and includes the authors' presentations tailored into chapters bringing together the cutting edge research for increasing our understanding and treatment of autism, a complex developmental disorder, with dramatically increasing prevalence reported internationally in recent years.

In this new millennium, more than in the past, there is a growing awareness that in the development of the new frontiers in science, public health, and the arts, all are dependent on increased collaboration, not only between nations, but also between different disciplines. The explosive increase in the volume of communication, and at higher rates of Internet speed, has provided both the need and the means for increased collaboration. In the area of developmental disabilities and autism this trend has brought with it the potential for decreasing the existing gap between disseminated knowledge and the implication of such information for improved quality of life and health. However, this potential has also gone in the opposite direction when the media and others have prematurely heralded new scientific explorations as new scientific breakthroughs.

Both Israel and North Carolina are well positioned to contribute to the growing body of knowledge and intervention in this developmental disorder. Israel has had the advantage of having had as the Chair of the National Autism Society Mrs. Lea Rabin, wife of their eminent and martyred Prime Minister, Yitzhak Rabin. She fostered a nationally supportive climate for researchers and clinicians in this area. Likewise, North Carolina is the first state in the U.S. to legislate a statewide program, based at the University of North Carolina, mandated to study and to develop cost effective services across the life span of individuals in this diagnostic category. The Division for the Treatment and Education of Autistic and Communications Handicapped CHildren (TEACCH) was established at the University of North Carolina in 1972, and has provided educational research and interventions, replicated in many countries (Schopler, 2000). The collaboration between our two states has resulted in joint research and intervention initiatives represented in part by this volume and by the research symposium on which it is based.

Because a significant proportion of our collaboration during the past two decades was directed toward intervention, we were especially interested in focusing on the relationship between research intervention outcomes. In both states we have had direct experience with new therapy techniques achieving sudden popularity, but lacking in supporting data, with anecdotal reports of remarkable outcome results. Likewise, there have been intriguing results reported from scientific studies, conducted under controlled experimental conditions. Some of these findings, even when replicated in other controlled studies, did not seem to be confirmed in the freestanding clinical situation.

In an effort to improve our understanding of the occasional gap between research and clinical application, we asked each of our chapter authors, reporting on latest research directions in their areas, also to identify direct and indirect implications of research for interventions.

Because our joint collaboration has involved both intervention and basic research, this volume represents both of these enterprises. This book is based on the first Cooperative Scientific Workshop funded by The North Carolina–Israel Scientific Research Program. The workshop, "Research Frontiers in Autism: Genetics, Behavior and Intervention" took place in June 1999 in Jerusalem, Israel. This landmark event could not have been launched without the able and energetic help of many people.

ACKNOWLEDGMENTS

Idit Aviram served as the workshop coordinator and administrator and handled countless details with efficiency. Sigal Tidhar and Tammy Pilowsky ably lent assistance. The Schools of Education and Social Work and the Department of Psychology at The Hebrew University of Jerusalem were supportive of this project. In North Carolina, we are grateful to Edward Brooks, Associate Provost, and Don Bailey, Director of the Frank Porter Graham Child Development Center at the University of North Carolina, who provided guidance and support in obtaining matching funds to enable our North Carolina scholars to participate in the workshop. Our collaboration with Israeli colleagues could not have been carried out without the support of Robert Golden, Chair of the Department of Psychiatry, and Gary Mesibov, Director of Division TEACCH. The role of the North Carolina–Israel Partnership under the leadership of Bill Cassell, Jane Patterson, and Professor Ephraim Katzir was instrumental in creating the opportunity for the cooperative scientific workshop program. We appreciate their interest and support in our work in autism. Hamutal Meiri, the Israel Executive Director of NCIP has been a tireless worker and constant supporter of the autism projects in Israel and we could not have accomplished our workshop without her. Merritt Mulman, the North Carolina Executive Director, was very helpful in providing logistical support. We are grateful to Dr. Yona Ettinger and Yakov Bartura, the Director and Deputy Director of the U.S.–Israel Bi-National Science Foundation for administering the program and for their useful advice throughout the process. Lastly, we are deeply appreciative of the efforts of Kathie Barron, editorial assistant, who helped keep us on track and cheerfully handled many technical details of the organization of this book.

REFERENCE

Schopler, E. (2000) International priorities for developing autism services via the TEACCH model. *International Journal of Mental Health*, *29*(1,2), 1–97, 1–88.

Contents

Chapter 6

FRAGILE X SYNDROME AND AUTISM   75

Deborah D. Hatton and Donald B. Bailey, Jr.

Chapter 7

ANALYSIS OF THREE CODING REGION POLYMORPHISMS IN AUTISM:
EVIDENCE FOR AN ASSOCIATION WITH THE SEROTONIN
TRANSPORTER   91

Nurit Yirmiya, Tammy Pilowsky, Lubov Nemanov, Shoshana Arbelle,
Temira Feinsilver, Iris Fried, and Richard P. Ebstein

Chapter 8

AUTISM, STRESS, AND CHROMOSOME 7 GENES   103

Michael Shapira, David Glick, John R. Gilbert, and Hermona Soreq

Section III: Communication and Social Issues

Chapter 9

COMMUNICATIVE INTENT IN AUTISM   117

Cory Shulman, Odette Bukai, and Sigal Tidhar

Chapter 10

ISSUES IN EARLY COMPREHENSION DEVELOPMENT OF CHILDREN
WITH AUTISM   135

Linda R. Watson

Chapter 11

THE EXPERIENCE OF LONELINESS AND FRIENDSHIP IN AUTISM:
THEORETICAL AND PRACTICAL ISSUES   151

Nirit Bauminger and Connie Kasari

Section IV: Education and Interventions

Chapter 12

ISSUES IN EARLY DIAGNOSIS AND INTERVENTION WITH YOUNG
CHILDREN WITH AUTISM   171

Lee M. Marcus, Ann Garfinkle, and Mark Wolery

Chapter 13

EVALUATING TREATMENT EFFECTS FOR ADOLESCENTS AND ADULTS
WITH AUTISM IN RESIDENTIAL SETTINGS   187

Mary E. Van Bourgondien and Nancy C. Reichle

Chapter 14

PSYCHOPHARMACOLOGIC TREATMENT STUDIES IN AUTISM   199

Linmarie Sikich

Chapter 15

SLEEP PROBLEMS IN AUTISM   219

Shoshana Arbelle and Itezhak Z. Ben-Zion

Chapter 16

CONCLUDING COMMENTS   229

Cory Shulman, Robert Zimin, and Edna Mishori

THE RESEARCH BASIS FOR AUTISM INTERVENTION

I

Theoretical and Developmental Framework

Introduction

Eric Schopler, Nurit Yirmiya, Cory Shulman, and Lee M. Marcus

As this book came from a collaborative workshop dealing with both basic research and intervention, we hoped to use this spirit for cooperation to shed some further light on the occasional gaps between research and clinical application. We urged each of our chapter authors, reporting on latest research directions in their areas, to identify direct and indirect implications of research for interventions or conversely, implications of current intervention for research.

The first section deals with the theoretical framework for our book. In Chapter 1, Schopler offers an interesting historical explanation for the recurring gap between research and clinical intervention. He suggests that this gap plays an important role in the marketing of treatment techniques that may be based on science, pseudo-science or anti-science. To reduce this gap he sketched out an ingenious remedy of adapting the different scientific methods as appropriate for different categories of intervention.

In Chapter 2, Burack et al. present a scholarly view of the importance of development, not only for typical children, but also for those with autism and related developmental disorders. The developmental process is best studied not only vertically across the life span of individuals, but also horizontally in cross-sectional comparisons. For autism, such studies show that certain social and language skills may improve with age, while other skills, such as communicative skills in Asperger's syndrome, show qualitative decreases as social communication demands become more complex in adolescence and adulthood. Implications for intervention are especially important for individual understanding and for selecting developmentally appropriate interventions.

Bilu and Goodman, in Chapter 3, present a fascinating paradox in terms of the research evidence for treatment outcome effectiveness. They take on the remarkable therapy phenomenon of facilitated communication (FC) as employed in one sector of the ultra-

ERIC SCHOPLER and LEE M. MARCUS • Division TEACCH, School of Medicine, University of North Carolina at Chapel Hill, Chapel Hill, North Carolina 27599-6305.   NURIT YIRMIYA • Department of Psychology and School of Education, The Hebrew University of Jerusalem, Jerusalem, 91905 Israel.   CORY SHULMAN • School of Social Work and School of Education, The Hebrew University of Jerusalem, Mount Scopus, Jerusalem, 91905 Israel.

The Research Basis for Autism Intervention, edited by Schopler, Yirmiya, Shulman, and Marcus. Kluwer Academic/Plenum Publishers, New York, 2001.

orthodox community in Israel. Perhaps more than any other treatment technique for autism, FC has been shown ineffective for improving the communication skills of individuals in the severe end of the autism spectrum. Improvement in communication skills according to most studies was shown to be the function of the facilitator rather than the client's improved communication. However, in spite of the overwhelming evidence produced by formal research, there was an increasing use of FC by the ultra-orthodox Haredi community in Israel. This community continued to use FC to reinforce their community values and to produce more positive attitudes toward the child. Thus they ignored scientific evidence and continued to use FC with unabated enthusiasm. This chapter demonstrated that FC may be ineffective according to the methods of experimental science, yet showed positive effects according to the methods of cultural anthropology, an apparent paradox addressed in Schopler's chapter.

Biological Perspectives in Section II include a range of issues from behavior genetics and genetics. In Chapter 4, Yirmiya, Shaked, and Erel report on a meta-analysis of studies comparing siblings of individuals with autism with siblings of children with other diagnoses. This statistical review suggests that siblings of children with autism are more vulnerable to autism. When the "lesser variant" or "broad phenotype" of autism is considered, the data are not clear cut. Some researchers suggest that siblings of children with autism fare less well than siblings of children with diagnoses other than autism whereas others fail to find differences. The authors of this chapter conclude that the "lesser variant" of autism should be more clearly operationalized. Furthermore, future studies should compare the well being and functioning of siblings of children with autism to those of siblings of children with other known and unknown genetic-based disorders to delineate the unique phenotype of siblings and to assist in finding the relationship between behavior and genes. In Chapter 5, Hatton and Bailey offer an interesting summary of the literature and their own work on the association between fragile X syndrome and autism. In one study, they conducted an intragroup comparison between boys diagnosed with both fragile X and autism and boys diagnosed with only fragile X. They report that boys diagnosed with fragile X and autism compared to those diagnosed only with fragile X fared less well on measures of relating and communication, imitation, and using of objects. In another study comparing boys with fragile X syndrome (without autism) to boys with autism (with fragile X), they found that although the developmental levels were comparable, social development was more impaired in the autistic sample. These data are important for the connection between behavior and genes. The last two chapters in the section focus on pure genetics. In Chapter 6, Yirmiya et al. investigated the involvement of three coding region polymorphisms in autism and found evidence for an association between the serotonin transporter promoter region (5-HTTLPR) and autism. These two genetic studies demonstrate the complexity involved in searching for the genetic basis of autism and the far-reaching potential of locating autism-related chromosomes. In Chapter 7, Shapira, Glick, Gilbert, and Soreq report on the possible association between stress, autism, and chromosome 7 genes. They suggest that some genes on chromosome 7 have been found to be associated with autism and they set out to explore whether the *ACHE* gene that encodes the enzyme acetylcholinesterase is involved and failed to demonstrate its involvement in their current study.

In Section III, connections between communication and social interaction are discussed. In Chapter 8, Shulman, Bukai, and Tidhar focus on communicative intent. They offer a scholarly tour through the definition and some important differences in the expression of such intent between typical children and those with autism. In this context they report an interesting observational study defining both quantitative and qualitative aspects of communicative intent. Clinical implications of improved understanding of the expression of communicative intent in autism are both diagnostic and educational. The potential for subtyping according to communicative intent is noted, as is the importance of context in a structured setting for motivating children to respond to social and communicative stimulation.

In Chapter 9, Watson offers a thoughtful review of problems in comprehension, widely recognized as a central problem affecting both communication and social interactions in both the amount and quality of such interactions. As the previous chapter provided deeper insights by comparing developmental differences of typical children and the problems with communicative intent in autism, so Watson makes a parallel comparison between typical children and those with autism in the achievement of comprehension. Although it is widely recognized that typical children's comprehension evolves with development, there is no consensus regarding the process by which typical children understand the communicative acts of their culture. Yet, at both the typical and the autistic ends of the continuum, it is widely believed that meaning is developed and constructed in the context of early social interaction.

From her survey of the research on comprehension for the autism spectrum, Watson concludes that there is no research support for the effectiveness of attempts to improve comprehension by improving speech perception skills as with auditory integration training. Likewise, training in improving discrimination between consonants and vowels has only limited support. By contrast, substantial evidence supports the conclusion that interventions designed to improve social–cognitive functions have also improved comprehension. These include strategies for improving attention, imitation, and joint attention. For very young children with more severe language impairment, augmented communication strategies with visual cues facilitate communication.

In Chapter 10, Bauminger and Kasari survey a primary consequence of the autism syndrome, the experience of loneliness and of friendship, a problem more often referred to than studied. As in the other chapters, they use the developmental context of typical children for understanding and differentiating the experience of loneliness and friendship for those in the autism spectrum. The overlap between social impairment on the one hand and cognitive–communication problems on the other has made the distinction between these primary features of autism difficult, especially in formulating operational research measures. The authors have reduced this problem by focusing on attachment, intimacy, and social emotional factors, while recognizing the primacy of friendship based on emotional factors leading to intimacy; on the other hand, friendship based on the more cognitive factors relates to companionship often relevant for autism. They also review the importance of the social environment for forming and maintaining friendship and the influences of peers, parents, and teachers. The authors suggest interesting implications for intervention, taking into account developmental factors. Children in the high functioning end of the autism spectrum can improve their friendship with interventions linked to speech, language, cognition, and play skills, while children on the more impaired end of the continuum can make use of social skills training. The authors caution against the overuse of social skills training while ignoring the indirect, more holistic friendship qualities necessary for more highly evolved relationships involving social–emotional understanding. Their review has useful implications for interventions at different levels of development including those able to develop friendship with attachment and intimacy, social and behavioral skills leading to companionship, and supportive interventions that bolster the formation of friendship.

Section IV includes reviews of several important areas of intervention including pre-school education, residential treatment for adults, treatment with drugs, and treatment of sleep problems. All four chapters consider the relationship between diagnosis and under-standing of the individual and the intervention implemented.

In Chapter 11, Marcus, Garfinkle, and Wolery present current trends and findings about valid factors for predicting autism with early diagnosis. The problem of predicting autism in preschool children is still in its beginning phase, and becomes less predictable the younger the child. Problems of learning and cognition are linked to intervention strategies for clarifying information, organization, and generalizing across settings with directive instructions, individualized visual supports, and other autism-related educational princi-ples. The chapter includes important components of preschool programs, derived from a review of existing preschool programs. An early intervention program for children under 3 years old utilizing this information is outlined.

In Chapter 12, Van Bourgondien and Reichle deal with the needs of adolescents and adults in the more severe range of the autism spectrum, who may be best served in a residential program. Although empirical research on the residential modality is limited, this chapter reviews both program goals and evaluation research leading to an outcome study conducted with TEACCH's Carolina Living and Learning Center. The evaluation was conducted from both the perspective of the program as a home and also as a learning environment, a setting in which residents can express preferences and engage in preferred activities. Changes in the individual should encompass both the acquisition of adaptive skills and also the reduction of inappropriate behaviors.

In Chapter 13, Sikich presents a scholarly review of the current psychopharmacologic therapies used extensively with autism. It includes a summary of current research meth-odologies for treatment efficacy. Criteria are delineated for grouping therapies as unsup-ported but potentially useful, possibly efficacious, probably efficacious, and well estab-lished. These criteria are applied to a range of drug interventions along with the known negative side effects. These include: neuroleptics, a traditional antipsychotic group; the atypical antipsychotics developed to minimize negative dyskinesia side effects; serotonin reuptake inhibitors, first used for depression and obsessive–compulsive behaviors; se-cretin, a hormone secreted by the small intestine; megavitamins; biopterin; Ritalin; and immunoglobulin therapy. With her survey, Sikich concludes that there is currently no drug therapy for dramatically changing the core symptoms or course of autism. On the other hand, there is good evidence that many different pharmacologic therapies may improve overall functioning or have benefits by enhancing other behavioral and educational inter-ventions. Age is a factor in that some medications have some support of efficacy with adults but not children, and also the reverse. This review concurs with past reviews in suggesting both caution and individualized variability in drug reactions. The gap between research and clinical application discussed in Chapter 1 has narrowed only slightly. The use of drug therapy is still more an art than a science, best decided on individual bases by collaboration between physician, parents, and involved professionals.

A brief review of sleep problems is presented in Chapter 14. Sleep problems are on a continuum of severity, estimated at 25% of typical children and over twice as many children in the autism spectrum. The report offers a summary of the types of sleep problems, their etiology and treatment. Arbelle and Ben-Zion's report is useful as information on sleep problems of autism is sparse.

The research represented in this volume has implications for intervention that are still often only indirect. That is, the findings contribute to the understanding of the disorder and help to shape treatment structures. In this manner, research has narrowed the gap between research and clinical application discussed in Chapter 1, but it continues to exist. We hope that by continuing to join multidisciplinary knowledge and clinical expertise we may be able to advance in our understanding and treatment of the enigma of autism.

2

Treatment for Autism

From Science to Pseudo-Science or Anti-Science

Eric Schopler

Some would argue that science and faith are irreconcilably opposed to each other. Most of us would probably agree that raising and teaching a child with autism requires both faith and science; nevertheless there seems to be a structural conflict between the social role of parenting versus the social role of professional research clinicians. Parents whose child has been diagnosed with autism are usually under great pressure. They need to know what the diagnosis means, what options they have, and what the possible consequences may be. After the interpretation of their child's diagnostic evaluation or their own study of the disorder they hear that autism is a developmental disorder with no known cure. At the same time they may hear that a potential cure has been identified—a drug, an intensive behavior therapy, or some other technique. Their search for the most effective intervention intensifies, and they often become involved with a new, experimental technique on the basis of personal testimony or anecdotal accounts of remarkable improvement. Their advocacy for using such a technique may encounter skepticism from their professional consultants if scientific verification for this technique does not exist. When parents expect guidance and support for determining the best treatment backed by scientific evidence, they are often frustrated by inconsistency and disagreement among professionals. Such uncertainties add to the stress of learning their child's diagnosis.

However, the roots of professional disagreements follow a fault line through the history of clinical psychology. In this chapter I trace the history of the uneasy relationship between science and pseudo-science. I review how the basic problem of intervention outcome has special relevance from the parents' perspective, and also from the growing number of professionals who have recognized that children are best helped through good parent–professional collaboration (Schopler, 1997). The concepts ᵤ
are defined, as is the nature of autism. The ever-growing inventory o

ERIC SCHOPLER • Division TEACCH, School of Medicine, University of Nort
Chapel Hill, North Carolina 27599-7180.

The Research Basis for Autism Intervention, edited by Schopler, Yirmiya, Shulr
Academic/Plenum Publishers, New York, 2001.

is reviewed with special attention to the evidentiary basis of outcome claims, ranging all the way from science to pseudo-science and anti-science. This chapter cites a profusion of treatment techniques, with outcome claims nurtured more often by enthusiasm than empirical evidence of effectiveness. The basis for the confusion is identified, along with suggestions for the direction of a more appropriate design for research evidence of treatment effectiveness.

HISTORICAL BACKGROUND

At the turn of the 20th century, scientific interest in the physical sciences and the natural sciences, based primarily on deduction, increased while psychology and the so-called social sciences were not considered sciences, but rather a branch of philosophy relying more on inferential, than deductive reasoning. At universities, psychology was studied as a branch of philosophy. However, with the advent of World War II and the need for ever more advanced military technology, Defense Department contracts were farmed out to major U.S. universities to develop the most effective military destruction and defense technology. Their development depended on the methods of the physical sciences for isolating variables in a controlled laboratory situation. As this scientific technology won the war, a more broadly funded federal research program evolved. The celebrated scientific methods were applied to the social sciences devoted to the study of complex cultural and social interactions, defined and mediated by political and human aspirations and behavior. The result was frequently flawed research with results that were either self-evident or irrelevant outside the experimental laboratory. The gap between the "hard" and the "soft" sciences has been carried forward in psychology. So-called "laws of human behavior" were formulated from misapplied methods such as rat running experiments, repetition of nonsense syllables, and measurement of galvanic skin response, to name only a few. This research did build up a body of experimental knowledge replicated in other laboratories, but was usually unable to predict complex human behavior outside the controlled laboratory. However, with its computational emphasis on observed behavior, behaviorists such as Lovaas (Lovaas, Koegel, Simmons, & Long, 1973) played an important role in rescuing autism as defined by Kanner (1943) from the untested assumptions of psychodynamic theories that had produced a widespread misunderstanding of autism as a social withdrawal from emotionally cold parenting (Schopler, 1971). At the same time, the practice of operant conditioning and discrete trial training also produced concerns of missing the child in behavioral reductionism.

This led to the rise of a theoretical orientation less bound to specific behavioral responses, sometimes called the "cognitive revolution" (Gardner, 1985), bringing renewed interests in the "mind" including the work of psycholinguistics, brain modelers, and computer scientists. For this group of researchers, primary interest in stimulus strength and response patterns was replaced by mental actions such as thinking, attending, comprehension, imagining, remembering, feeling, knowing the minds of others, and executive functioning. The relevance of these broader concepts to social intervention and special education is perhaps self-evident, but the demonstration of the effectiveness of the resulting intervention still relied on methods derived from experimental methodology.

The parallel research trends in behaviorism, information processing, and neurobiological specificity have also been linked with risks of reductionism, prompting Bruner (1996) to promote a new direction, "cultural psychology," composed of selected information and shared values, conveyed by oral history. In the context of these important historical trends it is not surprising that attempts at prioritizing therapies according to supporting research evidence have been less than successful.

PERPETUATION OF THE RESEARCH–CLINIC GAP

An American Psychological Association (APA) Task Force (1995) was convened to develop guidelines for the selection of therapies for mental disorders and psychosocial aspects of physical disorders. The Task Force tried to bridge the aforementioned research gap by making a fine distinction between treatment *efficacy* and *effectiveness*. The latter term was applied to treatments supported by the methods based on the physical sciences, while the term *efficacious* was confined to clinical application with variable interventions and comorbidity of diagnosis. The similarity in sound between efficacy and effectiveness did not disguise the fact that clinical trial research did not provide guidance for actual clinical practice (Goldfried & Wolfe, 1996). The criteria for "good science" research are quite different from the criteria for a good clinical or service program. Scientific demonstrations of treatment effectiveness are expected to be tested according to criteria derived from experimental methods. These include random assignment of subjects to the experimental group and to a matched control group. Both inclusion and exclusion criteria are to be specified. These may include age groups, gender, language levels, and intelligence test scores— in other words, variables appropriate to the intervention and its outcome claims. The length and frequency of the intervention must be specified, as treatment dosage is likely to affect outcome. If the intervention is designed for a particular disorder, such as autism, it is important that all the subjects meet the same diagnostic criteria and that these are not confounded by dual diagnoses. When all these criteria are met in a treatment outcome study, compelling evidence for effectiveness is shown. Unfortunately this rarely happens, and has not yet occurred in the case of autism (Rogers, 1998).

On the other hand, clinical or public service programs cannot readily meet such research criteria. They may come into existence by special legislative or service mandate, for a broad diagnostic category such as developmental disorders, with parent involvement and diagnostic assessment for individualized treatment and educational structures fitting the individual child. These complex variables are not easily controlled for, especially with a low-incidence disorder. In such a program random assignment of subjects to a treated and an untreated control group may not be legal or feasible. A fixed length of intervention is not consistent with individualized treatment requirements, and the exclusion of dual diagnoses can violate the right to an appropriate intervention. Superimposing artificial research criteria on such programs may not result in the most useful measures of treatment effectiveness. In short, such programs have valid differences in the selection, treatment, and study of their populations. Recognizing this state of affairs, the chairs of the APA Task Force, Lonigan, Elbert, and Johnson (1998), acknowledged that "treatments are never fully validated, and validation of any sort would imply that the mechanism for the effectiveness of the intervention were known—a condition that exists for few child or adult interventions" (p. 139).

A second contribution to the gap between research and clinical application was identified by J. Detweiler (2000) when he reviewed the most recent compendium of effective treatments for both pharmacological and psychosocial therapies. He noted that reports of effectiveness varied greatly according to whether they addressed researchers, clinicians, educators, or consumers.

Although the Task Force Chair had published the suggestion that most treatments have not been fully validated, a member of the Task Force representing services for children stated that it is the responsibility of professionals to be knowledgeable about validated treatment effectiveness and to provide families with such information (Rogers, 1998, p. 169). Reviewing the Lovaas Early Intervention Project (Lovaas, 1987), Rogers recognized that he had not yet met the Task Force criteria for treatment effectiveness. Yet she made the difficult-to-interpret assertion that his Early Intervention Project used "the strongest scientific design" (Rogers, 1998, p. 169). Perhaps she did not have access to all of the published shortcomings of his research methods and procedures (Feinberg & Beyer, 1997; Gresham & MacMillan, 1998; Schopler, Short, & Mesibov, 1989). Possibly she merely confused the term *scientific* with empirical evidence. She then selected seven additional programs approximating the same kind of experimental research criteria as being "probably efficacious," criteria not designed to fit clinical service programs. There is no reason to doubt that these programs are probably efficacious, but not because they almost met inapplicable experimental laboratory criteria.

BRIDGING THE GAP BETWEEN RESEARCH AND SERVICE

Both parents and professionals have a need to bridge the research–service gap. But different materials are available to each group. Parents newly initiated to the challenges of autism soon learn that autism is usually a lifelong disorder, with no known cure. On the other hand, a great many treatment techniques are disseminated on the Internet. In addition, pilot research, often attended by anecdotal reports of dramatic improvement, receives premature publicity. Many such pilot studies are disseminated in the news on television, or published in a convincing account of recovery written by an enthusiastic parent.

Some of the questions raised by research professionals also occur to some of the parents. Was the recovery attributable only to the use of this technique, or to one of the many other influences on the child's life? Was recovery due to the intensity or duration of the treatment? Was the diagnosis reliably established, or are there other conditions or variations of the disorder? Will the recovery last over time? Both parents and professionals recognize that dramatic improvement occurs in individuals, without scientific evidence and without answers to many of the questions raised.

There are many sources of possible error from questions of research design, control groups used, and subject selection applicable to the controlled clinical trial phase of intervention effectiveness research. However, the most important question for bridging this gap is the relationships between outcome claims and evidence for such outcome claims.

Such evidence can be divided into three categories. The first is referred to as science— the process by which questions are answered using an appropriate source of evidence. The process is objective in the sense that the research is based on the criteria of the APA Task Force, and the positive results can be replicated by different investigators using different groups of children. Such replication gives the results of scientific investigation relative independence from the investigating scientist.

The second category is pseudo-science, the process in which major errors are made in the selection and interpretation of the evidence. For example, frontal lobotomies were first developed by an eminent Portuguese neurologist, E. Moniz. For developing the surgical techniques believed to be a cure for schizophrenia, he received the Nobel Prize in 1949. Premature general use, without adequate replication of this technique in the United States, showed that it turned psychiatric patients into living vegetables. This inhumane practice was discontinued after the needless crippling of thousands of schizophrenic patients. It had not even been used in Russia or China, countries frequently criticized for human rights violations.

The third category of anti-science is reserved for flagrant perversion or disregard of evidence. Examples can be selected from different sources including Freud's tendency to regard his intuition as science. An example was cited by M. A. Hagen (1997, p. 21); Freud had a patient with whom he discovered connections between depression, sinus pain, constipation, and coitus interruptus. Because the patient's wife wanted no more children, they practiced coitus interruptus. Freud's diagnostic formulation was that this caused his system to back up psychologically and physiologically, inducing blockage. For treatment he prescribed both cocaine and nose surgery. This absurd treatment was applied to similar patients with no testing of falsifiable hypotheses and no controlled conditions of observations, and no replicable results were produced. It is unnecessary to review all the misunderstanding of autism produced by inappropriate application of Freudian theories. However, these all can be used to illustrate the use of anti-science.

In the latter part of this chapter various popular treatment techniques for autism will be reviewed to see how it is possible to slide from science to pseudo-science and anti-science. However, before discussing the degree of scientific evidence demonstrated by advocates of various treatment techniques, it is useful to review the nature of autism and the associated therapies in a continuous spectrum.

AUTISM AS A SPECTRUM DISORDER

In recent years increasing numbers of professionals refer to autism as a spectrum disorder (Wing, 1997). This comes from a growing understanding that autism is not a single condition. It involves a range of disabling behaviors, both in intensity and frequency. Moreover it is increasingly recognized that these behavior problems vary and change with development. This is reviewed in Burack's chapter in this volume. Autism is defined as a spectrum of social impairments, ranging from mute lack of awareness when autism and mental retardation coexist, to the high functioning autism or Asperger syndrome end of the continuum, in which a computer specialist has no interest in social interaction outside his computer screen. A similar spectrum can be found in the area of communication ranging from muteness and limited language skills to normal-sounding speech. Autism also involves restricted interest—from repetitive body motions and interests in parts of toys to special interest in plane schedules, higher mathematics, and computer technology.

Lorna Wing (1997) conceptualized the autism features in a different but related fashion. She referred to four groups: (1) aloof, (2) passive, (3) active but odd, and (4) overformal. In spite of the difference in definition, she also considered autism a spectrum disorder. For research purposes autism is frequently considered a unitary category, especially if the study hopes to identify a specific chromosome location or neurological locus.

However, it is unlikely that anyone having seen individuals of varying ages and developmental functions with the diagnosis of autism would not also consider it a spectrum disorder.

INTERVENTION SPECTRUM

The autism spectrum is complex, with considerable individual variation. From a medical perspective, it does not yet have either a specific established cause or treatment. Under these conditions it is not surprising that a great volume of different treatment techniques have been developed, ranging from a host of drug therapies to special diets, intensive behavior therapy, educational approaches, and cultural corrections. These techniques are as different from each other as are the individuals who have developed or advocated them. Yet, they also share certain commonalities:

1. In most every instance the initiator was convinced that his or her new technique is a good and plausible treatment. Often the technique had been tried with different subjects or different purposes. (For example, before fenfluramine was used for autism in the hope of correcting the syndrome by correcting an imbalance of the serotonim neurotransmitter, it had been used for weight reduction in Europe.)
2. The initiator then conducts a pilot study. The probability of funding for a full-scale study is usually improved if the pilot study shows promising positive results. Under this kind of pressure any positive change in the child is likely to be attributed to the experimental technique, even though anecdotal observations do not usually answer questions such as specific treatment effect. From the parents' perspective their own child's improvement is of greater interest than accurate identification of causal connections. This often results in an anecdotal account expanded to a book, picked up by the media, and disseminated before any formal study has been completed.
3. No specific treatment technique has been found to be effective with all or even most children in the autism spectrum. Moreover, costs and negative side effects are not considered, predicted, or discussed initially. Because of this process, many specific techniques are used excessively during the pilot phase. With prolonged use, they recede into short-lived fads.

The tasks of bridging the gap between pilot enthusiasm and long-range effectiveness, when applied to the larger diagnostic group, falls to the professional research/clinician's social role. However, these researchers have been committed to a scientific research methodology that has not yet bridged the gap between the controlled experimental laboratory and the parameters of clinical complexities—the gap between clinical trial and clinical application.

BRIDGING THE CONTROLLED RESEARCH TO SERVICE GAP

Scientific studies of treatment effectiveness are often evaluated by outcome claims referred to as "recovery," "cure," and "indistinguishable from normal." The application of experimental research methods coupled with such outcome claims has cast the gap between research and service into concrete spanning the last half century.

To reduce this gap without resorting to chaos theory, and while maintaining a scientific commitment to the rules of evidence, it is necessary to recognize that all interventions do not fit the same mold and cannot be conveniently studied with the same research methodology without committing pseudo-science. Three categories of intervention are defined, each with somewhat different outcome study requirements. These are reviewed as: (1) medical approaches, (2) habilitation approaches, and (3) autism culture and related interventions. The distinction between these three intervention categories involves important differences in diagnostic formulation, professional disciplines involved, outcome claims, and corrective procedures used. Although there is overlap between these three categories, important distinctions can readily be defined.

As autism includes a great spectrum of disabling conditions and treatment interventions, so it also involves the concerns of a spectrum of professionals. The medical approaches are usually represented by professionals with a medical or Ph.D. degree. They tend to have the longest educational preparation including exposure to scientific methodology. This educational background is conducive to a mandate for finding the cause and/or cure for a disorder.

MEDICAL MODEL

The medical model involves an emphasis on the etiology, or underlying causal mechanism, for autism. Like the disease model, it carries an assumption of a causal mechanism as has been demonstrated for many diseases, and carried over to a syndrome such as autism. Even when the investigator recognizes that the condition is a multiply-determined syndrome, the research strategy tends to focus on a specific mechanism, related treatment techniques, and treatment outcome identified as cure or recovery, that is, removal of the disease. Interventions in this category usually include various biochemical agents such as fenfluramine, secretin, and a variety of drugs discussed in Chapter 13 of this book. However, this category also includes behavioral or cognitive techniques such as intensive early intervention.

Such treatments may share with medical interventions the expectation of identifying an explicit treatment technique for a specific disorder or disease, derived from a demonstrated causal mechanism, with outcome expectations of cure or recovery. This most valued aspiration has not been achieved to date for the autism spectrum, although the breakthroughs in genetic engineering, alluded to in Chapter 7 of this book, hold such potential.

Specific behavioral interventions have been shown effective for a variety of autism problems. For example, aerobic exercise has been shown to reduce aggression (Gabler-Halle & Chung, 1993), disruptive behavior (McGimsey & Favell, 1988), and stereotyped and self-injurious behavior (Baumeister & McLean, 1984; Morressey, Franzini, & Kosen, 1992); it also improved attention span and on-task behavior (Powers, Thibadeau & Rose, 1992) and a score of other behaviors (Koegel & Koegel, 1995). Such specific behavioral changes are useful, and their achievement has been demonstrated with methods adopted from laboratory science. However, these behavioral changes are a far cry from treatment claims of "cure," recovery, or "return to normal functioning" for the individuals whose specific behavior has been modified. When such global treatment claims are made, they should be supported by the same kind of evidence used for demonstrating any behavioral change. This is especially important when such treatment is to be converted into social policy through judicial or legislative action. It is the treatment developers' desire to produce the political pressure needed for converting personal access to a specific treatment technique into social policy that increases the tendency to drift into pseudo-science. A few examples are given in the following sections.

Fenfluramine

It is generally agreed, at this time, that no one drug can cure or even improve all or even most cases of autism. In her scholarly review, Lin Sikich (Chapter 13, this book) summarizes the efficaciousness of the most recently studied drug therapies. The neuroleptic group is considered probably efficacious in the improvement of hyperactivity, aggression, and peer relatedness. However, negative side effects such as stiffness and involuntary movements have been found in increasing severity with long-term usage.

Fenfluramine seemed an attractive alternative to the standard neuroleptics not too long ago. Fenfluramine therapy was revealed with a dramatic flourish, reporting the surprising effect of almost doubling the IQ of a hospitalized young child during the course of the experiment (Geller, Ritvo, Freeman, & Yuwiler, 1982). Moreover, a rational basis for fenfluramine treatment known to lower serotonin levels in the brain was suggested. Some autistic children were known to have low blood levels of serotonin, whereas the majority seemed to have excessively high levels. If this was the primary mechanism in the development of autism, fenfluramine could be a corrective for children with high serotonin levels.

The dramatic IQ increase in one subject was heralded as a major breakthrough, not only in the prestigious *New England Journal of Medicine* (Ciaranello, 1982), but also on television and in newspapers. This resulted in thousands of parents requesting fenfluramine treatment for their autistic child. On the basis of the excited and premature publicity, a costly multicenter grant was funded. Beneficial effects, when they occurred, appeared only in a small proportion of subjects, and had no correlation with the treatment levels of blood serotonin. Many subjects showed negative or no effects, and in not a single case was the near doubling of IQ effect replicated. Campbell (1989) concluded that fenfluramine may be helpful for an individual autistic child, but cannot be recommended for the group. Gualtieri, Evans, and Patterson (1987) recommended that human trials of fenfluramine be delayed until the long-term neurotoxicity already reported in laboratory animals was tested more thoroughly. Here then is an example where the gap between trial study and clinic application was ignored or drowned out by publicized expectations, resulting in a pseudo-scientific process and needless costs and disappointments. Because it is a highly socially valued goal, based on the successful methods of scientific technology, claims of recovery or cure by such treatments must stand or fall by the experimental laboratory methods from which they were derived. It is these treatment techniques that have the greatest tendency to drift into pseudo-science. When the consequences of such pseudo-science also produce negative social effects, it may be described as anti-science.

ABA and the Early Intervention Project

The Early Intervention Project, also referred to as Families for Intensive Autism Treatment (FIAT), was heralded by a pilot project (Lovaas, 1987) requiring 40 hours per week of behavior therapy, administered by graduate students in various settings using primarily discrete trial learning reinforced with rewards, and undesirable behaviors suppressed with aversives such as slaps and loud no's. Aversives were subsequently discontinued. The study's outcome claim was that 47% (of 19 children studied) recovered their normal functions, while the remainder improved.

This study raised a number of important, unresolved research questions: Can these dramatic recovery claims be replicated with a random sample of autistic children? Does the outcome of "normal function" represent recovery? Is the outcome of "normal function" a result of a child's experience in the mainstream or is it a reflection of the classroom's adaptation to the child? Will IQ increase in a random sample? When aversives are discontinued, how is replication affected? Is 40 hours of intensity needed? If not, how can children who need less intensity be identified? What training is required for therapists? Can therapy be done at home or at school?

However, before replication research could answer these questions, the early intervention promoters denied all criticism of their research methods. Parents were told if they did not use this treatment their child's future would be poor. They were also told to demand this treatment technique and workshops taught parents how to sue school systems. This resulted in many parents and school systems in court asking a judge to decide issues that clearly belonged in the province of replication research. The results of this misplaced process enhanced the prospect of promoting pseudo-science.

This has led to negative consequences including the promotion of a distrustful environment between school and parents, loss of public credibility for professionals, and denial of the most appropriate intervention for individual children if different from the court-designated Lovaas method. A backlash against special needs programs is encouraged when funds are funneled into the legal system. In addition, accountability by empirical research is made irrelevant and legitimate class action initiatives have been undermined. Such negative and frequently unintended consequences are consistent with the pursuit of pseudo-science.

HABILITATION APPROACH

In this category interventions are based on the recognition that autism is not a disease or mental illness, but a lifelong disorder in which negative effects can be improved and even reversed into socially useful activities performed by individuals living a positive quality lifestyle. Both research and intervention are in the realm of education, using the most appropriate individualized techniques derived from cognitive, behavioral, and special education theory.

The primary purpose of these interventions is not so much directed at connecting cause and cure as it is to help each individual to achieve optimum adaptation. This is achieved by improving the skill level of each individual. Where there is an autism-related obstacle or delay in specific skill acquisition, environmental accommodations to the deficit are made. Both skill acquisition and environmental accommodation are essential components for optimum adaptation. The successful outcome of habilitation interventions may be quite different, depending on the individual's placement in the autism spectrum. Optimum adaptation may be in the form of successful attendance in graduate school, living independently with supported employment, or effectively participating in a sheltered workshop.

Outcome can be appropriately measured with methods different from the experimental paradigm applied in the medical approach. Skill acquisition can be measured according to the realization of the Individualized Educational Program (IEP). Questions about the effectiveness of environmental accommodation can be assessed by observational methods and peer review.

The spectrum of professionals usually working under this approach include teachers and allied health professionals such as psychologists, speech therapists, occupational and physical therapists, social workers, and rehabilitation workers. This group includes professionals with educational preparation of Master's degrees in the Western educational system. They see themselves as advocates for the individual's education and welfare, mandated to teach adaptive skills and to make appropriate environmental accommodations. Examples of the habilitation approach include augmented communication, the TEACCH Program, and mainstreaming.

Augmented Communication

Many useful techniques have been developed in recent years to enable individuals with various communication handicaps to minimize and overcome obstacles. These have included typewriters, computerized voice enhancement, pointers, and facilitated communication (FC). These techniques are usually helpful. However, it is only the promoters of FC who have tried to promote it as a means for enabling individuals previously considered with severe disability of autism or mental retardation to express remarkable cognitive skills in philosophic reflection and declaration of love (Biklen, 1990). Proponents of FC declared this a scientific breakthrough although dozens of studies (Jacobsen, Mulick, & Schwartz, 1995) demonstrated that the communication originated in the facilitator and not in the client. In spite of the lack of research evidence, FC advocates called for a redefinition of autism as motor apraxia rather than a problem of social reciprocity or communication. In Chapter 3 of this volume, Bilu shows that adherents to an orthodox, unquestioning religious ideology embrace the use of FC regardless of the evidence of its ineffectiveness.

This example of pseudo-science was leveraged to new heights when FC promoters used it as evidence for accusing parents or caretakers of physical or sexual abuse of their handicapped child. Such cases multiplied rapidly; most were usually thrown out of court for lack of appropriate evidence. But even when acquitted, the accused parents' community life was destroyed. Other negative consequences included the consumption of large sums of money by the legal system instead of services for children with special needs. Advocates prescribing FC on a routine basis deny the client's right to the most appropriate form of augmented communication. It spreads misinformation, confusion, and distrust in the absence of evidence. Such unambiguous antisocial consequences would appear to be clear markers of anti-science.

TEACCH Program

The North Carolina program for the Treatment and Education of Autistic and related Communication Handicapped CHildren (TEACCH) has been described in detail elsewhere (Campbell, Schopler, Mesibov & Sanchez, 1995; Mesibov, 1995; Schopler, 1997; Schopler, 1986). It is the only statewide program offering comprehensive services in the community from preschool age to adulthood, serving individuals in the autism spectrum. Services include: diagnosis, individualized assessment, parent–professional collaboration, public school classrooms, and supported employment. The published program descriptions also include the program goal for each client: achieving optimum adaptation by improving skills and by accommodating the environment to any remaining deficits. TEACCH offers an interesting example of a habilitation intervention that has met outcome criteria different from those considered essential by the APA Task Force (Lonigan et al., 1998). Numerous outcome studies have been published, some of which conform to the criteria applicable to medical intervention and cited by the APA Task Force. These included formal studies, published in peer-reviewed journals to demonstrate improvement in skill acquisition for children and their parents (Mesibov, 1997; Schopler, 1997). Other data demonstrated changes to accommodate remaining autism deficits in the environment at home, at school, and in the wider community (Dawson & Osterling, 1997; Ozonoff & Cathcart, 1998; Sheinkopf & Siegel, 1998). Although some of these outcome data do not conform to the criteria specified by the APA Task Force, they are appropriate to the goals and mandates of a Clinical Service program as discussed previously. The generalization of research methods from the experimental laboratory to clinical trial research has consistently produced a gap between such research and clinical service application.

As discussed in the preceding, a habilitation program such as TEACCH, with different outcome criteria, should generate evidence for both positive change in the children and in modification of the environment to accommodate unresolved autism deficits. Schopler (1997) and Mesibov (1997) have published evidence of improvement in children and the effectiveness of environmental change in the public school classroom offering structured teaching individualized for the autism spectrum. There are also descriptive data demonstrating program effectiveness that are not part of the experimental research legacy.

For example, over the 30 years' existence of the Program, the North Carolina State Department of Public Instructions increased its request for 10 public school TEACCH affiliated classrooms to about 300 such classrooms. The state increased its request from three regional TEACCH centers to eight. The Program was replicated not only within North Carolina, but also in other states and in every continent around the globe (Schopler, 2000). In addition, instructional treatment manuals have been published and revised in the series Individualized Assessment and Treatment for Autistic and Developmentally Disabled Children (Schopler, Lansing, Reichler, 1980; Schopler, Lansing, & Waters, 1983; Watson, Lord, Schaffer, & Schopler, 1989). Such evidence for service clinical program effectiveness is arguably more scientifically true than evidence from an experimental methodology that does not bridge the gap between clinical trial research and clinical application.

THE AUTISM CULTURE

With this orientation autism is seen as a cultural phenomenon. Mesibov and Shea (in press) have discussed the commonly defining features of autism as producing a culture parallel to the culture of the deaf. Consistent with this perspective, there are elements in the mainstream that match the autism culture and produce a connective link for the individuals involved. An example is introduction of visual structure into the classroom to promote learning and independent functioning for a student with autism. In addition, some individuals use their autistic characteristics to develop important products for the mainstream community. These may be in the form of art, animal science, or computer technology. Individuals who promote improvement through cultural changes do not always have special educational preparation and may include artists, computer specialists, and scientists, who, like Temple Grandin, elect to identify themselves publicly with the autism diagnosis because they recognize it as a part of their own identity. Some illustrations from art, science, and public opinion are listed in the following paragraphs.

The Squeeze Machine

Temple Grandin is a talented individual with a Ph.D. degree in animal science and a diagnosis of autism. Grandin thought that her autism developed from insufficient tactile experience during her infancy. Possibly she had a low threshold for touch, or adults refrained from such touching. From her subjective understanding of this experience, she resolved that the anxiety she experienced from tactile deprivation might be remediated by a squeeze machine in which she could control the amount of tactile contact she desired. After extensive use she claimed it made her feel better. She did not claim it would cure autism or even make all users feel better. She allowed interested buyers to try it out. If it made them feel better she would sell them a copy of her machine. Without outcome claims, no scientific outcome study seemed warranted. Instead the squeeze machine may be regarded as a kind of furniture of potential interest to individuals in the autism culture.

Grandin's subjective experience of autism also led her to produce changes in the mainstream culture. She applied her subjective autism-tactile experience to the design of the chute through which cattle move for processing (Grandin, 1992b). She designed the sideboards of the chutes of a width and height that touched the animals on both sides so they could feel secure while passing through and avoid frightening visual distractions. This design resulted in a better quality of meat and a more humane way of processing beef cattle. Her design has been exported and used in many other countries. She also has been very effective in explaining autism to professionals and the larger community (Grandin, 1992a), and she has been a popular lecturer. The changes made by Grandin's contributions have been of help to other individuals with autism by making better connections for them with the mainstream through improved popular acceptance and understanding of autism.

Paintings

Another example is Jessy Park, whose autism is brilliantly observed and described by her mother (Park, 1992, 2001). Jessy has a lovely sense of color, which she uses for expressing her artistic talents and special interests in astronomy shown in many paintings of the façade of houses against a starry night sky. These paintings have been purchased with increasing interest by professionals working with autism. By converting her autistic preoccupations into attractive paintings, Jessy Park has achieved sufficient popularity to have a one-man show in New York City for an audience well beyond the "autism community."

Pony Therapy

Pony therapy is another example of cultural intervention. It first came to my attention in England when a group of parents informed me that they had all successfully used pony therapy, or taking a child with the autism diagnosis to learn horseback riding. This seemed quite feasible, as many children with autism are quite strong in motor skills and coordination. However, it was not immediately apparent why they referred to it as "therapy." It had not been formally studied in professional journals. On interviewing this parent's group it appeared that horses were an important part of the British culture. When a child with autism was able to ride and enjoy this activity, he became part of the family interest, forming a bond that was not impeded by problems of social reciprocity. If a pony therapy advocate insisted that the social reciprocity problems were "cured" by this activity, then a study employing the methods discussed under medical intervention might have to be implemented. In the meantime it can be an effective bonding activity for the family, without elaborate evidence. A parallel development could be traced for "dolphin therapy" in locations in Israel and Florida.

Facilitated Communication

Facilitated Communication (FC), a technique shown to illustrate anti-science as a habilitation intervention, can also be reviewed for its cultural effects. Although virtually no research evidence supported the sophisticated levels of communication claimed by FC advocates, and even though FC was used for specious lawsuits alleging sexual abuse, Bilu and Goodman (Chapter 3, this book) showed this technique to have some positive cultural effects in the ultra-orthodox community. Using interview methods appropriate to cultural anthropology, they learned that FC offered the children's families a new, highly positive perception of autism, while at the same time reaffirming the validity of core values of an ultra-orthodox community. The community celebrated this positive cultural effect, while being aware that this technique did not change the children as claimed by FC advocates. Clearly, then, FC can be a failure by the research criteria of habilitation intervention categories, and still have positive cultural effects for an extreme subculture. But these unique effects can be understood only with research methods appropriate to cultural anthropology.

IMPLICATIONS FOR INTERVENTION BY SOCIAL POLICY

Which of the three intervention categories discussed here is most important to be supported with social policy or public funds? The answer is not self evident and depends on who is involved in the discussion. For individuals, parents, and professionals who see autism primarily as a disease, a condition too devastating to be tolerated, with symptoms to be suppressed or eliminated, the medical model is of the greatest interest. This group will sponsor or participate in the testing of many new experimental techniques, even when they are aware that the intervention is untested and is likely to mean high costs and unknown or negative side effects. Interventions in this category also have the advantage of being considered as part of the tradition of miraculous discoveries produced by science and technology during the past century. It has produced genetic mapping with its potential for the cure of many genetic diseases, hailed by many as the greatest scientific breakthrough of this past century. However, the potential for negative social consequences is ever present. New DNA testing may be used to deprive people of insurance coverage. Private business interests have patented promising chromosomal sites, thus controlling knowledge important to the mapping of genes. The potential for pseudo- and anti-science is clearly present.

The habilitation category is most important to families and professionals who have accepted autism as a chronic developmental disorder that, with appropriate education and community acceptance, can lead to a satisfying life. At this time the majority of individuals and their families probably belong to this group. They seek for their children the best adaptation possible, and the best quality of life, regardless of existing handicap. This is very much like the goal they have for their typical children, even though it is difficult to measure. It is not readily measured by research methods derived from experimental science, but rather by questions answered in the context of relevant environmental accommodation.

The cultural change approach has been shown to occur at several levels. The commonalities of autism have produced a culture of autism parallel to the culture of the deaf. The emphasis in these interventions is on accepting autism traits, and matching aspects of the main culture with certain autism characteristics. It can involve training and employment that match special interests of autism with related activities. Interests in routines can be matched with sorting and cleaning tasks; interests in numbers (instead of people) can be channeled into a wide range of accounting and computer tasks. This kind of cultural matching can be beneficial to both autistic and typical groups.

At the higher level of functioning in the autism spectrum are the artists and scientists, individuals such as Jessy Park, Temple Grandin, and maybe even Bill Gates and Einstein. They are able to use their special interests, preferred to social interactions, and convert their autism experience into a useful or original product. Unless these individuals run into special problems, they require only that their personality idiosyncrasies are accepted or approved by the community. Questions of cultural treatment outcomes are best measured by the methods of cultural anthropology.

While the interventions from different treatment categories cannot be shown effective by the same research criteria, all three intervention categories form an integral and necessary part of the intervention enterprise. The medical research category seeks cause and cure. The habilitation effort seeks to apply optimum adaptation, and the cultural end of the spectrum makes special contributions by changing the environment. Although this group is perhaps the smallest in number, it holds a most important promise both to the remaining individuals in the autism spectrum and to the general society. The few with the most talent serve to remind the others that it is possible to move along the autism spectrum to improvement and better adaptation. For the general public, these individuals with autism serve as an especially important reminder that they can make a special contribution to social change. Because they are unfettered by preoccupations of social reciprocity and competing interests, it is easier for them to engage in divergent thinking than it is for more typical individuals. They may be able to join the talented few who throughout history produced sociocultural change through new technology, art, and science. The acceptance of individuals in the autism spectrum is important not only to members of the spectrum, but also to the remainder who are beneficiaries of divergent thinking.

Professionals engaged in turf struggles about scientific validity of the knowledge from different disciplines should develop compassion for each other's access to the true nature of autism. We might remember that to the extent to which any of our methods have enabled us to glimpse better knowledge of course, treatment, and outcome, what we have seen is based on images floating upside down on each of our retinas, an image less precise than the constructs of our models and our quantifications of behaviors.

REFERENCES

American Psychological Association, Task Force on Psychological Intervention Guidelines (1995). Template for developing guidelines: Interventions for mental disorders and psychosocial aspects of physical disorders. Washington, DC: Author.

Baumeister, A., & MacLean, W. E., Jr. (1984). Deceleration of self injurious and stereotypic responding by exercise. *Applied Research in Mental Retardation. 5*, 385–393.

Biklen, D. (1990). Communication unbound: Autism and praxis. *Harvard Educational Review, 60*(3), 291–314.

Bruner, J. (1996). *The Culture of Education.* Cambridge, MA: Harvard University Press.

Campbell, M. (1989). Pharmacotherapy in autism: An overview. In C. Gilberg (Ed.), *Diagnosis and Treatment of Autism* (pp. 203–218). New York: Plenum.

Campbell, M., Schopler, E., Mesibov, G. B., & Sanchez, L. E. (1995). Pervasive developmental disorders. In G. O. Gabbard (Ed.), *Treatment of Psychiatric Disorders: The DSM-IV Edition* (pp. 151–178), Washington, DC: American Psychiatric Press.

Ciaranello, R. D. (1982). Hyperseratonemia in early infantile autism. *New England Journal of Medicine, 307*, 181–183.

Dawson, G., & Osterling, J. (1997). Early intervention in autism. In J. J. Guralnick (Ed.), *The Effectiveness of Early Intervention.* Baltimore, MD: Brooks.

Detweiler, J. B. (2000). A guide to treatment that works. *APA Review of Books, 45*(2), 148–151.

Feinberg, E., & Beyer, J. (1997). Creating public policy in a climate of clinical indeterminacy: Lovaas as the case example du jour. *Infants and Young Children, 10*(3), 54–66.

Gabler-Halle, D., Halle, J. W., & Chung, Y. B. (1993). The effects of aerobic experience on psychological and behavioral variables in individuals with developmental disabilities, a critical review. *Research in Developmental Disabilities, 14*, 359–386.

Gardner, H. (1985). *The Mind's New Science: A History of the Cognitive Revolution.* New York: Basic Books.

Geller, E., Ritvo, E. R., Freeman, B. J., & Yuwiler, A. (1982). Preliminary observations on effects of fenfluramine on blood serotonin and symptoms in three autistic children. *New England Journal of Medicine, 307*, 165–169.

Goldfried, M. R., & Wolfe, B. E. (1996). Psychotherapy practice and research: Repairing a strained relationship. *American Psychologist, 51*(10), 1007–1016.

Grandin T. (1992a). An Inside View of Autism. In E. Schopler & G. B. Mesibov (Eds.) *High Functioning Individuals with Autism* (pp. 105–124), New York: Plenum.

Grandin, T. (1992b). Calming effects of deep touch pressure in patients with autistic disorders: College students and animal. *Journal of Child and Adolescent Psychopharmacology, 2*, 63–72.

Gresham, F. M., & MacMillan, D. L. (1998). Early intervention project: Can its claims be substantiated and its effects replicated? *Journal of Autism and Developmental Disorders, 28*, 5–13.

Gualtieri, T., Evans, R. W., & Patterson, D. R. (1987). The medical treatment of autistic people: Problems and side effects. In E. Schopler & G. Mesibov (Eds.), *Neurobiological Issues in Autism* (pp. 373–388), New York: Plenum.

Hagen, M. A. (1997). *Whores of the Court: The Fraud of Psychiatric Testimony and the Rape of American Justice* (p. 21), New York: HarperCollins.

Jacobsen, J. W., Mulick, J. A., & Schwartz, A. A. (1995). A history of facilitated communication: Science, pseudo science and anti science. *American Psychologist, 50*(9), 750–765.

Kanner, L. (1943). Autistic disturbances of affective contact. *Nervous Child, 2*, 227–250.

Koegel, R. L., & Koegel, L. K. (1995). *Teaching Children with Autism.* Baltimore: Brookes.

Lonigan, C. J., Elbert, J. C., & Johnson, S. B. V. (1998). Empirically supported psychosocial interventions for children: An overview. *Journal of Clinical Psychology, 27*(2), 138–145.

Lovaas, O. I. (1987). Behavioral treatment and normal educational and intellectual functioning in young autistic children. *Journal of Consulting and Clinical Psychology, 55*, 3–9.

Lovaas, O. I., Koegel, B. L., Simmons, J. O., & Long, S. J. (1973). Some generalization follow-up measures on autistic children in behavior therapy. *Journal of Applied Behavior Analysis, 6*, 131–166.

McGimsey, J. F., & Favell, J. E. (1988). The effects of increased physical exercise on disruptive behavior in retarded person. *Journal of Autism and Developmental Disorders, 18*, 162–179.

Mesibov, G. B. (1995). A comprehensive program for serving people with autism and their families: The TEACCH model. In J. L. Matson (Ed), *Autism in children and adults: Etiology, assessment, and intervention* (pp. 85–97), Belmont, CA: Brooks, Cole.

Mesibov, G. B. (1997). Formal and informal measures on the effectiveness of the TEACCH Program. *Autism, 1*(1), 25–35.

Mesibov, G. B., Schopler, E., & Hearsey, K. A. (1994) Structured teaching. In E. Schopler & G. B. Mesibov (Eds.), *Behavioral Issues in Autism* (pp. 195–207), New York: Plenum.

Mesibov, G. B. & Shea, V. (in press) The culture of Autism. In G. B. Mesibov & E. Schopler (Eds.), *The TEACCH Approach to Autism.* New York: Plenum.

Morressey, P. A. Franzini, L. R., & Kosen, R. L. (1992). The salutary effect of light calisthenics and relaxation training on self-stimulation in the developmentally disabled. *Behavioral Residential Treatment, 7,* 373–386.

Ozonoff, S., & Cathcart, K. (1998). Effectiveness of a home program intervention for young children with autism. *Journal of Autism and Developmental Disorders, 28,* 25–32.

Park, C. (1992). Autism and art: A handicap transfigured. In E. Schopler & G. B. Mesibov (Eds.), *High Functioning Individuals with Autism* (pp. 250–259), New York: Plenum.

Park, C. (2001). *Exciting Nirvana.* Boston: Little Brown & Co.

Powers S., Thibadeau, S., & Rose, K. (1992). Antecedent exercise and its effects on self-stimulation. *Behavioral Residential Treatment. 7,* 15–22.

Rogers, S. J. (1998). Empirically supported comprehensive treatments for young children with autism. *Journal of Clinical Child Psychology, 27*(2), 168–179.

Rogers, S. J., & Dilalla, D. L. (1991). A comparative study of a developmentally based preschool curriculum on young children with other disorders of behavior and development. *Topics in Early Childhood Special Education, 11,* 29–48.

Schopler, E. (1971). Parents of psychotic children as scapegoats. *Journal of Contemporary Psychotherapy, 4,* 17–22.

Schopler, E. (1986). Relationship between university research and social policy: Division TEACCH. *Popular Government, 51*(4), 23–32.

Schopler, E. (1997). Implementation of TEACCH Philosophy. In D. J. Cohen & F. R. Volkmar (Eds.), *Handbook of Autism and Pervasive Developmental Disorders*, 2nd edition (pp. 787–789), New York: John Wiley & Sons.

Schopler, E. (2000). International priorities for developing autism services via the TEACCH Model. *International Journal of Mental Health, 29,* 1&2.

Schopler, E., Lansing, M. D., & Reichler, R. J. (1980). *Teaching Strategies for Parents and Professionals* (Vol. II, 2nd ed.), Austin, TX: PRO-ED.

Schopler, E., Lansing, M. D., & Waters, L. (1983). *Teaching Activities for Autistic Children.* Austin, TX: PRO-ED.

Schopler E., Short A., & Mesibov, G. B. (1989). Relation of behavioral treatment to "normal functioning." Comment on Lovaas. *Journal of Consulting and Clinical Psychology, 57,* 162–164.

Sheinkopf, S. J., & Siegel, B. (1998). Home based behavioral treatment of young children with autism. *Journal of Autism and Developmental Disorders, 28,* 15–23.

Watson, L., Lord, C., Schaffer, B., & Schopler, E. (1989). *Teaching Spontaneous Communication to Autistic and Developmentally Handicapped Children.* Austin, TX: PRO-ED.

Wing, L. (1997). The autistic spectrum. *Lancet, 350,* (9093) 1761–1766.

3

Applying Developmental Principles to the Study of Autism

Jacob A. Burack, Luigi Pastò, Mafalda Porporino, Grace Iarocci, Laurent Mottron, and Dermot Bowler

One paradox of traditional developmental theory is that growth is dependent on periods of reorganization that are often associated with apparent regressions in behavior (Bever, 1982; Zigler & Glick, 1986). Within this framework, development is not continuous but occurs in a succession of qualitative changes that emerge from periods of relative upheaval. Although this pattern of development is typically associated with the cognitive development of humans, it can also be seen in the development of inanimate things. For example, this notion might be applied to the development of a scientific discipline or subdiscipline, as periodic challenges to the prevailing thinking and reconceptualizations of accepted tenets are necessary for theoretical, methodological, and/or empirical advances. Consistent with this framework, we contend that the developmental study of autism is a subdiscipline that experienced considerable growth during the past two decades but, in its budding maturity, must be reconsidered within the context of increasingly precise theory and methodology. This task is doubly challenging for the developmental study of autism as issues relevant to both the study of normal development and of psychopathology must be considered. This task of merging domains is most problematic owing to basic differences in underlying world views and methodologies (Burack, 1997). Whereas developmental theory is based on establishing universal patterns, the essence of the study of psychopathology is the identification of specific impairments in certain clearly delineated groups and not in others. The rapprochement of these perspectives is the goal of the emergent discipline of developmental psychopathology, in which atypical and typical populations are viewed as mutually informative (Cicchetti, 1984; Sroufe & Rutter, 1984).

JACOB A. BURACK, and MAFALDA PORPORINO • McGill University, Montreal, Quebec, H3A 1Y2 Canada. LUIGI PASTÒ • Defence and Civil Institute of Environmental Medicine, North York, Ontario, M3M 3A9 Canada.   GRACE IAROCCI • Simon Fraser University, Burnaby, British Columbia, V5A 1S6 Canada. LAURENT MOTTRON • Hôpital Rivière des Prairies, Montreal, Quebec, H1E 1A4 Canada. DERMOT BOWLER • Department of Psychology, City University, London, EC1V OHB United Kingdom.

The Research Basis for Autism Intervention, edited by Schopler, Yirmiya, Shulman, and Marcus. Kluwer Academic/Plenum Publishers, New York, 2001.

The severity and pervasiveness of the associated problems manifested by persons with autism might suggest that they are so different from other people that the application of the typical blueprint of development might not be appropriate. However, the application of developmental principles provides a framework for understanding the emergence of both typical and atypical behaviors that is informed by decades of study of children with varied abilities and backgrounds. The hallmarks of the traditional developmental approach include issues of sequences, rates, and levels of development, and cross-domain relationships in level of functioning. In this chapter, we examine both the advantages and difficulties in using these developmental tenets for the study of autism within the context of questions that are intrinsic to the discipline of psychopathology and raise issues relevant to diagnosis and treatment.

DEVELOPMENTAL PRINCIPLES IN THE STUDY OF PERSONS WITH AUTISM

In our review of a developmental approach, we focus on principles of cognitive development that are associated with traditional developmental theorists such as Jean Piaget and Heinz Werner. During the past three decades, these frameworks were trans-formed considerably by developmentalists who sought to provide theoretical frameworks that were better able to incorporate both individual differences and the effects of external influences such as family, environment, and culture. Accordingly, they are not inclusive of the expanding realm of developmental thought, and their centrality to contemporary devel-opmental thinking is considerably diminished (Kessen, 1984). However, these early theo-ries provide a still helpful and commonly used framework for initial discussions of the development of behavior within and across different domains of functioning, or, as we will refer to them, the "vertical" and "horizontal" stories of development (for discussions of the merits of traditional developmental theories, see Chandler, 1997; Enns, Burack, Iarocci, & Randolph, 2000; Frye, 1991). The vertical stories refer to the progression of development through the paths of milestones associated with each domain of functioning or skill, and the horizontal stories to the relationships across areas of functioning. These types of story represent central tenets of classic developmental thought that are distinct but not entirely unrelated. The vertical stories derive from the notion of development as universally teleo-logical and the horizontal stories from the concept of systemically organized development.

Sequences of Development

The premise of teleological development is that the sequence of development, or attainment of milestones and abilities, is universal, regardless of rate of development. The theoretical necessity of this phenomenon can be argued from perspectives of biological commonalities, theoretical logic, linguistic and information-processing universals, or cul-tural and environmental similarities (Hodapp, 1990). The empirical evidence is seen within the consistency in sequences in the attainment of Piaget's problem-solving skills and other ve and language behavior across children from different cultures and with typicalities, including mental retardation (Weisz, Yeates, & Zigler, 1982; 979). The essential question is whether the sequences of development d domain of study are the same for a specific group as compared to the general population. This is informative for understanding developmental theory as it addresses issues of universality and the necessity of developmental milestones (Hodapp & Burack, 1990), and for assessing the performance and behavior of a group as it provides a guide for the expected order of acquisition of skills and behaviors.

From a methodological viewpoint, adherence to this assumption of similar sequence permits inter-individual and cross-group comparisons for all aspects of development as it prescribes a common metric for the essential notion of progression through stages. Thus, comparisons of rate of development are meaningful as the course of development is the same across persons. Similarly, comparisons with regard to level of functioning become significant as the various levels are maintained within a constant ordering. Thus, a specific level of functioning, Y, is always preceded by the same number of levels, $Y-1$ ($Y-2$, $Y-3$ ...), that occur consistently in the same order. Evidence that persons with autism traverse typical or universal developmental sequences is cited with regard to receptive and expressive communication (Burack & Volkmar, 1992; Wenar, Ruttenberg, Kalish-Weiss, & Wolf, 1986), Piagetian tasks (Morgan, 1986; Morgan, Cutrer, Coplin, & Rodrigue, 1989), and theory of mind (e.g., Baron-Cohen, 1989; Happé, 2001; Tager-Flusberg, 2001), although evidence of atypical sequences is also cited, especially in the social realm (Wenar et al., 1986).

Developmental Level

Developmental level, the distance traveled, refers to the level of functioning of the individual and is associated with the acquisition of skills and abilities and levels of efficiency in performance. Each developmental level is characterized with distinct developmental histories and issues (Sroufe & Rutter, 1984). This may be seen at a micro-level with regard to specific areas of functioning or at a macro-level with regard to general developmental level. In both cases, time is again often used as a metric with which to communicate levels of functioning—within the psychometric tradition, these are commonly discussed in terms of the average age at which the level of functioning is commonly displayed. In contrast to these age-related designations, developmental level is described in Piagetian operational terms of specific abilities and functions and more accurately reflects the functional independence between developmental level and age. This distinction is best exemplified by the general disassociation between level and age among persons with mental retardation (with and without autism). As the cognitive functioning of the majority of persons with autism is in the range of mental retardation, performance deficits that were initially thought to characterize the functioning of these persons are often simply a function of lower developmental level (Volkmar, Burack, & Cohen, 1990).

Developmental disassociations are also evident in the discrepancies among domains that are characteristic even among higher functioning persons with autism. These disassociations between developmental level and expected concomitant age are evidenced at every stage of development of an ability or skill from initial emergence to eventual attainment. However, the patterns are not consistent throughout development. For example, the manifestation of social communicative difficulties among persons with autism may change substantially during the course of development. Among younger children with autism, profound deficits are common in social communicative skills, such as eye contact, nonverbal communication through the use of gestures, and joint attention. By school age, however, children with autism manifest some selective attachments to their parents and generally improved communicative skills. Conversely, behavior problems (e.g., self-stimulatory behaviors) may become more marked over the course of development (Piven, Harper, Palmer, & Arndt, 1996). Similarly, increased discrepancies in levels of social communicative functioning and adjustment between persons with and without autism are typically observed during adolescence, the period in development when social communication skills become more complex and maintaining social relationships requires more sophisticated abilities, including initiating and sustaining conversations, socioemotional reciprocity, and empathy (Sigman & Ungerer, 1984). Thus, understanding the unique relationships between specific difficulties and developmental level requires longitudinal or cross-sectional studies in which functioning is considered at various developmental levels.

Rate of Development

In typical developmental contexts, rate is discussed with regard to two independent constructs that are used to measure speed of travel—the distance already traveled over the amount of time that passed since the commencement of the "journey." This equation is, of course, the commonly used one of kilometers or miles per hour. In development, the distance traveled is the level of functioning that in Piagetian terms is discussed with regard to milestones or abilities already attained and in psychometric frameworks with regard to mental age or developmental level. The time passed component of the equation is, of course, the individual's age. The relevance of time to development is typically overstated, as development is largely independent of time (Hodapp, Burack, & Zigler, 1990). As evidenced in the literature on sequences of cognitive development among persons with mental retardation, the integrity of development is not contingent on time. This is best expressed by Werner (1948, 1957), who demonstrated inherent similarities between microgenic development that is measured in milliseconds and orthogenic development that is measured across years (for a review, see Enns et al., 2000). Despite the inconsequentiality of time to developmental progress, it provides a metric for calculating the rate of development, a useful index for evaluating individuals' developmental precocity in relation to their same-aged peers and to predict future levels of functioning.

This relationship of rate between distance traveled and chronological age is the hallmark of traditional measures of the psychometric notions of IQ and DQ. Although psychometric measures tend to be relatively reliable predictors of future behavior, the rate of development cannot be seen as constant throughout development. The depiction of a constant rate is an illusion that results from the plotting of development over extended periods of time and the ignoring of variations within shorter time frames. Rather, specific periods of development vary considerably with regard to rate as some are associated with the rapid acquisition of abilities and others with apparently long intervals of little movement (Fischer, Pipp, & Bullock, 1984).

The Association between Developmental Level and Impairment: Early Deficits

The charting of a comprehensive picture of development at either the micro- or macro-level is dependent on assessments at different ages or levels of functioning. This type of charting is necessary, as constancy of impairments can vary. Thus, some difficulties evident early on in development may persist throughout development, whereas others may fade later in development when performance of the task is eventually mastered. For example, gaze avoidance is fairly typical in young children with autism, but is not evident later in development (Fecteau, Mottron, Berthiaume, & Burack, in preparation; Piven et al., 1996). Similarly, higher functioning persons with autism routinely attain the first level of theory of mind (ToM), albeit at a much later mental age than typically developing persons and those with mental retardation (Yirmiya, Erel, Shaked, & Solomonica-Levi, 1998), and even attain second-order ToM by adulthood (Bowler, 1992).

The extent to which eventual attainment of a skill or ability can be considered "catching up" needs to be evaluated within the context of several issues related to the nature of the developmental process and its outcome. The eventual attainment of an ability or skill does not ensure that the developmental process is typical but just delayed, or that the processes used in displaying the attained skill are similar to those used by others. One alternative is that, with experience, strategies usually not associated with a task can be adapted for its performance. A second concern regarding "catching up" is that the delay in attaining the skill may be associated with other problems that arose because of the delay in attaining the skill. For example, whereas persons with autism may finally be able to complete first-order ToM tasks, the more compelling question is, What are the effects of the delay in attaining it? A direct consequence may be a delay or an inability to attain higher order ToM tasks. A less directly observable, but possibly more problematic, outcome is that that they missed out on considerable social information from their environment during the extended period in which they were less likely to learn from, succeed in, and feel rewarded by social interactions.

The Association between Developmental Level and Impairment: Late Deficits

In another scenario, development may appear typical at young ages when all that is required is simple behaviors or understanding, but become deficient later in development when more complex behaviors or understanding is required. The example of ToM is relevant here as most higher functioning persons with autism display first-order ToM but considerably fewer display second-order ToM. Similarly, persons with Asperger syndrome acquire language skills at the expected ages but display qualitative abnormalities in pragmatic language beginning soon thereafter and continuing throughout development (APA, 1994).

In addition to the manifestation of lower developmental levels, late deficits can also be associated with maladaptive and idiosyncratic behaviors as exemplified by ritualistic statements, such as repetitive questioning, that appear only among persons with autism once language development is sophisticated enough for the verbalization of questions (Fecteau et al., in preparation; Piven et al., 1996). Similarly, the commonly observed circumscribed pattern of interests among typical children older than 4 years that entails the collection of, interest in, and questions about, is evident among persons with autism but with considerably more intensity, higher levels of expertise, and less integration with broader context (Lord, Rutter, & LeCouteur, 1994). Thus, these late deficits may represent the "plateauing" of the development of a certain type of behavior, or a more complex interplay between level of functioning, that may even be intact, and other sources of maladaptive development. For example, the increasingly sophisticated demands of social interactions associated with adolescence, such as socioemotional reciprocity, may be problematic for certain persons who were able to successfully navigate the simpler social demands of childhood, such as parallel play.

Cross-Domain Relationships

The concepts of level and rate of development are also pertinent to intra-individual differences in performance across domains of functioning (i.e., developmental structure). In this manner, developmental structure is characterized both by the relationships among domains of functioning and the relative rates of development across these domains. No two individuals display the exact same profile, as variability across levels of functioning are so common that Fischer (1980) notes "that unevenness is the rule of development." Yet, across both the general and atypical populations, specific and consistent profiles emerge for individuals within each grouping. Thus, researchers are able to describe general developmental structures that are common across typical children or structures that are unique to specific groups of children that are categorized according to a salient characteristic, such as gender, or by the type of atypicality, such as autism. With regard to these groupings, the prevailing question pertains to the relative strengths and weaknesses of each group. A caveat to this question is that the horizontal profile may remain relatively static or may change, even dramatically, through the course of development (Fecteau et al., in preparation; Hodapp & Zigler, 1990, 1995).

The horizontal story, or profile of development, is particularly pertinent to the study of persons with autism as it is the basis of the diagnosis of all psychological disorders that are based on the identification of unique clustering of behavioral characteristics. Because autism is a disorder of behavior, for which no reliable physiological or genetic markers are yet available, the characterization of persons with autism as a meaningful grouping and as reliably distinguished from other groups is solely dependent on a unique profile of behavioral development. As with other groups, the profiles vary considerably across all individuals diagnosed with the disorder but are sufficiently convergent that a pattern of both weaknesses and strengths emerges. In relation to developmental level and relative to the performance of typically developing children or to other etiologically homogeneous groups of persons, task performance among children with autism may appear delayed with respect to some skills, appropriate for others, and even advanced on yet others. The patterns of similarities among these profiles are the basis of the "lumping" of these persons into a single diagnostic category, whereas the differences reflect the individuality of each person and may be informative about the multilinearity of development of the disorder.

The issues of patterns of development are relevant to the level of synchrony between individual development and the changing criteria for diagnosis at the various developmental periods. For each individual, all aspects of development including those relevant to the diagnosis of autism evolve, although the extent of the change for each specific area varies across persons. These changing patterns result in at least three possibilities that arise from these transformations (Towbin, 1997). One, the typical pattern of autism is maintained throughout development. Two, persons with autism need to be rediagnosed as experiencing pervasive developmental disorders not otherwise specified. Three, the initial diagnosis of autism spectrum disorder is seen as erroneous due to improvements in areas of functioning that preclude this diagnosis. These potential differences in naturally occurring developmental outcomes associated with autism are essential both to considerations of the efficacy of diagnostic systems and to the evaluation of treatment programs.

The role of these developmental issues in diagnosis and conceptualizations of autism is evident in the Autism Diagnostic Interviews (ADI) criteria (Lord, Rutter, & LeCouteur, 1994), the leading research tool for the diagnosis of the disorder. The ADI system is largely based on the presence of behaviors at 4 to 5 years of age, as the algorithm is constructed with two basic principles. One, behaviors that disappear before 4 years of age are not relevant for a diagnosis of autism and, two, behaviors that are apparent after 5 years of age, even if they eventually fade or disappear, are relevant. This type of strategy is consistent with a developmental framework as it is based on the notions of behaviors changing over time, even with regard to problematic or atypical behaviors.

The Application of a Liberal Developmental Framework

The traditional notion of a tightly organized and interdependent developmental organism is challenged by the unusual, and often relatively extreme, patterns of behavioral strengths and weaknesses among persons with autism. This unevenness is clearly discrepant with the traditional conceptualization of consistent and universal profiles. In an effort to reconcile these unique characteristics within a developmental framework, we adapt a liberal developmental approach, as initially articulated by Cicchetti and Pogge-Hesse (1982), in which the concept of developmental structure is provided considerable flexibility in order to accommodate findings of different rates of development across domains. They suggested that the uneven patterns of development evident in atypical populations reveal the limits to which certain developmental links might be stretched, but still maintained, within an organized developing system. From this perspective, different areas of functioning can be interrelated even when developmental profiles are uneven, because the variability across areas is still subject to the organizational principles of the overarching developmental system (Burack, 1997; Cicchetti & Pogge-Hesse, 1982). Domains of functioning are connected, but these connections are elastic rather than rigid and static. Within this liberal understanding of developmental structure, variability in the rate of development across domains of functioning is evidence that these domains can be linked in some loose, but systematic, way (Burack, 1997).

Both the principles that link different areas of function and the linked areas may be different from those that are commonly identified with typical developmental sequences. For example, Hodapp and colleagues (Hodapp & Burack, 1990; Hodapp, Burack, & Zigler, 1990, 1998; Hodapp & Zigler, 1995) describe local homologies of shared origin (Bates, Benigni, Bretherton, Camaioni, & Volterra, 1979), which involve two or more behaviors that share a single underlying scheme or cognitive function, and consequently are subject to developmental changes that occur relatively synchronously. Consistent with this viewpoint, the development of means–end behaviors with objects is related to early intentional communication in typically developing children as well as in children with autism and children with mental retardation (Hodapp & Zigler, 1995). Similarly, changes in level of early language (one-word utterances to multiword sentences) are associated with changes in symbolic play (single-schemed play to multischemed play) in all three groups (Hodapp & Zigler, 1995).

With regard to lessons for developmental theory, cross-domain variability in functioning among persons with autism provides information about the relatedness or interdepen-
dence of domains that is not available when typical developmental histories are examined.
For example, contrasting performance between expressive and receptive language skills
among persons with autism provides a unique opportunity to assess the relationships among
these language domains.

SPECIFICITY, NORMALCY, AND UNIQUENESS: ISSUES FROM PSYCHOPATHOLOGY

The primary contributions of the discipline of psychopathology to the endeavor of the
developmental study of persons with autism are in the form of questions that are antithetical
to the "big story" of traditional universal developmental approaches. They highlight the
"small story" of specific impairments within clearly delimited groups, and differences
among subpopulations of persons. These questions include those of specificity, normalcy,
and uniqueness (Wagner, Ganiban, & Cicchetti, 1990; Yirmiya et al., 1998; Zelazo, Burack,
Benedetto, & Frye, 1996). The specificity question refers to the nature of the impairment as
it asks whether one or more specific impairments are at the core of the disorder. The
normalcy question refers to group comparisons as it asks whether the performance of
persons with autism on one or more criteria is different than that of typically developing
individuals. The uniqueness question is the extension of the normalcy question as it asks
whether the atypical behavior is found only in that group or is also evidenced among other
persons with atypical developmental histories.

The Specificity Question

The specificity question is at the core of the "medical model" for study of populations
who are atypical in any way including psychological, behavioral, or physiological. It is
directed at precisely isolating the problem or problems as central to or even responsible for
the general atypicality. This orientation is favored by many researchers of autism that is
characterized by spikes in the profiles of development that are often independent of general
developmental level of functioning (Ehlers et al., 1997), and may reflect specific deficits
that are considered integral to the unusual patterns of behaviors. Within the behavioral
study of autism, this question was central to the focus on deficits in theory of mind,
executive function impairments, and Weak Central Coherence (WCC), among others, as
the core problem in autism.

This type of question is consistent with modular systems of cognition, in which
domains of functioning are thought to develop independently of one another. The impairment in theory of mind tasks in relation to other areas of functioning among persons with
autism is often cited as evidence for an independent module (Baron-Cohen, 1989). However, this is difficult to ascertain because of the possibility that some more general mechanism may account for the data (Frye, Zelazo, & Burack, 1999; Zelazo, Burack, Boseovski,
Jacques, & Frye, 2001). For example, Frye, Zelazo, and Palfai (1995) found that the ToM
abilities in typically developing children depend on a more general mechanism that allows
children to use rules of a particular complexity, and similar developmental associations are

found among persons with autism and Down syndrome (Frye et al., 1999; Zelazo et al., 1996).

The specificity question does not have to be aimed solely at identifying the core impairment, but rather simply at finding one or more areas of deficits that are characteristic of this disorder. These impairments may be universal to persons with the disorder but, consistent with the notion of behaviorally based developmental disorders, this is not necessary. Rarely is any single impairment universal among persons with a developmental disorder and conversely, individuals with developmental disorders rarely manifest all the characteristics of the disorder.

An alternative to the specificity approach of finding one or a few impairments within a group is the delineation of a developmental profile of strengths and weaknesses across domains of functioning that is generally characteristic of a group. This framework provides a more comprehensive portrayal of the horizontal structures associated with the group and diminishes the focus on the notion of core deficits. Furthermore, the use of within-group analyses to establish the horizontal profiles avoids the methodological problems associated with matching when the determination of specific problems is based on cross-group comparisons (these are discussed later in the chapter).

The "Normalcy" Question

The normalcy question is the essence of the determination of whether the target group is atypical. Although atypicality is not necessarily problematic and may even represent valuable strengths and adaptive behaviors, the normalcy question is intrinsic to issues of diagnosis and intervention. The determination of normalcy or atypicality can be based on any one of several methodologies including statistical, societal consensus, or professional judgment (for reviews of this topic, please see Gorenstein, 1992; Lilienfeld & Marino, 1995).

Typically developing individuals are used to address the question of normalcy—is the performance of the target group (i.e., persons with autism) typical compared to that of the comparison group? When addressing the normalcy question in studies of persons with autism, higher functioning persons with autism (i.e., with average IQ scores) are compared with typically developing persons of the same chronological age and IQ. However, the choice of an appropriate comparison group becomes more complicated when the target group includes lower functioning person with autism. The performance of low functioning persons with autism cannot be compared with the performance of typically developing peers, as differences may reflect a generally slowed rate of development rather than autism per se. By definition, lower functioning persons will be found deficient on most tasks if compared to typically developing persons of the same chronological age. To address the normalcy question, therefore, low functioning persons with autism must be matched with typically developing children of the same mental age (MA). By matching the groups on a measure of overall functioning, researchers can control for differences among groups on rate of development and, more meaningfully, ascertain problematic domains of function among persons with autism.

The performance of low functioning persons with autism can also be compared to the performance of other persons with mental retardation and matched for IQ and chronological age (CA). Although this strategy may reduce concerns about discrepancies in rate of development and life experiences between groups, it remains problematic, as a "typical" group of persons functioning in the range of mental retardation is unattainable. Persons with mental retardation make up a heterogeneous group with approximately 1000 different etiologies (e.g., chromosomal abnormalities, congenital defects, prenatal infections, and neurologic insult), each of which is associated with a different developmental profile (Burack, 1990; Burack, Hodapp, & Zigler, 1990; Dykens, 1998). These differences in developmental profiles among etiological groups indicate that heterogeneity in etiology among the persons in the comparison groups may lead to inconsistent conclusion of "normalcy" across studies, even when groups are matched on mental age. The number of persons from any given etiological group will bias the findings toward the strengths and weaknesses of that group. Therefore, the findings will be dependent on the unique etiological makeup of each comparison group. For example, a comparison group with 10 persons with Down syndrome and 2 with Williams syndrome will show a different profile than a comparison group with 6 persons with fragile X and 6 persons with Williams syndrome, thereby leading to potentially different findings in group comparisons. The distinctions between the etiological groups limits the notion of assessing normalcy for lower functioning persons with autism.

The "Uniqueness" Question

The normalcy question refers to whether a group is somehow different than the norm, but does not address whether this difference is unique to the target group or is also found among other groups of individuals. Thus, a uniqueness question is necessary to assess the extent to which characteristics, either at the macro-level (e.g., socioemotional domain) or at the micro-level (e.g., visual selective attention) are unique to a particular group of persons. This question is integral to the differentiation among groups, and thereby to the development of more precise diagnostic, empirical, and intervention strategies.

As with the question of specificity, the issue of uniqueness, even if that term was not always mentioned explicitly, was discussed most commonly with regard to the theory of mind deficit. For example, Baron-Cohen (1989, 1993) and others argued that impairments in theory of mind and mentalizing were unique to persons with autism. This notion was called into question, however, with evidence that certain groups of persons with mental retardation also showed impaired performance on theory of mind tasks (e.g., Zelazo et al., 1996; Zelazo et al., 2001). Yirmiya et al. (1998) clarified this apparent discrepancy when they demonstrated, with a meta-analysis, that ToM deficits are not unique to autism but that the severity of the delay is. Their analysis highlights the need to consider issues such as severity, intensity, and frequency of a problem and length of delay when assessing deficits within a developmental framework.

In studies addressing the "uniqueness" question, the target group and the comparison group are matched for general developmental level. As the performance of persons with autism is characterized by variability across domains of functioning, any composite measure of general developmental level is insufficient. If the domain of study is a relative strength for persons with autism, then matching for general developmental level will entail that the comparison persons will be at a lower developmental level on the target domain. Conversely, if the domain of study is a relative weakness for persons with autism, then the comparison persons will likely be at a higher developmental level on the target domain.

One strategy that can be used to correct for this difficulty is to match the groups on a measure that is related to the ability that is being tested. This strategy minimizes the likelihood of finding group differences, but maximizes the accuracy of findings of impaired or superior performance

The uniqueness question cannot be answered with certainty until every possible population and subpopulation is tested. A more efficient strategy, however, would be to compare groups that are conceptually related in some way. For example, specific clinical groups of children with aphasia and developmental language disorder (DLD) display impairments in language functioning that resemble those of persons with autism. Similarly, persons with fragile X syndrome and persons with autism demonstrate similar impairments in the socioemotional domain. This strategy of comparing those groups that are most similar with respect to the domain of study is a conservative one that may mask deficits and differences in relation to the general population. However, the finding that a specific impairment is unique to or most severe among persons with autism, as compared to a similar group, provides more precise evidence both about autism in general and about the specific aspect of functioning in relation to domain-general development. Comparisons to relatively dissimilar groups will provide more examples of deficits or differences, but will provide less exact information with regard to cause of the deficit or its place in the more general organization of development.

The primary drawback associated with the use of etiologically specific groups in addressing the uniqueness question is that relevant findings are not generalizable to larger populations. For example, if the comparison is made up of persons with Down syndrome, then the implications of the findings cannot extend beyond this specific population (Burack, Evans, Klaiman, & Iarocci, 2001; Yirmiya et al., 1998). The implications cannot be extended to all persons with mental retardation, as the performance of persons with Down syndrome is not representative of that larger population. Despite these inherent limitations, the increased methodological precision is essential to conceptualizing unique aspects of various disorders.

Developmental Considerations in Matching Groups: Methodological Issues in the Quest to Assess Normalcy and Uniqueness

The integrity of conclusions regarding both the normalcy and uniqueness questions is based on comparisons with other populations and, therefore, largely dependent on matching strategies that continue to be widely debated in the study of persons with developmental disabilities (Burack, Evans, Klaiman, & Iarocci, 2001; Mervis & Robinson, 1999). Matching for developmental level, however, is complicated by the large variability in performance across domains of functioning among persons with autism. One approach to resolving this difficulty is the use of multiple measures of developmental level to assess global developmental level. A major obstacle to this approach is the inadequacy of current standardized tests for assessing developmental level. Standardized tests of persons with autism typically reveal a unique behavioral profile of strengths and weakness. This complicates the matching process by undermining the validity of general or composite measures of global developmental level. For example, composite measures of functioning that are biased toward verbal skills (e.g., WISC-III-R) will underestimate the developmental level of persons with autism who are relatively stronger in nonverbal domains. Conversely, measures that disproportionately reflect visual spatial skills (e.g., Ravens Progressive Matrices), a relative strength among persons with autism, may overestimate their developmental level (Shah & Frith, 1993). The associations among the issues of unique group profile, developmental level, and standardized tests are further complicated by the variability in the relationships among scores across the various domains for typical as well as for atypical populations (Mervis & Robinson, 1999). Thus, strategies and tools appropriate for matching at one developmental level may not be appropriate at another.

The impact of the matching measures on the findings and conclusions regarding group differences highlights the need to rethink the implications of comparison studies and strategies. They are certainly necessary but they may need to be presented in a more precise manner. The inconsistencies among matching measures are evident in the finding that performance of persons with autism, as compared to that of typically developing persons, is impaired when the groups were matched on nonverbal MA but not when they are matched on mean length of utterance (Ozonoff, Pennington, & Rogers, 1991). This type of evidence indicates that the notion of matching is not a definitive method for evaluating group strengths and/or weaknesses, but simply provides a heuristic context for approximate comparisons of level of performance among domains of functioning. Thus more informative strategies might include the use of more than one comparison group with each matched to the target group on performance on specific domains of functioning rather than a single one matched on a single composite measure of global developmental level. For example, the target group may be matched with one comparison group on a nonverbal measure of performance, with another comparison group on a specific measure of language abilities (e.g., expressive language), and yet with another comparison group on general developmental level. This strategy enables increased precision in evaluating the level of functioning in specific domains within a more comprehensive developmental framework.

Interpreting Nonsignificant Findings

The developmental premise that groups of persons matched on mental age should show similar abilities or level of performance on many aspects of functioning led to an interest in studies of nonsignificant findings in which no differences are found between the persons with autism and their matched peers. In areas of suspected deficit, findings of no differences with appropriate matching suggest that the apparent problem may be an artifact of the generally delayed development among lower functioning persons with autism or a function of some broader area of difficulty. However, the failure to find differences between groups matched at a certain MA does not preclude the possibility of a syndrome-specific problem; rather it denotes that at a certain point (or points) in development the groups do not differ on a specific task.

The relevance of findings of no differences is contingent on two basic developmental premises. One premise is that the identification of group differences at one or a few points in development is not sufficient for the argument of "no differences." Rather, the task is to show that differences between the groups were never apparent. This entails assessing levels of performance at the appropriate developmental transition points when the ability in question first emerges, since that is the point in time when differences are most likely to be apparent. An even more extensive strategy includes the use of cross-sectional or longitudinal studies across a wide range of developmental levels, including those prior to, concurrent with, and after the emergence of the ability. This strategy provides a more precise depiction of the level of functioning on certain tasks at specific developmental levels, and minimizes the possibility that developmental or group differences might be obscured, as often happens when findings from persons of different developmental levels are grouped together for statistical purposes (Burack, 1997).

A second issue is that an argument for no differences is contingent on evidence that similar performance on a task reflects similarities in the underlying processes. Regardless of when in development the behavioral outcome appears among persons with autism, the underlying processes or mechanisms may not be identical to those seen in typically developing children at that developmental level. As already discussed, the delayed attainment of a particular ability may be due to the individual's capacity to compensate for his or her weakness by using some alternative strategy or ability rather than by actual attainment of that skill. In this case, the behavioral outcome of similar performance does not accurately reflect the underlying processes or the inherent impairments that delayed the acquisition of the skills.

These difficulties in interpreting findings of no differences between groups do not diminish the value of this type of evidence, as all information about functioning is essential to providing a thorough account of the behavioral profile of persons with autism. However, they reflect the need, as when examples of impairment are found, for increased precision in delineating the nature of the target behavior and the developmental period for which conclusions can be drawn.

CONCLUSIONS: IMPLICATIONS FOR INTERVENTIONS

The application of developmental principles to the study of persons with autism provides a context for organizing knowledge concerning the functioning and behaviors of this population across the life span. This framework is helpful for assessing the basic questions relating to psychopathology, including specificity of problem, normalcy, and uniqueness of disorder to the population. Similarly, the developmental principles, both the vertical and horizontal stories, provide a context for the implementation and assessment of interventions with persons with autism.

The issues of order, rate, and level of development, associated with the vertical stories, are informative with regard to circumscribed abilities or aspects of behavior, whereas the developmental profiles associated with horizontal stories are relevant to understanding the complex relations across domains of functioning or behavior. The developmental profiles across domains are independent of general rate of development or IQ level, but are based on comparisons of developmental rates within domains. They provide initial guidance with regard to identifying both areas of impairment, such as language and play, that need to be the focus of intervention and domains of strength, such as rote memory and word decoding, that can be utilized in the intervention process and in other endeavors to maximize individuals' levels of adaptation. The areas of impairment generally cannot be "fixed," but enhancement of behavioral level, especially those relevant to social adaptation, may considerably enhance quality of life. As with any population, the maximization of the benefits associated with strengths is likely to foster feelings of positive self-regard and

accomplishment, although the exclusive focus on areas of strengths can impede development in other areas (Mottron & Burack, 2001).

Once the specific aspect of behavior for intervention is identified, knowledge of the
relevant developmental sequences and current level of functioning in that specific domain
are essential to determining the program to be implemented. The focus of intervention
needs to be commensurate with level of functioning in the specific domain and generally
consistent with developmental sequences. For example, symbolic play, which is the use of
one object to represent a different object; the use of a doll as an agent of action; and acts that
suggest the existence of imaginary objects may all require prior experience with functional
and conventional use of actual toys. Thus, attempts to facilitate development in a domain
are enhanced by the process of building upon prior foundations of abilities that are essential
within typical developmental progression. Similarly, the horizontal story of both the
facilitative and interfering effects of developmental level of certain domains on others need
to be considered in developing intervention programs. Sigman, Dissanayake, Arbelle, and
Ruskin (1997) argued that spontaneous symbolic play was more likely to occur in children
with autism whose language abilities were comparable to those of 5-year-old typically
developing peers and only when it was necessitated by a given task. The abandonment of
the consideration of these developmental stories in devising treatment programs represents
a haphazard approach that is akin to seeking growth where there are no roots or other type
of foundation.

Developmental interpretations of clinical phenomena are informative for the implementation and choice of interventions. Within this framework, the ability to perform a
specific task, especially when it occurs later than expected with regard to general developmental level, does not imply that the same processes are involved nor does it guarantee the
emergence of abilities that typically follows successful attainment. This necessitates the
reconsideration of specific skills within the broader framework of evolving developmental
pathways and organization when considering the implementation of treatment. For example, interventions aimed at improving the social behavior and adaptation of children with
autism by teaching them to pass false-belief tasks are likely less beneficial than those
focused on more basic abilities such as switching attention across all aspects of a scenario
and thinking before acting. In addition to its benefits for passing false-belief and other ToM
tasks, this latter strategy might also facilitate the emergence of those skills that typically
follow the attainment of ToM and related areas of functioning.

The application of developmental principles to the study of autism represents a useful
and necessary framework for studying and treating persons with autism. This endeavor,
however, is far from complete as issues of theory, methodology, and interpretation still
need to be refined. Our goal in writing this chapter was to initiate further consideration of
relevant issues, as the success of this approach is dependent on the collaboration among
scholars with different areas of expertise in providing a comprehensive mosaic of the
development of persons with autism.

REFERENCES

American Psychological Association (1994). *Diagnostic and Statistical Manual of Mental Disorders* (4th edition).
    Washington, DC: Author.

Baron-Cohen, S. (1989). The autistic child's theory of mind: A case of specific developmental delay. *Journal of Child Psychology & Psychiatry, 30,* 285–297.

Baron-Cohen, S. (1993). From attention-goal psychology to belief-desire psychology: The development of a theory of mind, and its dysfunction. In S. Baron-Cohen, H. Tager-Flusberg, & D. Cohen (Eds.), *Understanding Other Minds: Perspectives from Autism* (pp. 59–82). New York: Oxford University Press.

Bates, E., Benigni, L., Bretherton, I., Camaioni, L., & Voltera, V. (1979). *The Emergence of Symbols: Cognition and Communication in Infancy.* New York: Academic Press.

Bever, T. G. (1982). *Regressions in Mental Development: Basic Phenomena and Theories.* Hillsdale, NJ: Erlbaum.

Bowler, D. M. (1992). 'Theory of Mind' in Asperger's syndrome. *Journal of Child Psychology and Psychiatry, 33,* 877–893.

Burack, J. A. (1990). Differentiating mental retardation: The two group approach and beyond. In R. M. Hodapp, J. A. Burack, & E. Zigler (Eds.), *Issues in the Developmental Approach to Mental Retardation* (pp. 27–48). New York: Cambridge University Press.

Burack, J. A. (1997). The study of atypical and typical populations in developmental psychopathology: The quest for a common science. In S. S. Luthar, J. A. Burack, D. Cicchetti, & J. R. Weisz, (Eds.), *Developmental Psychopathology: Perspectives on Adjustment, Risk and Disorder* (pp. 139–165). New York: Cambridge University Press.

Burack, J. A., Evans, D. W., Klaiman, C., & Iarocci, G. (2001). The mysterious myth of attentional and other defect stories: Contemporary issues in the developmental approach to mental retardation. *International Review of Research in Mental Retardation, 24,* 299–319.

Burack, J. A., Hodapp, R. M., & Zigler, E. (1990). Technical note: Toward a more precise understanding of mental retardation. *Journal of Child Psychology and Psychiatry, 31,* 471–475.

Burack, J. A., & Volkmar, F. R. (1992). Development in high and low functioning autistic children. *Journal of Child Psychology and Psychiatry, 33,* 607–616.

Chandler, M. (1997). Stumping for progress in a post-modern world. In E. Amsel & K. A. Renninger (Eds.), *Change and Development: Issues of Theory, Method, and Application.* Mahwah, NJ: Erlbaum.

Cicchetti, D. (1984). The emergence of developmental psychopathology. *Child Development, 55,* 1–7.

Cicchetti, D., & Pogge-Hesse, P. (1982). Possible contributions of organically retarded persons to developmental theory. In E. Zigler & D. Balla (Eds.), *Mental Retardation: The Developmental-Difference Controversy.* Hillsdale, NJ: Erlbaum.

Dykens, E. M. (1998). Maladaptive behavior and dual diagnosis in persons with genetic syndromes. In J. A. Burack, R. M. Hodapp, & E. Zigler (Eds.), *Handbook of Mental Retardation and Development.* New York: Cambridge University.

Ehlers, S., Nyden, A., Gillberg, C., Sandberg, A. D., Dahlgren, S. O., Hjelmquist E., & Oden, A. (1997). Asperger syndrome, autism and attention disorders: A comparative study of the cognitive profiles of 120 children. *Journal of Child Psychology and Psychiatry, 38,* 207–17.

Enns, J. T., Burack, J. A., Iarocci, G., & Randolph, B. (2000). Issues of microgenesis, ontogenesis, and psychopathology in global-local processing: A Wernerian story of development. *Journal of Adult Development, 7,* 41–48.

Fecteau, S., Mottron, L., Berthiaume, L., & Burack, J. A. (in preparation). Developmental transformations of autistic symptoms.

Fischer, K. (1980). A theory of cognitive development: The control and construction of a hierarchy of skills. *Psychological Review, 87,* 477–531.

Fischer, K., Pipp, S., & Bullock, D. (1984). Detecting developmental discontinuities. In R. N. Emde & R. J. Harmaon (Eds.), *Continuities and Discontinuities in Development.* New York: Plenum.

Frye, D. (1991). The end of development? In F. S. Kessel, M. H. Bornstein, & A. J. Sameroff (Eds.), *Contemporary Constructions of the Child: Essays in Honor of William Kessen.* New York: Erlbaum.

Frye, D., Zelazo, P. D., & Burack, J. A. (1999). Cognitive complexity and control: Implications for theory of mind in typical and atypical populations. *Current Directions in Psychological Science, 7,* 116–121.

Frye, D., Zelazo, P. D., & Palfai, T. (1995). Theory of mind and rule-based reasoning. *Cognitive Development, 10,* 483–527.

Gorenstein, E. E. (1992). *The Science of Mental Illness.* San Diego: Academic Press.

Happé, F. G. E. (2001). Social and nonsocial development in autism: Where are the links? In J. A. Burack, T. Charman, N. Yirmiya, & P. R. Zelazo (Eds.), *The Development of Autism: Perspectives from Theory and Research* (pp. 235–252). Mahwah, NJ: Erlbaum.

Hodapp, R. M., & Burack, J. A. (1990). What mental retardation teaches us about typical development: The examples of sequences, rates, and cross-domain relations. *Development and Psychopathology, 2,* 213–225.

Hodapp, R. M., Burack, J. A., & Zigler, E. (1990). The developmental perspective in the field of mental retardation. In R. M. Hodapp, J. A. Burack, & E. Zigler (Eds.), *Issues in the Developmental Approach to Mental Retardation.* New York: Cambridge University Press.

Hodapp, R. M., Burack, J. A., & Zigler, E. (1998). Developmental approaches to mental retardation: A short introduction. In J. A. Burack, R. M. Hodapp, & E. Zigler (Eds.), *Handbook of Mental Retardation and Development.* New York: Cambridge University Press.

Hodapp, R. M., & Zigler, E. (1990). Applying the developmental perspective to individuals with Down syndrome. In D. Cicchetti & M. Beeghly (Eds.), *Children with Down Syndrome: A Developmental Perspective.* New York: Cambridge University Press.

Hodapp, R. M., & Zigler, E. (1995). Past, present, and future issues in the developmental approach to mental retardation and developmental disabilities. In D. Cicchetti & D. J. Cohen (Eds.), *Developmental psychopathology,* Vol. 2: *Risk, Disorder, and Adaptation* (pp. 299–331). New York: John Wiley & Sons.

Kessen, W. (1984). Introduction: The end of the age of development. In R. Sternberg (Ed.), *Mechanisms of Cognitive Development.* San Francisco: Freeman.

Lilienfeld, S. O., & Marino, L. (1995). Mental disorder as a Roschian concept: A critique of Wakefield's "harmful dysfunction" analysis. *Journal of Abnormal Psychology, 104,* 411–420.

Lord, C., Rutter, M., & LeCouter, A. (1994). Autism Diagnostic Interview -- Revised: A revised version of a diagnostic interview for caregivers of persons with possible pervasive developmental disorders. *Journal of Autism and Developmental Disorders, 24,* 659–685.

Mervis, C. B., & Robinson, B. F. (1999). Methodological issues in cross-syndrome comparisons: Matching procedures, sensitivity, and specificity. *Monographs of the Society for Research in Child Development, 64,* 115–130.

Morgan, S. B. (1986). Autism and Piaget's theory: Are the two compatible? *Journal of Autism and Developmental Disorders, 16,* 441–457.

Morgan, S. B., Cutrer, P. S., Coplin, J. W., & Rodrigue, J. R. (1989). Do autistic children differ from retarded and normal children in Piagetian sensorimotor functioning? *Journal of Child Psychology and Psychiatry, 30,* 857–864.

Mottron, L., & Burack, J. A. (2001). Enhanced perceptual functioning in the development of autism. In J. A. Burack, T. Charman, N. Yirmiya, & P. R. Zelazo (Eds.), *The Development of Autism: Perspectives from Theory and Research* (pp. 131–148). Mahwah, NJ: Erlbaum.

Ozonoff, S., Pennington, B. F., & Rogers, S. J. (1991). Executive functioning deficits in high-functioning autistic individuals: Relationship to theory of mind. *Journal of Child Psychology and Psychiatry, 32,* 1081–1105.

Piven, J., Harper, J., Palmer, & Arndt, S. (1996). Course of behavioral change in autism: A retrospective study of high IQ adolescents and adults. *Journal of the American Academy of Child and Adolescent Psychiatry, 35,* 523–529.

Shah, A., & Frith, U. (1993). Why do autistic individuals show superior performance on the block design task? *Journal of Child Psychology and Psychiatry, 34,* 1351–1364.

Sigman, M., Dissanyake, C., Arbelle, S., & Ruskin, E. (1997) Cognition and emotion in children and adolescents with autism. In D. J. Cohen & F. R. Volkmar (Eds.), *Handbook of Autism and Pervasive Developmental Disorders,* 2nd ed. (pp. 248–265). New York: John Wiley & Sons.

Sigman, M., & Ungerer, J. (1884). Cognitive and language skills in autistic, mentally retarded, and normal children. *Developmental Psychology, 20,* 293–302.

Sroufe, L. A., & Rutter, M. (1984). The domain of developmental psychopathology. *Child Development, 55,* 17–29.

Tager-Flusberg, H. (2001). A re-examination of the theory of mind hypothesis of autism. In J. A. Burack, T. Charman, N. Yirmiya, & P. R. Zelazo (Eds.), *The Development of Autism: Perspectives from Theory and Research* (pp. 173–192). Mahwah, NJ: Erlbaum.

Towbin, K. E. (1997). Pervasive developmental disorder not otherwise specified. In D. J. Cohen & F. R. Volkmar (Eds.), *Handbook of Autism and Pervasive Developmental Disorders,* 2nd ed. (pp. 248–265). New York: John Wiley & Sons.

Volkmar, F. R., Burack, J. A., & Cohen, D. J. (1990). Deviance and developmental approaches in the study of autism. In R. M. Hodapp, J. A. Burack, & E. Zigler (Eds.), *Issues in the Developmental Approach to Mental Retardation* (pp. 246–271). New York: Cambridge University Press.

Wagner, S., Ganiban, J. M., & Cicchetti, D. (1990). Attention, memory and perception in infants with Down syndrome: A review and commentary. In D. Cicchetti & M. Beeghly (Eds.), *Children with Down Syndrome: A Developmental Perspective* (pp. 147–179). New York: Cambridge University Press.

Weisz, J. R., Yeates, K. O., & Zigler, E. (1982). Piagetian evidence and the developmental-difference controversy. In E. Zigler & D. Balla (Eds.), *Mental Retardation: The Developmental-Difference Controversy* (pp. 9–26). Hillsdale, NJ: Erlbaum.

Weisz, J. R., & Zigler, E. (1979). Cognitive development in retarded and nonretarded persons: Piagetian tests of the similar sequence hypothesis. *Psychological Bulletin, 86*, 831–851.

Wenar, C., Ruttenberg, B. A., Kalish-Weiss, B., & Wolf, E. G. (1986). The development of normal and autistic children: A comparative study. *Journal of Autism and Developmental Disorders, 16*, 317–333.

Werner, H. (1948). *Comparative Psychology of Mental Development* (revised.). New York: Follett.

Werner, H. (1957). The concept of development from a comparative and organismic point of view. In D. Harris (Ed.), *The Concept of Development*. Minneapolis: University of Minnesota.

Yirmiya, N., Erel, O., Shaked, M., & Solomonica-Levy, D. (1998). Meta-analyses comparing theory of mind abilities of individuals with autism, individuals with mental retardation, and normally developing individuals. *Psychological Bulletin, 124*, 283–307.

Zelazo, P. D., Burack, J. A., Benedetto, E., & Frye, D. (1996). Theory of mind and rule use in individuals with Down's syndrome: A test of the uniqueness and specificity claims. *Journal of Child Psychology and Psychiatry, 37*, 479–484.

Zelazo, P. D., Burack, J. A., Boseoviskij, J., Jacques, S., & Frye, D. (2001). A cognitive complexity and control framework for the study of autism. In J. A. Burack, T. Charman, N. Yirmiya, & P. R. Zelazo (Eds.), *The Development of Autism: Perspectives from Theory and Research* (pp. 193–216). Mahwah, NJ: Erlbaum.

Zigler, E., & Glick, M. (1986). *A Developmental Approach to Adult Psychopathology*. New York: John Wiley & Sons.

4

The Otherworldly Gifts of Autism

Mystical Implementation of Facilitated Communication in the Ultra-Orthodox Community in Israel

Yoram Bilu and Yehuda Goodman

THE CULTURAL CONSTRUCTION OF AUTISM

Facilitated communication (FC) is a set of techniques designed to improve the communicative skills of children suffering from pervasive developmental disorders. Widely used during the late 1980s and early 1990s, its validity became the subject of a heated controversy. Without seeking to reopen this controversy, in this chapter we highlight a peculiar application of these techniques in the Haredi (ultra-orthodox) community in Israel. This implementation of FC offers the children's families a new, highly positive, perception of autism, while at the same time serving to reaffirm the validity of core values of the community. We collected the data throughout 1995–1996 in the context of a larger study dealing with communication patterns and boundary maintenance in the Haredi community in Israel.

Our case study points to ways in which mental disorders are culturally constituted and historically situated (e.g., Gaines, 1992; Kleinman, 1988). Autism is culturally malleable to a fairly limited extent—given, indeed, the pervasiveness of "primary" biological and psychological malfunctions. Nevertheless, even in such a case the particular systems of local knowledge in which the malfunction is embedded might substantially reconstitute it. We seek to show how in a given historical moment, specific mental disorders are selected and transformed into highly ritualized and stylized performances in a dramatic morality

YORAM BILU • Department of Psychology and Department of Sociology and Anthropology, The Hebrew University of Jerusalem, Mount Scopus, Jerusalem, 91905 Israel.   YEHUDA GOODMAN • Van Leer Institute, Jerusalem, 93114 Israel.

The Research Basis for Autism Intervention, edited by Schopler, Yirmiya, Shulman, and Marcus. Kluwer Academic/Plenum Publishers, New York, 2001.

play encapsulating core dilemmas and contested values of the community (cf. Foucault, 1973). Thus by relying on a well-established sociological tradition originating in Durkheim, we try to highlight not only the individual implications of the usage of FC in the Haredi community, but also the ways this community (like other societies) relates to mental disorders as a form of social deviance and uses them to create integration, cohesion, and solidarity (Ben-Yehuda, 1985). Specifically, we are interested in the construction of autism as a rhetorical device and in the dialogical possibilities that this construction opens for reaffirming the core values of the society. Our focus is thus on the transactional process between center and periphery through which children suffering from severe disorders such as autism are appropriated and remade by central figures in the Haredi community in Israel.

Our case study demonstrates how bounded cultural enclaves (such as the Haredi community) become partially enmeshed in the interactive systems that constitute the modern world. This example also shows, however, the selective permeability of group boundaries in the age of global cultural flow. The fast (although not uncontested) adoption of augmentative communication aids by Haredim in Israel seems to support Appadurai's (1990: 8) contention that "technology… now moves in high speeds across various kinds of previously impervious boundaries." But this trafficking was not accompanied by a similar incorporation of the theoretical rationale underlying the original clinical use of FC. Rather, an extensive process of local adaptation or "indigenization" (Hannerz, 1989) reframed and realigned the technique and its rationale in keeping with the community's hegemonic values.

Our emphasis on interactive networks in the globalization model resonates with the multiple levels of communication generated by the introduction of FC to the Haredi community. Ostensibly, the technique is designed to improve the users' communication abilities. But beyond that, the networks provide the means for the intriguing dialogue aforementioned between moral agents of the social order and individuals suffering from autism, as well as for an intergroup dialogue with the secular world outside the community, and a metaphysical dialogue with the afterworld "above" it.

In what follows we present the controversy over FC and its implementation in the Haredi community, explain its unique novel religious rationale, examine the messages elicited in FC sessions in Haredi settings, and describe their relationship to core values and concerns of the community. Next, we turn to the clinical implications of FC for Haredi families. Lastly, we compare this form of FC with the clinical set of techniques from which it was borrowed, showing how the religious application may shed new light on clinical FC. The two versions are particularly similar, we argue, in their attempt to reconstitute the autistic children in a new, ostensibly more positive mold.

THE CONTROVERSY OVER FACILITATED COMMUNICATION

FC, first developed in the 1970s in Australia (Crossley, 1992), gained much popularity in the United States in the 1980s and early 1990s (Biklen, 1990). In FC sessions the facilitators provide a continuous physical assistance to the children, helping them to communicate by pointing to pictures or letters on a communication board, or by typing out messages on a computer keyboard. The mounting popularity of FC was counterbalanced by a subsequent wave of controlled experimental studies that failed to replicate the positive effects attributed to the technique in a naturally occurring context. Reviews of these studies have usually echoed the unequivocal conclusion reached by Eberlin, McConnachie, Ibel, and Volpe: "At the present time there has not been one scientifically valid confirmatory finding supporting the claims that FC produces independent client-generated communication" (1993: 528; see also Jacobson, Mulick, & Schwartz, 1995). Using effective modes of experimental control, many of the studies have demonstrated that the communicative outputs attributed to the handicapped persons were in fact produced by the facilitators, probably without intent or awareness (e.g., Dillon, Fenlason, & Vogel, 1994; Eberlin, Ibel, & Jacobson, 1994; Montee, Miltenberger, & Wittrock, 1995). To the critical eye, this ample documentation of "facilitator influence" has reduced FC to "unwitting ventriloquism" (Routh, 1994).The produced messages were thus explained as stemming not from the children but from their facilitators.

THE IMPLEMENTATION OF FC IN THE HAREDI COMMUNITY IN ISRAEL

Since the beginning of 1995, a succession of reports in Israeli newspapers depicted the growing use of and subsequent controversy over FC in Haredi circles. Israeli Jews are distributed along a wide spectrum, from complete atheists to devout observants (Sobel & Beit-Hallahmi, 1991), and Haredim (more than 10% of the population) are located at the uttermost religious pole of this continuum. Like other religious fundamentalist groups, Haredim are marked by deep opposition to secular lifestyles—augmented by deliberate attempts to retain sociocultural life patterns as crystallized in traditional communities of earlier centuries (Heilman & Friedman, 1991). Haredim's twin spiritual ideals are the strict fulfillment of all religious precepts and the study (by men) of Jewish sacred texts, in religious academies. Of immense importance are thus the spiritual leaders of the community, ordained rabbis, whose moral authority and advice is sought and accepted without challenge.

The entrepreneurial role of strictly observant individuals in promoting a recently introduced, controversial procedure such as FC and their readiness to examine to that end a large quantity of data published in specialized professional journals, from which the Haredim are usually estranged, cannot be taken for granted. The acquaintance with popular television programs on FC that this promotion involved is particularly remarkable, given the pernicious image of television in the Haredi community and the general proscription to watch it. All this unusual reaching out and barrier crossing may suggest that FC was believed to hold a special promise for religious believers (and for those standing on the boundary between the secular and the religious world)—beyond the ambitious goal of improving the communication skills of severely incapacitated individuals. The essence of this significance became crystal clear with the first media reports on FC in the Haredi settings. The communication was geared to otherworldly planes; the impaired children were perceived as mediums susceptible to supernormal agencies and able to impart knowledge derived from them.

According to Israeli religious newspapers, this esoteric use of FC had been cultivated in Haredi circles in the United States and was then imported to Israel. In the new surrounding it has been promoted by a group of committed individuals and voluntary associations situated in Jerusalem and Bnai Brak, the two urban strongholds of Israeli ultra-orthodoxy.

The individual advocates of the system, rabbis coming from a variety of orthodox back-grounds, have been primarily engaged in FC sessions conducted in private family settings. The voluntary associations, less inhibited in their eagerness to publicize the elicited communications, specialized in public displays of FC sessions in front of large audiences. In both settings the overwhelming majority of the message senders were children coming from observant families. Likewise, most of the facilitators were women from strictly religious backgrounds. The sessions were run by the religious promoters who presented the questions to the children. Mystically oriented rabbis and religious activists seeking to bring secular Jews back to religion were particularly instrumental in promoting FC. A wide plethora of tools has been employed to document and distribute the communications extracted in private and public performances, to expound their meaning, and to amplify their reverberations. These included posters, articles in newspapers and periodicals, bro-chures, lectures, and even audiocassettes and videocassettes for rent and sale.

This propagation of "metaphysical FC" in the Haredi community was not left un-answered. A series of critical articles in Haredi newspapers, bearing titles such as "autism and charlatanism" or "autism without mysticism," have cautioned against the esoteric use of FC by mobilizing against it venerated rabbinical figures, as well as observant physicians, psychologists, and educators. Many of the arguments of the religious professionals reso-nated with the methodological caveats in the scientific reviews of the phenomenon, while the rabbinical figures reacted to FC from the classic hyperconservative stance, claiming that any system of ideas or set of procedures not grounded in Jewish tradition should be shunned. These critical voices, however, have not been successful in discrediting the phenomenon and in stopping its spread. FC continues to thrive in religious circles, as children suffering from autism disclose through it messages from otherworldly planes.

THE RELIGIOUS RATIONALE OF FC IN THE HAREDI CONTEXT

Judging from their publications, the Haredi promoters of FC are well versed in the clinical literature on FC. But they promulgate it in a very selective way, focusing on the reported dramatic improvements in communication skills while seeking to minimize the wealth and weight of disproving data. In dealing with the alleged achievements of FC, the promoters confound scientific and religious discourses. The brochures and cassettes they distribute always start with detailed depictions of the professional history of the procedure. This introduction appears rigorous and sober minded as it focuses on the empirical evidence in support of FC and on the professional experience and academic background of its proponents. But the reliance on scientific status symbols appears as part of a rhetorical scheme hiding specious reasoning, since it always ends with a narrative twist. In the last analysis, the religious reports assert that the scientific–positivist paradigm, despite its enumerated achievements, fails to account for the entire gamut of FC effects. As phrased by one of the publications, "We are facing a phenomenon scientists have no idea how to cope with."

The shift from scientific to religious idioms is marked by reframing allegedly inexpli-cable FC effects as "miracles" which include anecdotal reports on advanced literacy without prior exposure to reading and writing, fluent communication in foreign languages, elicitation of coherent messages without staring at the keyboard, communication during states of deep coma, absorbing written material and conducting complex calculations in enormous speed, and knowledge of Divine Truth. All these "miracles," except the last one, are elaborations on arguments raised by facilitators (and popularized by the media) without manifest reference to otherworldly reality and metaphysical entities. The religious promulgations capitalize on these extraordinary anecdotal reports, presenting them as rigorous scientific findings, only to expose the limitations and short-sightedness of the empirical perspective.

Jewish texts are cited to support the Haredi exegesis of FC. One example is the legend about the embryo in its mother's womb that "looks and sees from one end of the world to the other." This amazing farsightedness is correlated with no less amazing insight or introspection, as the embryo is also believed to master the entire corpus of the Holy Scriptures. A metaphorical reading of another phrase—"A candle burns above its (the embryo's) head"—serves as a mediating link in accounting for these prodigal embryonic capacities. The candle stands for the soul, viewed as the Godly element in human existence, which, in the embryonic state, still enjoys a free-floating, extracorporeal position. As a Divine spark unconstrained by material limitations, nothing physical or spiritual is beyond the pale of the soul. This blissful state is short lived, however. From the moment of birth, the soul, encased in a limiting bodily habitat, is bereft of the prenatal spectacular faculties.

Following the erasure of the prenatal Platonic traces of erudition and unobstructed vision at birth, learning becomes strenuous and slow. The laborious process of secondary acquisition is mediated by the brain which, being a material organ, is more limiting than enabling. Cherished by science as the site of high mental processes, the generator of human intellect and creativity, the brain is pondered here as a confining device, a screen, which distances humans from their Divine source, the pure omniscient soul. The knowledge it can grasp, perforce constrained by human inherent fallibility, is but a small fraction of the endless primordial wisdom lost upon parturition.

This line of reasoning renders another Talmudic statement comprehensible: "Since the Temple was destroyed, prophecy has been taken from prophets and given to fools and children." The injured brains of children suffering from autism viewed in mundane life as the source of unending misery, constitute an asset from a mystical viewpoint, since they allow privileged access to their God-given soul. Dialectically, the more incapacitated the individual, as reflected in both physical and mental dysfunctioning, the more permeable the bodily screen which effectively separates normal people from their Divine, supernormal source. This dialectical process is responsible for the "miraculous" performances of children suffering from autism, in the Haredi FC sessions. From a mystico-religious perspective, the procedure is an effective tool for bypassing the afflicted body and making direct contact with the pure soul. Through this contact, extraordinary information from otherworldly spheres may be obtained which, as one of the brochures puts it, "enables us to get rid of any doubt regarding the foundations of our faith."

"WHAT DOES THE SOUL SAY" IN FC SESSIONS?

Cloaked in this metaphysical garment, the Haredi FC provides a meeting ground for the transcendental and the mundane—which is otherwise uncommon in Judaism. Jewish mystics have sought to induce themselves into ecstatic and contemplative states, in which they could experience the presence of the Divine (Idel, 1988). But these experiences were typically private events, limited to mystical virtuosi, and highly ineffable. FC sessions, in contrast, often take place in public settings, in front of a large audience, and their messages are lucid and easily conveyable. These messages, "the secrets of the soul," are disclosed by the impaired child with the facilitator's assistance in response to questions addressed by the rabbi in charge of the session.

The most compelling theme dealt with is divine providence. The children report that they are strongly aware of God's existence and, based on the experiences of their souls in the afterworld, are cognizant of his omnipresence and guidance. Having faith in God, loving and worshipping him, and following his will in learning and piety are depicted as the most important things in life. These objectives are not external prescriptions, but rather reflections of human intrinsic motivation. The children, stripped of the distorting constraints of base bodily desires, are able to articulate through the facilitation the genuine wishes of their souls—thus providing evidence as to the innate spirituality of human nature.

Once God's immanence and omnipresence (in the world as well as in humans) has been established, it is important to reconcile it with the miserable fate of the children. Since the notion of divine providence, based on the moral principle of divine restitution as individually geared to each believer is a cardinal pillar of faith in Judaism, the agony and pain of the children and their families must be accounted for. This is particularly true in the case of autism, in which early onset discredits any explanation focusing on the victim's sins. One of the publications responded to this moral challenge with the following generalization, based on repeated messages from the children: "All the brain-damaged without exception know that they had lived in this world before, know their former name and parents' names, and *know the sin for which they came to this world in such a miserable form*. They all know that they did not come to this world to do penance, since they know the ultimate truth and do not have (the option of free) choice. They came to the world simply and solely to endure this anguish, which for them is a rectification of the sin for which they came into being" (italics added).

As in other religious systems, the notion of reincarnation, or the transmigration of souls serves to account for apparent aberrations in the principle of divine retribution, embodied, in this case, in the mutilation of innocent children. The possibility of rectification makes the Jewish variant of reincarnation a demonstration of divine grace, given the opportunity imparted on the transmigrated soul to improve its transcendental status in the hereafter. The vicissitudes of the souls in their former incarnations and in afterlife were minutely portrayed in the FC sessions with special emphasis on their sins. Among the transgressions responsible for the message senders' present wretchedness, moral breaches on the interpersonal level were particularly noticed. Of these, verbal misbehaviors, from gossiping to vilifying and slandering, appeared as a cardinal sin. The salience of this category of misdeeds in the context of autism reflects (and further reinforces) the principle of divine retribution: those who had sinned with their mouth were doomed to suffer from gross communication impairments in their new reincarnation. Other reported sins included adultery, embezzlement, and apostasy. The depictions of the souls' wanderings in the afterworld focused on the celestial jury and the penalties it imposed on the culprits.

The information regarding the children's former incarnations, vices, and punishments is elicited in the course of a staccato succession of questions and answers. The publications, claiming to bring an accurate documentation of the sessions, present these dialogues verbatim. Less typically, a coherent "autobiography" of an impaired person, presented as a confessional memoir, would be elicited in response to a request to relate a life (or rather former-life) story. In both genres the message senders express total acceptance of the impairment, presented as an opportunity to ameliorate the transcendental status of their souls, and beseech others in their vicinity to subscribe to this point of view. In unfolding the suffering they endure because of their deformities and limitations, however, the impaired launch pointed criticism against the rejection and contempt that are their share in the wider society. Their plea for human tolerance and compassion (rather than heavenly mercy) resonates with similar complaints raised by autistic and other afflicted children in non-religious FC sessions.

The privileged access of the impaired children to their souls endows them with special divinatory skills amply tested in FC sessions. Even though the publications admonish against engaging the children in petty matters, the personal sphere is represented in the communications in attempts to disclose the causes of individual life problems, from illness and economic misfortune to truancy, heavy smoking, and marred family relationships, or the unfolding of future events, such as winning in the lottery and success in the religious academy. The fact that the disclosed causes always pertain to the religious domain attenu-ates the relative insignificance ascribed to these mundane concerns. The wide spectrum of the questions in FC sessions, spanning the trivial and the sublime, is illustrated by the following passage taken from a dialogue with a 7-year-old autistic child.

Question: Is the presence of the Divine clear to you?
Answer: It is as clear to me as the reality of sunlight is clear to you.
Q: Why did you come to the world in this form?
A: There is no suffering without sin, and I sinned in forsaking the study of the Torah.
Q: Why have so many troubles been occurring recently?
A: Because of [the prevalence] of "evil tongue" and sexual relations with menstruat-ing women.
Q: Why are you crying?
A: Because I can see through you.
Q: Why have there been so many cases of divorce recently?
A: Because adultery breeds divorce.
Q: Is God with us now?
A: He is all over.
Q: What precept should be emphasized to draw the redemption nearer?
A: Showing love without expecting reward.
Q: When I reached Rabbi Elazar [a well-known charismatic rabbi] I went back and refused to receive his blessing. Why?
A: Your soul, contaminated by your body, drove you away.
Q: Is midnight prayer conducive to drawing the redemption nearer?
A: It is conducive to both personal rectification and (collective) redemption.
Q: Is it recommended to work and study at the same time?
A: [Yes]. It is correct to do both. Laboring hard on both of them may cast vices into oblivion.
Q: What about seances?
A: [The messages are] valid. But it is forbidden to conjure the dead.

Q: How to choose between schools?
A: The pupil should decide, following his own heart.
Q: Is it permitted to engage in Karate?
A: [No]. This is a vain entertainment of the gentiles.

The controversy over FC within the Haredi camp reverberates in the sessions as well. Some promoters, apparently ill at ease with the hostile approach of some renowned religious authorities, extract messages from the children that support the use of FC and praise its achievements.

Many of the sessions, particularly in public settings, are pervaded by strong apocalyptic and revivalistic tones. In fact, the disclosure of personal and political matters merely serves as a prelude to highly charged communications asserting that redemption is imminent and urging the people around to repent and thus facilitate its coming. Repentance, in the form of meticulous religious observance and moral awakening, is presented both as a prerequisite for the coming of the Messiah, without whom salvation will not unfold, and as a last-moment opportunity to be spared of God's wrath. These messages clearly constitute the emotional climax of the encounters and, in the eyes of the organizers, are their *raison d'etre*. Their significance is indicated by the disproportionate space assigned in the publications to gloomy depictions of the plights and predicaments dialectically preceding redemption, to spirited exhortations to go back to the fold and repent, to frightening admonitions portraying in vivid colors the terrible fate facing those who would not, and to shining promises about the eternal bliss expecting those who would. A special periodical, designated "The Last Words for the Last Generation," of which two issues have already appeared, is devoted almost exclusively to dispatching these messages. The quotations on the cover of the second issue, taken from recorded FC sessions, convey the sense of fervor and urgency imbued in these apocalyptic messages:

- We who look asleep come to wake up those dormant in deceitfulness.
- This is a frightening and sad situation that begs for redemption. The world in its present form is doomed to disappear in the near future and we must—a life or death matter—to make Jews repent. This is the task of the present generation.
- This is the end.
- In a little while the world will cope with the final ordeal.
- God saves the souls just before the very end.
- Those opposing our mission will not be able to stop us nor to extinguish the truth.
- You live like drunks, not paying attention to the signs God is sending to you.

While the *dramatis personae* in the sessions—the organizers and most of the facilitators and the children—were coming from religious backgrounds, the catchment population of "metaphysical FC" has been secular no less than religious. The repeated messages to repent, in particular, which make the public sessions akin to Evangelical churches' revivalistic meetings, are primarily outer-oriented, even though the function of invigorating those within the Haredi and larger religious fold should not be disregarded. Given that in their communications the children posit the unity and solidarity of the Jewish people as a key for salvation, their messages to the nonreligious alternate between beseechment and admonition. Addressed rather than excluded in order to expedite the coming of the Messiah, they are also threatened with eternal damnation if they do not yield to the messages.

CLINICAL IMPLICATIONS OF METAPHYSICAL FC

Beyond the social significance of FC in strengthening core values of the Haredi community as mentioned previously, metaphysical FC, while far from directly ameliorating the incapacitated children's pervasive dysfunctioning, might put them in a new, positive light in the eyes of their parents, caretakers, and the community at large. After all, the children are employed as mediums with superhuman divinatory capacities owing to their unmediated access to their pure soul. Empirically, however, it is still an open question whether this positive reframing of the children's situation affects their parents in a significant, enduring way. Does metaphysical FC performances cognitively restructure the parents' perceptions of and attitudes toward their children and consequently make their handling of the children easier in any significant way?

Our study did not include observations of autistic children in their home environments, nor did we interview parents or relatives of autistic children in the Haredi community. Fortunately, however, we now have access to preliminary data based on a set of 30 in-depth interviews with such parents (primarily mothers) carried out by Michal Shaked, a doctoral student in the department of psychology at the Hebrew University. From this material, we have a better glimpse of the parents' evaluations of FC effects on both clinical and metaphysical levels, although it should be noted that these data convey the Haredi parents' discourse regarding their experiences with the children. We do not have empirical data based on observations to corroborate these verbal articulations.

All but four interviewees were familiar with FC and most of them referred to it spontaneously in the course of the interview. This may be taken as an indication of how ubiquitous and salient FC had become in the Haredi community. Moreover, half (15) of the interviewees reported actual attempts to communicate with their own children through this technique. However, only seven of these interviewees reported that FC was successful in some way, and most of them qualified this success to the spiritual, metaphysical level. Only three have maintained that FC was effective clinically, in improving somewhat the children's communication skills. The heated controversy regarding FC in the Haredi community was also reflected in this sample, as six of the parents expressed ambivalence or unequivocal opposition to the technique. Some of these parents based their skepticism on disappointing FC sessions in which the credibility of the facilitator could be easily put into question. Still, we should not disregard the positive effects metaphysical FC might have on some parents by the positive reframing of the children's status. Two mothers even reported that the FC experience had radically transformed their perception, attitude, and relationship with the child. This is how the first of them described this change:

> I think that this (FC) generated a huge transformation in my attitude towards him (her autistic son). People kept saying that he could understand ... that perhaps there is something in him. But I couldn't see anything. This really broke my heart, it was very depressing. But when they started with FC, he started saying things (in a FC session) ... he said it very nicely, and I suddenly discovered... it was a kind of a pathway to his inner essence, I discovered what was in him. Since then, I started loving him very much.

The second argued that

> [T]his (FC) gave me much strength ... it is encouraging that I have a girl that I can understand, that she is not merely ... (an object) ... That there is something real here ... that she is capable of understanding ... this gives me a feeling that I deal with a human being. It made me love her more, it made me more attached to her.

Despite these reported effects of metaphysical FC, the overall data gathered from the Haredi parents seem to indicate that for most of them the "triumph of the pure soul" ostensibly manifested in FC sessions served only as a limited resource in day to day coping with the harsh reality of the children's pervasive deficits.

BETWEEN CLINICAL AND METAPHYSICAL FC

As a peculiar mystical elaboration, "metaphysical FC" may be taken as a measure for the cultural distinctiveness of the Haredi community. At the same time, however, it also serves as a reminder that even a religiously fundamentalist enclave does not altogether insulate itself from the wider secular society within which it is uncomfortably situated. Ambitious as the objectives of clinical FC may appear, particularly in the context of dramatic displays of improved communicative skills and rich inner lives of severely incapacitated children, they seem pale in comparison with the paranormal claims of mystically induced FC. And yet, notwithstanding the gap between pseudo-scientific FC and its metaphysical counterpart, the similarities between the systems transcend common procedure and administration. Particularly, the emergence of metaphysical FC may shed light on the "mystico-religious" aspects of clinical FC. In both settings FC is used to bypass gross physical deficits to give voice to hidden aspects of the psyche. This basic resemblance is clouded by epistemologically divergent rationales. According to the psychological model underlying clinical FC, the hidden psychic aspects to be retrieved are located in the brain-mind, whereas the mystical model separates between the disembodied divine soul and the brain-mind and assumes that the more damaged the brain the louder and clearer the voice of the omniscient soul. It might be suggested that the two systems use different idioms of transcendence, hidden and internal in the clinical case (cf. Shweder, 1991), exteriorized and cosmological in the metaphysical case. Yet the boundary between the two may at time become blurred, as terms prevalent in the professional discourse indicating transcendence in the first sense (e.g., "silent wisdom" in the case of autism) may be imbued with "spiritual" overtones.

The near-miraculous accomplishments claimed for FC in clinical settings, the strong emotions and moral concerns that the procedure has instigated, and the "*veritable religiose adherence by its most extreme proponents*" (Jones, 1994: 492; italics added)—all these serve to cloak clinical FC in a near-mystical atmosphere. It might be argued that in the secularized version of transcendence reflected in clinical FC the mystique of the mute self—creatively intelligent, poetically sensitive, yet trapped in a broken body and bereft of the means to articulate and express the richness of its inner life—resonates with the divine spark that constitutes the soul in metaphysical FC. In the same vein, the image of clinical FC as an empowering technique put forth to liberate autistic children from the dark recesses of their mental prison by assisting them to communicate and realize their inner potentials resonates with the soteriological messages that the children convey in metaphysical FC, related to their imminent salvation from the sins they had committed in previous incarnations, their happy compliance with God's harsh verdict, and their exalted status as prophetic messengers.

It is interesting to note that in both settings, the children's messages are marked by a strong sermonizing accent. This moralizing draws the communications in the clinical setting closer to the religious exhortations of the children in the Haredi context. Moral complaints over the ill treatment of invalids and misfits are prevalent in both forms of FC. In clinical settings allegations of physical and sexual abuse have become particularly noted, further embittering the controversy over FC. Without going into the specific contents of these allegations, it might be argued that in the context of psychological (inner and hidden) transcendence, the retrieval of covert sexual traumas appears as the secularized equivalent of the unraveling of mystical secrets in metaphysical FC. In Haredi settings the allegations against abusers have been generalized to charges lamenting the growing moral deterioration and nonobservance and denouncing many religious transgressions. Intriguingly, in an oft-quoted case study of sexual abuse allegations, made through facilitation (Bligh & Kupperman, 1993: 532) "a religious value system and mention of God was evidenced even though the child had received no religious education." It might be concluded that in both settings, FC enables disabled children to appear as resolute moral critics of their respective milieus.

The optimistic and humanitarian tenor of clinical FC has been retained and even enhanced in the religious setting. Secular and observant proponents alike emphasize, beyond the technical improvement in communication that facilitation brings forth, favorable change in the children's status and stronger acceptance by their parents. But beyond that, metaphysical FC endows the children with a distinctive transcendental aura, highlighting their access to their omniscient souls and their exalted stance as intermediaries with the hereafter. In secular settings FC is viewed as conducive to disclosing human potentials which, at best, may put disabled children on a par with normal ones. Metaphysical FC further magnifies the position of the children, reframing their afflictions as an innate moral asset that even great rabbinical figures do not naturally possess. The religious publications amply depict the favorable attitudinal transformation that parents of disabled children have undergone once they became aware of their children's privileged mediational status and superhuman abilities. The humane, benevolent orientation toward autism that the supporters of metaphysical FC display stands at odds with the traditional attitude toward mental disorders and physical stigma in the Haredi community characterized by shame, denial, and concealment. The change may be viewed as the tacit influence of modern life facilitated by the tremendous toll that physical and mental stigma cast on the ultra-orthodox family. Traditionally, the exposure of such blemish could tarnish all family members and particularly harm the prospects of finding a worthy spouse through matchmaking (Goshen-Gottstein, 1987).

Whether clinical or metaphysical, the redemptive presumptions of FC have met with a fierce opposition in both settings. The scientific skepticism regarding the efficacy of FC was reiterated in Haredi circles. And in both settings the moral preaching of FC proponents, emphasizing the humane aspects of the procedure and the hope it has been giving to the afflicted and their families, was countervailed by criticism accentuating the damage that unrealistic expectations regarding the children's abilities might cause their families. The public sessions of metaphysical FC have drawn most of the fire in the religious camp. They were denigrated as circus-like performances in which the children's precarious well-being was put at additional risk because of their harsh exposure to the limelight. Judging from the interviews of Haredi parents of autistic children, it seems that the enthusiastic claims of the entrepreneurs of metaphysical FC are overstated. Most of the parents reported that the improvement following FC session was modest at best. In a few cases, however, parents reported a dramatic change in their attitude toward the children following their participation in the sessions. In any case, it should be noted that although some of them had severe doubts as to the validity of FC, none reported negative effects as a result of exposing the children to FC.

The metaphysical halo that FC gained in the Haredi community situates the controversy over the technique in a broad cultural context—which goes beyond the question of sheer scientific validity. The juxtaposition of autism and Jewish ultra-orthodoxy constitutes a dramatic encounter between nature and culture. Autism, one of the least penetrable human ailments, is a pervasive, biologically based ("natural") disorder. In contrast, the Jewish ultra-orthodox community, with its profound commitment to the all-encompassing Law, hardly leaves any aspect of life outside the pale of culture. What happens when autism strikes this community? In this chapter we tried to show that, while the multiple disruptive behaviors of the children do not disappear, the metaphysical rationale of FC opens unexpected possibilities for reframing these behaviors in a novel, more positive cast.

ACKNOWLEDGMENTS

We thank Israel Bartal, Nachman Ben-Yehuda, Kimmy Caplan, Zeíev Klein, Mel Spiro, and Nurit Yirmiya for their helpful comments. We also thank Michal Shaked for sharing with us the interviews' transcriptions concerning the issue of metaphysical facilitated communication. We are grateful to the Schein Foundation of the Social Science Faculty at the Hebrew University of Jerusalem for supporting this project.

REFERENCES

Appadurai, A. (1990). Disjuncture and difference in the global cultural economy. *Public Culture*, 2, 1–24.

Ben-Yehuda, N. (1985). *Deviance and Moral Boundaries*. Chicago: The University of Chicago Press.

Biklen, D. (1990). Communication unbound: Autism and praxis. *Harvard Educational Review*, 60, 291–314.

Bligh, S., & Kupermann P. (1993). Brief report: Facilitated communication evaluation procedure accepted in a court case. Journal of Autism and Development Disorders, 23, 553–557.

Crossley, R. (1992). Getting the words out: Case studies in facilitated communication training. *Topics in Language Disorders*, 12, 29–41.

Dillon, K. M., Fenlason, J. E., & Vogel, D. J. (1994). Belief in and use of a questionable technique, facilitated communication, for children with autism. *Psychological Reports*, 75, 459–464.

Eberlin, M., Ibel, S., & Jacobson, J. W. (1994). The source of messages produced during facilitated communication with a boy with Autism and severe mental retardation: A case study. *Journal of Pediatric Psychology*, 19, 657–671.

Eberlin, M., McConnachie, G., Ibel, S., & Volpe, L. (1993). Facilitated communication: A failure to replicate the phenomenon. *Journal of Autism and Developmental Disorders*, 23, 507–530.

Foucault, M. (1973). *Madness and Civilization*. New York: Vintage Books.

Gaines, A. D. (1992). From DSM I to III-R; Voices of self, mastery and the other: A cultural construction of psychiatric classification. *Social Science and Medicine*, 35, 3–24.

Goshen-Gottstein, E. (1987). Mental health implication of living in an Ultraorthodox Jewish subculture. *Israel Journal of Psychiatry*, 24, 145–166.

Hannerz, U. (1989). Notes on the global ecumene. *Public Culture*, 1, 66–75.

Heilman, S. C., & Friedman, M. (1991). Religious fundamentalism and religious Jews. In M. E. Marty, & S. R. Appleby (Eds.), *Fundamentalisms Observed*. Chicago: University of Chicago Press.

Idel, M. (1988). *Kabbalah: New Perspectives*. New Haven, CT: Yale University Press.

Jacobson, J. W., Mulick, J. A., & Schwartz, A. A. (1995). A history of facilitated communication. *American Psychologist*, *50*, 750–765.

Jones, D. P. H. (1994). Autism, facilitated communication, and allegations of child abuse and neglect. *Child Abuse and Neglect*, *18*, 491–537.

Kleinman, A. (1988). *Rethinking Psychiatry*. Berkeley: University of California Press.

Montee, B. B., Miltenberger, R. G., & Wittrock D. (1995). An experimental analysis of facilitated communication. *Journal of Applied Behavior Analysis*, *28*, 189–200.

Routh, D. K. (1994). Commentary: Facilitated communication as unwitting ventriloquism. *Journal of Pediatric Psychology*, *19*, 673–675.

Shweder, R. (1991). *Thinking Through Cultures*. Cambridge, MA: Harvard University Press.

Sobel, Z., & Beit-Hallahmi, B., Eds. (1991). *Tradition, Innovation, Conflict*. New York: SUNY Press.

II

Biological Perspectives

5

Comparison of Siblings of Individuals with Autism and Siblings of Individuals with Other Diagnoses

An Empirical Summary

Nurit Yirmiya, Michal Shaked, and Osnat Erel

The aim of the current study is to summarize the data regarding different characteristics, or outcome measures (including autism, the broad phenotype of autism, cognitive development, and psychological well-being) of siblings of individuals with autism as compared to siblings of individuals with normal development or with diagnoses other than autism. Analysis of the data was conducted using meta-analytic procedures. Meta-analysis combines outcomes of numerous studies to examine the association between variables, almost as though the participants from each individual study are now participating in a single experimental design. Thereby the larger sample size permits greater inferential power (Johnson, 1989). In addition, the procedure of meta-analysis enables researchers to test hypotheses that were not included in the individual articles (Hale & Dillard, 1991).

In 1960, Creak and Ini published a study on families of children with autism, or as then called, psychotic children. This was the first large-scale family study of children with autism. They reported that in the 79 families who had more than one child (149 siblings), two families had another child with autism, four families had another child with mental retardation, and 19 families had another child who was maladjusted. Creak and Ini concluded that "whilst the great majority of the siblings were normal, there are suggestions that for them, the risk for psychosis and/or mental defect is higher than the risk for the general population" (p. 174). Folstein and Rutter (1977) translated the aforementioned suggestion into a genetic hypothesis and conceptualized a continuum of underlying genetic liability for autism, with the full syndrome of autism as the most severe phenotype.

NURIT YIRMIYA, MICHAL SHAKED, and OSNAT EREL • Department of Psychology and School of Education, The Hebrew University of Jerusalem, Mount Scopus, Jerusalem, 91905 Israel.

The Research Basis for Autism Intervention, edited by Schopler, Yirmiya, Shulman, and Marcus. Kluwer Academic/Plenum Publishers, New York, 2001.

The data regarding possible differences between siblings of individuals with autism and siblings of individuals with diagnoses other than autism and normally developing individuals are not consistent. According to some studies, siblings of individuals with autism showed an elevated rate of autism (i.e., higher frequency of occurrence) and related difficulties (e.g., emotional, social, cognitive, linguistic) compared to siblings of individuals with other handicaps, and siblings of normally developing individuals (e.g., August, Stewart, & Tsai, 1981; Piven, Palmer, Jacobi, Childress, & Arndt, 1997). However, no significant differences between siblings of individuals with autism and siblings of individuals without autism were found in other studies (e.g., Boutin, Maziade, Merette, Mondor, Bedard, & Thiviege, 1997; Gillberg, Gillberg, & Steffenburg, 1992; Szatmari, et al., 1993). Some of the conflicting findings may be a result of theoretical and methodological differences among the studies such as employment of different comparison groups and the focus on various outcome measures with siblings of different ages.

Most researchers examined differences in the rate of autism and other outcome measures by comparing siblings of individuals with autism with siblings of individuals with Down syndrome and normally developing individuals. Only a few studies in which comparisons between siblings of individuals with autism and siblings of individuals with mental retardation (MR) of unknown etiology, with learning disabilities (LD), with psychiatric syndromes, or with other conditions have been published.

The issue of the comparison group to which siblings of individuals with autism are compared is important because different comparison groups "control" for different aspects associated with having a sibling with autism. Each comparison group has methodological advantages and disadvantages. For example, comparing siblings of individuals with autism to siblings of individuals with normal development does not "control" for whether some or all of the characteristics examined have a genetic basis, or an environmental basis such as a response to the condition of being a sibling of a child with autism.

Down syndrome is a specific chromosomal disorder, and therefore relatives of individuals with Down syndrome are not expected to be at a greater genetic risk (Piven et al., 1997). Thus, from a genetic risk perspective, a comparison group of siblings of individuals with Down syndrome is similar to that of normally developing individuals. However, the stress involved in growing up with a sibling with Down syndrome may affect different aspects of coping and well-being in siblings, and thus this comparison group may "control" for some of the environmental effects of having a sibling with a handicap. Learning disabilities have a genetic basis (DeFries, Fulker, & LaBuda, 1987; Faraone, Biederman, Krifcher, & Lehman, 1993; Wadsworth, DeFries, Fulker, & Plomin, 1995), and, therefore, comparing siblings of individuals with autism to siblings of individuals with LD may help determine whether there is a specific phenotype for the genetic basis of autism that differs from the phenotype associated with LD. However, individuals with LD most typically do not manifest mental retardation and in many ways are easier to care for than individuals with mental retardation or autism. Thus, a comparison group of siblings of individuals with LD enables some "control" of genetic risk, but the "control" for environmental effects is less than optimal. Finally, comparisons between siblings of individuals with autism and siblings of individuals with psychiatric conditions (e.g., schizophrenia) are important because they may clarify whether the risk for certain impairments is unique to autism or is general to families who already have one child with a psychiatric condition.

In addition to including different comparison groups, researchers have examined various outcomes when assessing the functioning of the siblings. These outcomes included the rate of autism, the rate of the broad phenotype, of nonverbal and verbal communication difficulties, anxiety, depression, cognitive abilities in general, social competence, and more. Therefore, results may vary as a function of both the comparison group studied and of the specific outcome measures examined.

Methodological as well as theoretical issues are involved in examining different outcome measures. Whereas the diagnosis of autism is well defined, and most researchers adhere to strict diagnostic procedures, there is no agreement about the definition and measurement of the lesser variant (also referred to as the broad phenotype) of autism. Some researchers focused on cognitive measures (e.g., Fombonne, Bolton, Prior, Jordan & Rutter, 1997; Szatmari et al., 1993), others emphasized communication abilities (e.g., Leboyer, Plumet, Goldblum, Perez-Diaz, & Marchaland, 1995; Plumet, Goldblum, & Leboyer, 1995), and still others examined aspects of social development and psychological well-being (e.g., Gold, 1993; Piven et al., 1997). The measures used to assess these outcomes also vary considerably, ranging from standard tests such as the Wechsler intelligent tests (1963, 1974, 1981), to questionnaires and clinical interviews regarding developmental history.

Furthermore, some outcomes were examined only with certain comparison groups. For example, the rate of autism in siblings of individuals with autism was examined in comparison to the rate of autism in siblings of individuals with Down syndrome, MR of unknown etiology, and children born with low birth weight. However, it is unknown whether more children diagnosed with autism are born to families who already have one child with autism than to families who already have one child with a psychiatric disorder other than autism. This is due to the fact that the rate of autism was not examined in siblings of individuals with autism as compared to siblings of individuals with other psychiatric diagnoses.

Similarly, in characterizing the broad phenotype or the lesser variant, most investigators employed comparison groups of sibling of individuals with Down syndrome and/or siblings of individuals with normal development (August et al., 1981; Bolton, Macdonald, Pickles, Rios, & Goode, 1994; Gillberg et al., 1992; Piven et al., 1997; Plumet et al., 1995; Smalley & Asarnow, 1990). Comparison groups of siblings of individuals with LD (Gillberg et al., 1992), and siblings of individuals with MR (but not Down syndrome) (Boutin et al., 1997), were each employed only once when examining the outcome relating to the broad phenotype of autism. In this chapter, we provide an empirical summary of the literature pertaining to siblings of individuals with autism as compared with siblings of nonautistic individuals while examining the potential contribution of different comparison groups (e.g., Down syndrome, MR of unknown etiology) and outcome measures (e.g., autism, broader phenotype) to the emerging findings.

METHOD

The PsychINFO, PsychLIT, ERIC, Social SciSearch, and Medline computerized systems were used to identify relevant published studies. The search included all published studies included in these systems, until May 1999. The key words used for the search were "autism and genetics," "autism and siblings," and "autism and brothers/sisters." Relevant studies were also gathered from reference lists of research papers, review articles, books, and book chapters focusing on autism and behavior genetics. The criteria for inclusion of a study in the sample were: (1) journal publication and (2) inclusion of siblings of at least one comparison group in addition to siblings of individuals with autism. The comparison group had to include a specific sample (i.e., not a comparison to a population without specification of sample size); (3) examination of behavioral data (i.e., biological markers and behavior toward the affected child were not examined in the current meta-analysis). Eighteen studies comparing siblings of individuals with autism and siblings of individuals with other handicaps or of individuals with normal development were identified through this extensive literature research.

In meta-analysis, different variables examined in the individual studies, such as comparison group and outcome measure, are selected and reexamined on a larger sample. The variables in this study were selected according to: suggestions made by different authors in the field; frequency of their appearance in empirical literature; theoretical considerations; and methodological considerations. The variables selected included: comparison group and outcome measures discussed above, as well as the gender of the siblings of the individuals with autism, and the level of functioning of the proband with autism. Other variables such as ascertainment methods, gender of the probands, socioeconomic status, family size, birth order, spacing between children, younger versus older siblings, availability or lack of social support, and religiosity may also influence findings (Bristol, 1984; Henderson & Vandenberg, 1992; Jones & Szatmari, 1988; Piven, Gayle, Chase, Fink, & Landa, 1990; Piven et al., 1991; Simeonsson & McHale, 1981). Unfortunately, owing to the small number of studies, in which these variables were explicitly considered, it was impossible to examine their contribution to the behavioral phenotype of siblings of individuals with autism.

Comparison Groups

The comparison groups employed in the various studies included siblings of: (1) normally developing individuals; (2) individuals with Down syndrome; (3) individuals with MR of unknown (nonspecific) etiology; (4) individuals with LD or dysphasia; (5) individuals with psychiatric problems; and (6) individuals composing other comparison groups. This included one study employing a comparison group of siblings of individuals with tuberous sclerosis complex or other unspecified seizure disorder (Smalley, McCracken, & Tanguay, 1995), a study employing a comparison group that included both siblings of individuals with Down syndrome and siblings of children born at a low birth weight in the same group (Szatmari et al., 1993), and another study employing a comparison group of children with school phobia.

Outcomes

This category initially included 13 outcomes reported in the literature. However, the small number of published studies precluded meaningful analyses with these variables. The different outcome measures were therefore combined into four main categories: (1) autism; (2) broad phenotype or lesser variant, which included various measures of language disability and deficits in social and behavioral domains, as well as measurements of specific

Pervasive Developmental Disorder (PDD) diagnoses;* (3) cognitive abilities and neuro-psychological abilities; and (4) measurements of psychological well-being and psychiatric problems including depression, anxiety, and behavior problems as assessed by the Child Behavior Checklist (CBCL).

Additional Variables

In addition, we examined the contribution of two additional variables: siblings' gender and level of functioning of the probands with autism. These two variables were included frequently enough in the studies to allow for their coding and analyses. The examination of these variables is important because it may assist in identifying a group of siblings (e.g., siblings of low functioning individuals with autism compared to siblings of high function-ing individuals with autism, or female siblings versus male siblings) that is at a higher risk for atypical development.

Siblings' gender: This category included: (1) brothers, (2) sisters, and (3) siblings—when the study did not offer separate data for brothers and sisters.

Level of functioning of the probands with autism: This category included (1) no differentiation between probands based on their developmental levels/mental ability; (2) probands with mental retardation; (3) high functioning probands; and (4) no information provided about the developmental level/mental ability of the probands.

Statistical Analyses

To perform the meta-analytic procedure, all data were transformed into standardized effect sizes (*d*) using the D-STAT program (Johnson, 1989, 1993). Standardized effect sizes represent the magnitude of an effect, and may be derived from means and standard deviations, proportions, frequencies, and significance values (*p*-values). Reliability values calculated per category of moderator variable ranged from 88% to 100%, with a mean of 96%. All disagreements were discussed and resolved by all authors.

The standardized effect sizes are then combined into a composite mean weighted effect size and the significance of this composite mean weighted effect size is determined. Cohen's (1977) criteria is that an effect size (in the metric of *d*) of .20 is of small magnitude, an effect size of .50 is of medium magnitude, and an effect size of .80 is of large magnitude. The composite mean weighted effect size is considered significant if its confidence interval (CI) does not include zero. In addition to its significance, the composite mean weighted effect size is assessed for its homogeneity, that is, whether it is consistent across the studies included. If so, this composite mean weighted effect size can be considered as representa-tive of the population from which it was drawn and free from the moderating effect of other variables. Meta-analysis is considered complete when homogeneity is achieved. Usually, owing to the effects of moderator variables, the composite mean weighted effect size

---

*One study measuring PDD subtypes (Szatmari et al., 1993); one study investigating various aspects of social and cognitive disability, IQ, language abnormality, learning disability, and scholastic status (August et al., 1981); one study investigating aspects of emotion recognition (Smalley & Asarnow, 1990); one study investigating the following developmental disorders: Asperger syndrome, speech and language problems or reading and spelling problems (Gillberg, 1992); and one study measuring deficits in the realm of communication, social behavior, and stereotyped behavior (Bolton et al., 1994).

calculated from several independent studies is not homogenous. In this case, the third step in a meta-analysis, categorical model testing, is employed to identify moderator variables, that is, variables that explain the inconsistency. To identify potential moderator variables, studies are divided into groups according to the different categories of a certain potential moderator variable. Statistical tests can then be conducted to determine whether a group of studies with a common moderator level are homogeneous.

When at least two homogeneous groups of studies within a potential moderator variable are identified, the fourth step in meta-analytic research may be carried out. This step involves computation of contrasts between the different composite effect sizes that were found to be homogeneous. Differences in mean weighted effect sizes from homogeneous categories imply the existence of a moderator variable (Hedges & Olkin, 1985). Contrasts between homogeneous levels within a certain category were carried out only when there were at least three effect sizes within each one of the homogeneous levels. For more information regarding the meta-analytic procedure please see Erel and Burman (1995) and Yirmiya, Erel, Shaked, and Solomonica-Levi (1998).

In the meta-analytic procedure, each study itself is the unit of analysis. This procedure requires independence of units of analysis. Therefore, whenever there was more than one outcome for the same group of participants and the same category as defined in this study (i.e., autism, broad phenotypy, cognitive development, psycholgogical well-being) a combined effect size over the various measurements was computed, and this combined effect size was treated as the outcome of the study. Each effect size included in the meta-analysis was computed and coded independently by the first two authors.

RESULTS

Only a few studies pertained to the same comparison group and the same outcome measures, and most of the associated composite mean weighted effect sizes were homogeneous. Thus, categorical model testing and comparisons (steps 3 and 4; see previous section) were not necessary in most cases. Therefore, the composite mean weighted effect size is reported with its significance and homogeneity status, per comparison group and outcome measure. When necessary and feasible (at least two effect sizes within each group of studies) the possibility that siblings' gender and level of functioning of the individuals with autism explain the nonhomogeneous findings within each comparison group and outcome measure was explored.

Outcome: Autism

The differences in the rate of autism between siblings of individuals with autism and siblings of other individuals were examined in five studies, yielding five effect sizes. Jorde (1990) reported a significantly higher rate of autism in siblings of individuals with autism as compared with siblings of individuals with normal development ($d = . 59$, CI: .29/.90). August et al. (1981) and Bolton et al. (1994) found that more siblings of individuals with autism were affected with autism than were siblings of individuals with Down syndrome. In these two studies, siblings were not differentiated by gender, and the probands with autism were not separated into low versus high functioning. The mean weighted effect size representing these studies was homogeneous, and of a low and nonsignificant magnitude ($d = 0.21$, CI: $-.03/.45$). Boutin et al. (1997) compared the rate of autism in siblings of individuals with autism who were also mentally retarded versus siblings of individuals with MR of unknown etiology ($d = .15$, CI: $-.34/.64$). This comparison did not yield a significant difference. Szatmari et al. (1993) examined the rate of autism in siblings of individuals with PDD and siblings of individuals with Down syndrome and low birth weight. The effect size was homogeneous, of low magnitude ($d = .30$, CI: $-.07/.66$), and was nonsignificant.

In sum, the studies reviewed here indicated that more siblings of individuals with autism are affected with autism when compared with siblings of individuals with normal development, but not when compared with siblings of individuals with Down syndrome or MR of unknown etiology or other conditions. However, the failure to find differences between siblings of individuals with autism and siblings of individuals with other atypical development may be due to the small number of siblings in each study. The recurrence rate of autism, although extremely high compared to the rate of autism in the general population (3% versus 0.3%–0.5% life births), is still so low that any given sample is most likely too small to yield significant differences. It is important to note that the rate of autism in siblings of individuals with autism as compared to the rate of autism in siblings of individuals with learning disabilities and siblings of individuals with psychiatric conditions was not studied. These comparisons may clarify whether autism occurs in families who already have one child with autism more often than in families who have a child with a psychiatric disorder in general, and thus point to specificity of recurrence of autism and its genetic basis.

Outcome: Broad Phenotype

Differences in the rate of the broad phenotype in siblings of individuals with autism and siblings of other individuals were examined in six studies, yielding eight effect sizes. Three effect sizes yielded from studies by Gillberg et al. (1992) and Smalley and Asarnow (1990) represent comparisons between siblings of individuals with autism and siblings of normally developing individuals regarding the rate of the broad phenotype. The mean weighted effect size was homogeneous but of low magnitude ($d = -.20$, CI: $-.58/.18$) and was nonsignificant. Five effect sizes from four studies by August et al. (1981), Bolton et al. (1994), Piven et al. (1997), and Plumet et al. (1995) represent comparisons between siblings of individuals with autism and siblings of individuals with Down syndrome regarding the presence of the broad phenotype. Effect sizes regarding brothers (one effect size) and brothers and sisters combined (three effect sizes) were significant and homogeneous. The effect size representing comparisons of sisters did not yield a significant effect size. The overall mean weighted effect size was of medium magnitude ($d = .45$, CI: $.24/.66$), homogeneous, and indicated that siblings of individuals with autism are diagnosed with the broad phenotype significantly more than siblings of individuals with Down syndrome. The data were significant and homogeneous for the two effect sizes which represented probands with autism who were mentally retarded and for the remaining three effect sizes, which represented studies in which there was no differentiation between low and high functioning individuals with autism. Computation of contrasts did not reveal significant differences between these two groups of studies, suggesting that the differences between siblings of individuals with autism and siblings of individuals with Down syndrome (DS) are the same whether siblings of low or high functioning probands with autism are included.

The broad phenotype was examined in siblings of individuals with MR of unknown etiology by Boutin et al. (1997), who found no significant difference in the rate of the broad phenotype between siblings of individuals with autism and siblings of individuals with MR of unknown etiology (d = .11, CI: −.38/.60). The broad phenotype was examined by Gillberg et al. (1992), who compared siblings of individuals with autism and siblings of individuals with LD. No significant differences were found between brothers and sisters of individuals with autism (undifferentiated as to whether high or low functioning) and brothers and sisters of individuals with LD. The mean weighted effect size for both comparisons of brothers and sisters was nonsignificant (d = −.20, CI: −.62/.22). Finally, Szatmari et al. (1993) examined the broad phenotype in siblings of individuals with autism and siblings of children with low birth weight and Down syndrome. The results indicated a nonsignificant difference (d = .10, CI: −.24/.44).

In sum, significantly more siblings of individuals with autism, as compared to siblings of individuals with Down syndrome, were affected with the broad phenotype. No significant differences emerged between the number of affected siblings of individuals with autism and siblings of normally developing individuals, individuals with MR due to an unknown etiology, LD, and other conditions. The failure to find significant differences may result from the paucity of studies regarding these comparisons and from the small number of participants. In addition, no studies were available regarding the prevalence of the broad phenotype in siblings of individuals with autism as compared to siblings of individuals with other psychiatric conditions, a comparison that is relevant to understanding whether the broad phenotype is unique to autism or not.

Outcome: Cognitive

Differences in cognitive abilities between siblings of individuals with autism and siblings of other individuals were examined in five studies, yielding seven effect sizes. Smalley and Asarnow (1990) examined WISC-R and WAIS-R scores of siblings of individuals with autism and siblings of normally developing individuals. The associated effect size was nonsignificant (d = −.40, CI: −1.34/.53). Siblings of individuals with Down syndrome and siblings of individuals with autism were compared with respect to their cognitive development by Fombonne et al. (1997) and Leboyer et al. (1995). The associated mean weighted effect size was homogeneous but of a low magnitude (d = .11, CI: −.18/.40) and did not indicate a significant difference. Fombonne et al. (1997) found no significant differences between the groups when all siblings were included; however, siblings of the individuals with autism scored significantly higher (i.e., indicated better performance) than siblings of the individuals with Down syndrome once the affected siblings were removed from the analyses.

Only Narayan, Moyes, and Wolff (1990) examined the cognitive abilities of brothers and sisters of individuals with autism in comparison to those of siblings of individuals with MR of unknown etiology. Brothers and sisters of individuals with autism scored significantly higher than brothers and sisters of individuals with MR (d = −.80, CI: −1.33/−.28). Ozonoff, Rogers, Farnham, and Pennington (1993) examined the performance of siblings of individuals with autism and siblings of individuals with LD on the verbal comprehension and perceptual organization factors of the WISC-R and WAIS-R. The associated effect size was large ($d = .63$, CI: 0/1.35) and indicated that siblings of individuals with autism scored less well compared to siblings of individuals with LD.

In sum, significant differences emerged between siblings of individuals with autism and siblings of individuals with LD, with siblings of individuals with LD showing higher cognitive ability. In contrast, no significant differences emerged between siblings of individuals with autism and siblings of normally developing individuals or siblings of individuals with Down syndrome. The results regarding the comparison between siblings of individuals with autism and individuals with MR were mixed: Some studies did not yield significant differences whereas other studies actually reported that unaffected siblings of individuals with autism score higher on cognitive tests compared to siblings of individuals with Down syndrome and with MR due to unknown etiologies. Information was unavailable about the cognitive functioning of siblings of individuals with autism as compared to siblings of individuals with other psychiatric conditions or to siblings of individuals from other comparison groups.

Outcome: Psychological Well-being and Psychiatric Syndromes

Behavior problems in siblings of individuals with autism and siblings of normally developing individuals were examined in three studies (Fisman, Wolf, Ellison, Gillis, Freeman, & Szatmari, 1996; Gold, 1993; Rodrigue, Geffken, & Morgan, 1993), yielding four effect sizes. The mean weighted effect size was homogeneous, of low magnitude ($d = .28$, CI: $-.01/.57$), and was nonsignificant. Two effect sizes referred to psychiatric outcomes in comparing siblings of individuals with autism and siblings of individuals with Down syndrome (Fisman, et al., 1996; Rodrigue et al., 1993). The mean weighted effect size was of medium magnitude ($d = .39$, CI:.04/.73), homogeneous, and significant.

Smalley et al. (1995) examined the rate of depression (as assessed by the K-SADS-E) in siblings of individuals with autism (undifferentiated according to high versus low functioning), and found that siblings of individuals with autism score higher on depression than siblings of individuals with Tuberous Sclerosis (TSC) and unspecified seizure disorders ($d = .74$, CI: .16/1.31). Kolvin, Ounsted, Richardson, and Garside (1971) found no differences in the rate of schizophrenia, depression, and neuroses among siblings of individuals with autism as compared to siblings of individuals with school phobia ($d = -.17$, CI: $-.53/.18$).

In sum, different psychiatric outcomes were examined in the various studies with significant differences emerging only between siblings of individuals with autism and siblings of individuals with Down syndrome. No differences emerged between siblings of individuals with autism and siblings of normally developing individuals, and mixed findings emerged regarding the comparison with siblings of individuals with other (nonautistic) psychiatric conditions. The psychiatric symptoms of siblings of individuals with autism in comparison to siblings of individuals with MR of unknown etiology, or to siblings of individuals with LD have not been investigated.

Additional Analyses

Owing to the lack of clearly defined boundaries of the broad deficit (Rutter, Bailey, Simonoff, & Pickles, 1997) and the small number of studies within each category, we combined the two outcomes of "broad phenotype" and "cognitive" into a single category and reanalyzed the data. To maintain independence of the units of analysis, the two effect sizes from the Smalley and Asarnow (1990) study and from the Bolton et al. (1994) and Fombonne et al. (1997) study were averaged. These data were examined according to type of comparison group. For all comparison groups, effect sizes were homogeneous, yet only the effect size representing the comparison between siblings of individuals with autism and siblings of individuals with Down syndrome yielded a significant effect size of medium magnitude ($d = .35$, CI: 16/.54). Comparisons between siblings of individuals with autism and siblings of individuals with normal development, with MR, with LD, and with other difficulties did not yield significant differences.

DISCUSSION

The findings of this meta-analytic study assist in evaluating the genetic hypothesis of autism, which suggests that autism is the most severe phenotype in a continuum of behavioral phenotypes, which aggregates in families of persons with autism. When autism as an outcome in siblings is considered, twin and sibling studies offer strong support for the genetic hypothesis. The rate of autism in MZ twins is much higher than in DZ twins (36% to 95% versus 0% to 4.8%, respectively) and the recurrence rate of autism in siblings of individuals with autism is 50- to 100-fold the rate of autism in the general population (August et al., 1981; Bailey, Philips, & Rutter, 1996; Bailey et al., 1995; Bolton & Rutter, 1990; Bolton et al., 1994, Folstein & Rutter, 1977; Fombonne & Dumazaubrun, 1992; Gillberg et al., 1992; Minton, Campbell, Green, Jennings, & Samit, 1982, Piven et al., 1990; Smalley, 1991, 1997; Smalley, Asarnow, & Spence, 1988; Steffenburg et al., 1989). Although environmental effects cannot be completely ruled out, the findings that families with one child with autism are at risk for having another child with autism are accepted as evidence that genetic factors play an important role in the etiology of autism (Bailey et al., 1996). Thus, when the outcome of autism is considered, researchers studying families of individuals with autism provide ample evidence for a significantly higher recurrence rate of autism in families of individuals with autism. However, the crucial comparison between families with a child with autism and families with a child with a psychiatric disorder remains to be examined.

Most researchers report that the broad phenotype or as often called the lesser variant is also found in siblings of individuals with autism in studies with and without comparison groups. When the broad phenotype is considered, researchers typically use various operational definitions and employ a variety of instruments. From a genetic perspective, differences in the rate of the broad phenotype were expected between siblings of individuals with autism and siblings of individuals with Down syndrome and normal development because both of these groups do not carry any known genetic liability. Results of the current study indicate that significantly more siblings of individuals with autism are affected with the broad phenotype as compared to siblings of individuals with Down syndrome only. It may be that the nonsignificant difference between siblings of individuals with autism and siblings of individuals with normal development is due to the smaller number of available studies (three for comparisons with siblings of individuals with normal development versus five for comparisons with siblings of individuals with DS). Clearly, more studies comparing siblings of individuals with autism and siblings of normally developing individuals are needed to increase the number of participants included in the analyses to clarify this issue. As indicated by the results, rates of the broad phenotype did not differ between siblings of individuals with autism as compared to siblings of normally developing individuals, siblings of individuals with MR of unknown etiology, siblings of individuals with LD, or siblings of individuals with low birth weight and Down syndrome. Future studies should continue to investigate the prevalence of the broad phenotype in various groups and strive toward a more unified operationalization of this construct.

Studies in which the cognitive abilities of the siblings were assessed yielded ambiguous findings. Siblings of individuals with autism scored significantly lower than siblings of individuals with LD, but higher than siblings of individuals with Down syndrome. When the two outcomes (broad phenotype and cognitive) were combined, a significant effect size emerged only between siblings of individuals with autism and siblings of individuals with Down syndrome. When psychiatric outcomes were examined, once more the data yielded a significant effect size only for the comparison between siblings of individuals with autism and siblings of individuals with Down syndrome. Nonsignificant findings emerged between siblings of individuals with autism and siblings of individuals with normal development, and some psychiatric conditions. More studies regarding the well-being and psychiatric status of siblings of individuals with various disorders are needed to achieve a more in-depth understanding of the unique and specific clinical profile of siblings of individuals with autism.

In general, the few significant differences reported in the current analyses are surprising given the clinical and research data and impressions suggesting that siblings of individuals with autism show a high incidence of cognitive, social, emotional, and communication difficulties. The current analyses were based only on studies including a comparison group because we were interested in whether more siblings of individuals with autism are affected, and whether a specific phenotype for the genetic basis of autism can be identified. Based on our findings, it is suggested that at present, the behavioral database is too small to allow for firm conclusions to be made as to whether siblings of individuals with autism are more impaired than siblings of individuals with other diagnoses when outcome measures other than autism are examined.

In contrast to the known prevalence rate of autism in the population, the prevalence rate of the broad phenotype in the general population is unknown. The nonsignificant differences between siblings of individuals with autism and siblings of individuals with diagnoses other than autism reported in the current study may be a result of a low prevalence rate and of the limited number of participants and studies. Categorical model testing evaluating additional variables could not be carried out owing to the small number of published studies. The small number of studies comparing siblings of individuals with autism to siblings of individuals with diagnoses other than autism that have been carried out and published was unexpected. This stands in contrast to approximately three times as many studies comparing parents of individuals with autism with parents of individuals with diagnoses other than autism. Perhaps some of the findings from the parental literature influenced conceptions regarding siblings, when actually more research is needed in order to achieve an in-depth understanding of the behavioral phenotype characterizing siblings of individuals with autism. Furthermore, the behavioral broad phenotype in children may be different from that found for adults. Future research should carefully examine the operational definitions of the broad phenotype for persons of different ages.

Finally, autism is a complex syndrome with many causative pathways. There may be more than one behavioral phenotype associated with the broad phenotype or the lesser variant of autism. Future studies comparing siblings of individuals with autism to siblings of individuals with diagnoses other than autism, while taking into account variables such as gender, level of functioning, ascertainment methods, and so forth, could assist in clarifying whether siblings of individuals with autism reveal a specific and unique behavioral profile. In addition, research aiming at exploring whether different expressions of the autism genotype are associated with various behavioral broad phenotypes may also yield important information. The behavioral broad phenotype found in families with one child with autism may be different than that found in families who have two children with autism. The phenotype may also differ as a function of other intra- and interpersonal variables such as gender of the proband and sibling, level of functioning of the proband, and various familial characteristics (e.g., socioeconomic status, available social support).

IMPLICATIONS FOR INTERVENTIONS

Specifying behavioral profiles of the siblings may assist in identifying the genes associated with autism and PDD in general. Until such genes are identified, the specification of the behavioral phenotypes can assist in early identification of developmental difficulties and in implementing appropriate interventions for siblings, who in addition to facing possible genetic liability are experiencing the difficulties associated with living with a sibling with autism. In fact some researchers report that the well-being of the siblings is associated with parental marital satisfaction (Rodrigue et al., 1993), and with whether parents resolve their feelings of acceptance of their child with autism (McHale, Simeonsson, & Sloan, 1984; McHale, Sloan, & Simeonsson, 1986; Simeonsson & McHale, 1981). Furthermore, siblings who reported being less depressed also reported having someone to talk to about their sibling with autism in contrast to siblings who reported being more depressed and not having anyone to talk to about their sibling with autism (Gold, 1993).

The diathesis-stress model (Brown & Harros, 1989; Burke & Elliott, 1999; Gottesman, 1991; Rende & Plomin, 1992; Rosenthal, 1970; Walker & Diforio, 1997; Walker, Downey, & Bergman, 1989), integrates genetic and environmental components in the conceptualization of psychopathology. The genetic and environmental components may vary in different families, with one or the other contributing more or less. However, even if siblings are affected genetically, the environment may have an important role in exacerbating or lessening the behavioral manifestations. Therefore, it may be that "Nature proposes and Nurture disposes" (Gottesman, 1991) and that social support to the parents and the siblings can operate as protective factors. Programs for individuals with autism may thus benefit from including support and intervention components designed specifically toward the family as a whole and toward the siblings as a unique group. These efforts may benefit not only the siblings but also the children with autism themselves.

ACKNOWLEDGMENTS

We thank Dr. Ada Zohar, Tammy Pilowsky, Ilana Eisenmajer, Michal Herbsman, and our colleagues who shared their work with us.

REFERENCES

References marked with an asterisk indicate studies included in the analyses.

*August, G. J., Stewart, M. A., & Tsai, L. (1981). The incidence of cognitive disabilities in the siblings of autistic children. *British Journal of Psychiatry, 138,* 416–422.

Bailey, A., LeCoutcur, A., Gottesman, I., Bolton, P., Simonoff, E., Yuzda, E., & Rutter, M. (1995). Autism as a strongly genetic disorder: Evidence from a British twin study. *Psychological Medicine, 25,* 63–78.

Bailey, A., Philips, W., & Rutter, M. (1996). Autism: Towards an integration of clinical, genetic, neuropsychological, and neurobiological perspectives. *Journal of Child Psychology and Psychiatry, 37*(1), 89–126.

*Bolton, P., Macdonald, H., Pickles, A., Rios, P., & Goode, S. (1994). A case-control family history study of autism. *Journal of Child Psychology and Psychiatry, 35,* 877–900.

Bolton, P., & Rutter, M. (1990). Genetic influences in autism. *International Review of Psychiatry, 2,* 76–80.

*Boutin, P., Maziade, M., Merette, C., Mondor, M., Bedard, C., & Thiviege, J. (1997). Family history of cognitive disabilities in first-degree relatives of autistic and mentally retarded children. *Journal of Autism and Developmental Disorders, 27,* 165–176.

Bristol, M. M. (1984). Family resources and successful adaptation to autistic children. In E. Schopler & G. B. Mesibov (Eds.), *The Effects of Autism on the Family* (2nd ed., pp. 289–310). New York: Plenum.

Brown, G. W., & Harros, T. O. (1989). *Life Events and Illness.* New York: Guilford.

Burke, P., & Elliott, M. (1999). Depression in pediatric chronic illness: A diathesis-stress model. *Psychosomatics, 40,* 5–17.

Cohen, J. (1977). *Statistical Power Analysis for the Behavioral Sciences.* New York: Academic Press.

Creak, M., & Ini, S. (1960). Families of psychotic children. *Journal of Child Psychology and Psychiatry, 1,* 156–175.

DeFries, J. C., Fulker, D. W., & LaBuda, M. C. (1987). Evidence for a genetic aetiology in reading disability of twins. *Nature, 329,* 537–539.

Erel, O., & Burman, B. (1995). Inter-relatedness of marital and parent–child relations: A meta-analytic review. *Psychological Bulletin, 118,* 108–132.

Faraone, S. V., Biederman, J., Krifcher, B., & Lehman, B. (1993). Evidence for the independent familial transmission of attention deficit hyperactivity disorder and learning disabilities: Results from a family genetic study. *American Journal of Psychiatry, 150,* 891–895.

*Fisman, S., Wolf, L., Ellison, D., Gillis., B., Freeman, T., & Szatmari, P. (1996). Risk and protective factors affecting the adjustment of siblings of children with chronic disabilities. *Journal of the American Academy of Child and Adolescent Psychiatry, 35,* 1532–1541.

Folstein, S. E., & Rutter, M. L. (1977). Infantile autism: A genetic study of 21 twin pairs. *Journal of Child Psychology and Psychiatry, 18,* 297–321.

*Fombonne, E., Bolton, P., Prior, J., Jordan, H., & Rutter, M. (1997). A family study of autism: Cognitive patterns and levels in parents and siblings. *Journal of Child Psychology and Psychiatry, 38,* 667–684.

Fombonne, E., & Dumazaubrun, C. (1992). Prevalence of infantile autism in 4 French regions. *Social Psychiatry and Psychiatric Epidemiology, 27,* 203–210.

*Gillberg, C., Gillberg, I. C., & Steffenburg, S. (1992). Siblings and parents of children with autism: A controlled population-based study. *Developmental Medicine and Child Neurology, 34,* 389–398.

*Gold, N. (1993). Depression and social adjustment in siblings of boys with autism. *Journal of Autism and Developmental Disorders, 23,* 147–163.

Gottesman, I. (1991). *Schizophrenia Genesis: The Origins of Madness.* New York: Freeman.

Hale, J. L., & Dillard, J. P. (1991). The uses of metaanlysis—making knowledge claims and setting research agendas. *Communication Monograph, 58,* 463–471.

Hedges, L. V., & Olkin, I. (1985). *Statistical Methods for Meta-Analysis.* Orlando, FL: Academic Press.

Henderson, D., & Vandenberg, B.(1992). Factors influencing adjustment in the families of autistic children. *Psychological Report, 71,* 167–171.

Johnson, B. L. (1989). *DSTAT: Software for the Meta Analytic Review of Research Literatures.* Hillsdale, NJ: Erlbaum.

Johnson, B. L. (1993). *DSTAT 1.10: Software for the Meta-Analytic Review,* Upgrade Document. Hillside, NJ: Erlbaum.

Jones, M. B., & Szatmari, P. (1988). Stoppage rules and genetic studies of autism. *Journal of Autism and Developmental Disorders, 18,* 31–40.

*Jorde, L. B., Mason-Brothers, A., Waldmann, R., Ritvo, E. R., Freeman, B. J., Pingree, C., MacMahon, W. M.,

Peterson, B., Jenson, W. R., & Mo, A. (1990). The UCLA-University of Utah epidemiologic survey of autism: Genealogical analysis of familial aggregation. *American Journal of Medical Genetics, 36*, 85–88

*Kolvin, I., Ounsted, C., Richardson, L. M., & Garside, R. F. (1971). III. The family and social background in childhood psychoses. *British Journal of Psychiatry, 118*, 396–402.

*Leboyer, M., Plumet, M. H., Goldblum, M. C., Perez-Diaz, F., & Marchaland, C. (1995). Verbal versus visuospatial abilities in relatives of autistic females. *Developmental Neuropsychology, 11*, 139–155.

McHale, S. M., Simeonsson, R. J., & Sloan, J. L. (1984). Children with handicapped brothers and sisters. In E. Schopler & G. B. Mesibov (Eds.), *The Effect of Autism on the Family* (pp. 327–342). New York: Plenum Press.

McHale, S. M., Sloan, J. L., & Simeonsson, R. J. (1986). Sibling relationships of children with autistic, mentally retarded, and nonhandicapped brothers and sisters. *Journal of Autism and Developmental Disorders, 16*, 399–413.

Minton, J., Campbell, M., Green, W. H., Jennings, S., & Samit, C. (1982). Cognitive assessment of siblings of autistic children. *Journal of the American Academy of Child Psychiatry, 21*, 256–261.

*Narayan, S., Moyes, B., & Wolff, S. (1990). Family characteristics of autistic children: A further report. *Journal of Autism and Developmental Disorders, 20*, 523–535.

*Ozonoff, S., Rogers, S. J., Farnham, J. M., & Pennington, B. F. (1993). Can standard measures identify subclinical markers of autism? *Journal of Autism and Developmental Disorders, 23*, 429–441.

Piven, J., Chase, G. A., Landa, R., Wzorek, M., Gayle, J., Cloud, D., et al. (1991). Psychiatric disorders in the parents of autistic individuals. *American Journal of Academy of Child and Adolescent Psychiatry, 30*, 471–478.

Piven, J., Gayle, J., Chase, J., Fink, B., & Landa, R. (1990). A family history study of neuropsychiatric disorders in the adult siblings of autistic individuals. *Journal of the American Academy of Child and Adolescent Psychiatry, 29*, 177–183.

*Piven, J., Palmer, P., Jacobi, D., Childress, D., & Arndt, S. (1997). Broader autism phenotype: Evidence from a family history study of multiple-incidence autism families. *American Journal of Psychiatry, 154*, 185–190.

*Plumet, M. H., Goldblum, M. C., & Leboyer, M. (1995). Verbal skills in relatives of autistic females. *Cortex, 31*, 723–733.

Rende, R., & Plomin, R. (1992). Diathesis-stress models of psychopathology: A quantitative genetic perspective. *Applied and Preventive Psychology, 1*, 177–182.

*Rodrigue, J. R., Geffken, G. R., & Morgan, S. B. (1993). Perceived competence and behavioral adjustment of siblings of children with autism. *Journal of Autism and Developmental Disorders, 23*, 665–674.

Rosenthal, D. (1970). *Genetic Theory and Abnormal Behavior*. New York: McGraw-Hill.

Rutter, M., Bailey, A., Simonoff, E., & Pickles, A. (1997). Genetic influences and autism. In: F. Volkmar & D. Cohen (Eds.). *Autism and Pervasive Developmental Disorders: A Handbook*, 2nd edit. New York: Wiley-Interscience.

Simeonsson, R. J., & McHale, S. M. (1981). Review: Research on handicapped children: Sibling relationships. *Child Care and Health Development, 7*, 153–171.

Smalley, S. L. (1991). Genetic influences in autism. *Psychiatric Clinics of North America, 14*, 125–139.

Smalley, S. L. (1997). Genetic influences in childhood-onset psychiatric disorders: Autism and attention-deficit/hyperactivity disorder. *American Journal of Human Genetics, 60*, 1276–1282.

*Smalley, S. L., & Asarnow, R. F. (1990). Brief report: Cognitive subclinical markers in autism, *Journal of Autism and Developmental Disorders, 20*, 271–278.

Smalley, S. L., Asarnow, R. F., & Spence, M. (1988). Autism and genetics: A decade of research. *Archives of General Psychiatry, 45*, 953–961.

*Smalley, S. L., McCracken, J., & Tanguay, P. (1995). Autism, affective disorders, and social phobia. *American Journal of Medical Genetics, 60*, 19–26.

Steffenburg, S., Gillberg, C., Hellgren, L., Andersson, L., Gillberg, I. C., Jakobsson, G., & Bohman, M. (1989). A twin study of autism in Denmark, Finland, Iceland, Norway and Sweden. *Journal of Child Psychology and Psychiatry, 30*, 405–416.

*Szatmari, P., Jones, M. B., Tuff, L., Bartolucci, G., Fisman, S., & Mahoney, W. (1993). Lack of cognitive impairment in first-degree relatives of children with pervasive developmental disorders. *Journal of the American Academy of Child and Adolescent Psychiatry, 32*, 1264–1273.

Wadsworth, S. J., DeFries, J. C., Fulker, D. W., & Plomin, R. (1995). Cognitive ability and academic achievement in the Colorado Adoption Project: A Multivariate genetic analysis of parent-offspring and sibling data. *Behavior Genetics, 25*, 1–15.

Walker, E. F., & Difosiog, D. (1997). Schizophrenia: A neural diathesis–stress model. *Psychological Review, 104,* 667–685.

Walker, E. F., Downey, G., & Bergman, A. (1989). The effects of parental psychopathology and maltreatment on child behavior: A test of the diathesis-stress model. *Child Development, 60,* 15–24.

Wechsler, D. (1963). *WPPSI Manual: Wechsler Preschool and Primary Scale of Intelligence.* San Antonio, TX: Psychological Corporation.

Wechsler, D. (1974). *WISC-R Manual: Wechsler Intelligence Scale for Children-Revised.* San Antonio, TX: Psychological Corporation.

Wechsler, D. (1981). *WAIS-R Manual: Wechsler Adult Intelligence Scale-Revised.* San Antonio, TX: Psychological Corporation.

Yirmiya, N., Erel, O., Shaked, M., & Solomonica-Levi, D. (1998). Meta-analyses comparing theory of mind abilities of individuals with autism, individuals with mental retardation, and normally developing individuals. *Psychological Bulletin, 124,* 283–307.

6

Fragile X Syndrome and Autism

Deborah D. Hatton and Donald B. Bailey, Jr.

Interest in the relationship between fragile X syndrome (FXS), the leading genetic cause of inherited mental retardation, and autism was piqued in 1982 when Brown et al. suggested that FXS might account for a significant number of cases of autism. Controversy regarding the nature and magnitude of the relationship between FXS and autism followed (Cohen et al., 1991; Fisch et al., 1986). Within the past several years, researchers have again focused on examining the relationship between these two disorders in prospective studies of children with FXS. The purpose of this chapter is to examine the relationship between FXS and autism using recent research and to discuss implications for intervention. Before discussing that, we will describe FXS and the existing literature on the relationship between FXS and autism.

For 7 years we were engaged in a longitudinal study of the early development of boys with fragile X syndrome. Initially the focus of this research was on early developmental trajectories (Bailey, Hatton, & Skinner, 1998); temperament and behavioral style (Hatton, Bailey, Hargett-Beck, Skinner, & Clark, 1999); patterns of early identification and entry into early intervention programs (Bailey, Skinner, Hatton, & Roberts, 2000); and the services and intervention modifications deemed effective by teachers, therapists, and parents (Hatton et al., 2000). However, in the course of this research, it became apparent that a number of children in our sample exhibited autistic-like behavior. When parents expressed early concerns about their child's development, many were referred first for an autism evaluation, and a number of the children had been independently diagnosed as autistic or were being served in classroom settings primarily designed for children with autism. Because of these factors and the growing discussion in the literature about possible links between autism and fragile X syndrome, we designed a series of three studies to examine this relationship. The results of this research and the implications for intervention are the focus of this chapter.

Although confusion about the relationship between autism and FXS has been perva-

DEBORAH D. HATTON and DONALD B. BAILEY, JR. • Frank Porter Graham Child Development Center, University of North Carolina at Chapel Hill, Chapel Hill, North Carolina 27599-8180.

The Research Basis for Autism Intervention, edited by Schopler, Yirmiya, Shulman, and Marcus. Kluwer Academic/Plenum Publishers, New York, 2001.

sive, it appears that they are two distinct disorders with some overlap. The identification of the *FMR1* gene in 1991 and subsequent studies of gene, brain, and behavior prompted Reiss and colleagues (Baumgardner, Green, & Reiss, 1994; Feinstein & Reiss, 1998; Reiss, 1996) to describe FXS as a neurogenetic disease that is well defined and has a specific cognitive behavioral phenotype and a known biological cause. Therefore, the study of individuals with FXS holds particular promise for understanding the biological basis for behavior and brain/behavior relationships (Cohen, 1995; Feinstein & Reiss, 1998), a field of study labeled behavioral neurogenetics by Reiss (Baumgardner et al., 1994; Feinstein & Reiss, 1998; Reiss, 1996).

Although several candidate genes have been identified for autism, it appears to be a multifactorial disorder and may actually represent a collection of related syndromes (Cook, 1998; Feinstein & Reiss, 1998). While FXS is diagnosed through molecular DNA testing, autism is diagnosed using behavioral measures. Nevertheless, research reported during the past 15 years suggests that 4% to 5% of individuals with autism have FXS and that a subset of individuals with FXS have well-defined characteristics of autism.

FRAGILE X SYNDROME

Fragile X syndrome is the leading known cause of inherited developmental disability with an estimated prevalence of 1:4000 males and 1:8000 females (Mazzocco, 2000). Although the constellation of characteristics that are associated with the syndrome was first described decades ago, the gene itself was not identified until 1991. Fragile X syndrome results from a mutation on the fragile X mental retardation gene (*FMR1*) on the long arm of the X chromosome. For some reason, the number of trinucleotide repeats (CGG) in this gene becomes unstable and expands beyond that found in individuals without FXS (typically between 6 and 50 repeats). When observed under a microscope in a specific cultural medium, this area of the X chromosome appears to be long and spindly—as if it might break off—thus the term *fragile* X syndrome. FXS is currently diagnosed with DNA testing, typically with blood samples.

Premutation carriers of FXS have between 52 and 200 CGG repeats that are unstable and prone to expansion. When the number of repeats reaches 200, individuals are said to have *full mutation FXS*. Typically, an expansion of 200 repeats or more is associated with hypermethylation of the *FMR1* gene and subsequent loss of production of the FMR protein (FMRP). FMRP is believed to be necessary for normal brain development (Small & Warren, 1995; Weiler et al., 1997), and a reduction or absence of this protein is thought to result in the characteristics of FXS (Merenstein, Sobesky, Tayor, Riddle, Tran, & Hagerman, 1996; Tassone et al., 1999).

In some individuals with the full mutation, the *FMR1* gene is not totally methylated, resulting in some protein production. In other cases, individuals may demonstrate mosaic patterns. That is, some of their cells may carry the full FXS mutation while others may carry a premutation, again resulting in some protein production. Surprisingly, researchers have reported that even individuals with fully methylated full mutations may produce small amounts of FMRP (Bailey, Hatton, Tassone, Skinner, & Taylor, 2000; Tassone et al., 1999).

Both males and females may be premutation carriers or may be fully affected by FXS. Approximately 1:250 females and 1:350 males are estimated to be premutation carriers of

FXS (Mazzocco, 2000). The premutation expands to the full mutation only when transmitted through females, however. A premutation male carrier would transmit his premutation to all daughters because he only has one X chromosome, and he cannot pass the mutation to his sons because they would receive his Y chromosome.

The likelihood of expansion from a premutation to a full mutation when passed from mother to child is related to the number of repeats that the mother has. When she has 90 or more CGG repeats, expansion to a full mutation is more likely to occur (Brown, 1996). Because female carriers have two X chromosomes, the risk of transmitting the fragile X during any pregnancy is 50%.

All females have two X chromosomes, and one is randomly inactivated in every cell of the body, hence the term, *X-inactivation*. Activation ratio describes the percentage of normal cells, rather than cells with FXS, that appear active in a female with FXS. As would be expected, activation ratio has been found to be significantly related to impairment in females with the full mutation (Feinstein & Reiss, 1998).

Although premutation carriers have typically been considered unaffected by FXS, evidence that some carriers are affected is emerging. Mazzocco (2000) provides an excellent review of studies that suggest that some carriers may be affected and discusses why it may sometimes be difficult to distinguish premutations from full mutations. Males with full mutation FXS typically present with mental retardation, communication delays, and characteristic physical (i.e., long face, large prominent ears, narrow, high-arched palate, hyperextensible joints, and macroorchidism if post-pubertal) and behavioral (e.g., hypersensitivity to sensory stimuli, eye gaze aversion, hand flapping, perseverative speech) features. As we shall discuss in the remainder of this chapter, a number of males also exhibit autistic-like behaviors, and most studies report that a significant number of individuals with fragile X syndrome also meet the diagnostic criteria for autism.

Females with the full mutation exhibit a wider range of characteristics due to X inactivation; however, Hagerman (1996b) reports that about one third function in the normal range of intellectual function; one third function in the borderline range, perhaps with learning disabilities; and one third will experience mental retardation. However, good population data are not currently available and estimates do vary, as evidenced by Feinstein and Reiss (1998) and Mazzocco (2000), who suggest that perhaps half of females with the full mutation FXS have mental retardation. Females have been described as being shy and anxious. Mazzocco, Kates, Baumgardner, Freund, and Reiss (1997) found that girls with FXS displayed more autistic behaviors than a comparison group of girls (seen at the same neurodevelopmental clinic) matched on age and IQ. Autistic behaviors were not associated with IQ, but they were inversely correlated with activation ratio that, according to Feinstein and Reiss (1998), suggests a "direct behavioral neurogenetic effect, not attributable to lowered IQ" (p. 399).

FRAGILE X SYNDROME AND AUTISM: REVIEW OF THE LITERATURE

Researchers trying to understand the relationship between FXS, a single gene disorder diagnosed by DNA testing, and autism, a behaviorally defined syndrome that appears to have multifactoral causes, have taken several approaches. Early studies that generated the original controversy focused on rates of co-occurrence of the two disorders. Subsequently, a series of studies detailing specific similarities and differences in individuals with FXS with and without autism and/or autistic behavior were reported.

Estimated Rates of Co-Occurrence

Early attempts to study the two disorders revolved around the following two questions: (1) What proportion of individuals with autism also have FXS? and (2) What proportion of individuals with FXS also meet diagnostic criteria for autism? The answers to these two questions are quite different.

With regard to the first question, in an examination of studies that assessed the proportion of individuals with autism who have FXS and the proportion of persons with mental retardation that have FXS, Fisch (1992) found that approximately 5% of each group had FXS. More recently, Dykens and Volkmar (1997) reviewed 17 studies conducted over an 11-year period (1983–1994) and found the rate of FXS reported in samples of individuals with autism varied from 1% to 16%, with an average of 4%. Based on these two comprehensive reviews of literature, it appears that from 4% to 5% of individuals with autism may also have FXS.

With regard to the second question (prevalence of autism within the FXS population) in Dykens and Volkmar's (1997) review, the prevalence ranged from 5% to 60%; however, seven studies reported a prevalence of 20% or more. Those findings are consistent with the recent 25% prevalence rates reported by Bailey et al. (1998), Cohen (1995), and Turk and Graham (1997). More recently, Rogers and colleagues (in press) used multiple rigorous criteria for autism in a study of 2-year-olds and found that 40% (5 out of 13) met all four criteria for autism. However, the small number of subjects in this study limits generalizations. Consequently, a conservative estimated prevalence of autism of 20% to 25% in individuals with FXS seems most appropriate at the present time.

Similarities and Consequences of Co-Occurrence

Cohen (1995) reported studies of autistic and nonautistic males with FXS, and results suggest that these individuals with both autism and FXS have poorer developmental outcome and more problem behaviors. Cohen (1995) described a sample of 80 males under the age of 22 years who lived with their families. Twenty (25%) of those males had diagnoses of autism based on clinical observation, caregiver interviews, and record review using DSM III-R clinical criteria in addition to FXS. Caregivers were interviewed in order to score the Vineland Adaptive Behavior Scales (Sparrow, Balla, & Cicchetti, 1984), and IQ scores were obtained on some participants using record review. Visual inspection of plots of age equivalent scores for the communication, daily living skills, and socialization scales showed two apparent clusters of participants, those with and without autism. Across all four dimensions, the group with autism and FXS showed poorer functioning.

Although cross-sectional data were used, examination of the slopes revealed statistically significant differences across ages for communication, daily living, motor, and social functioning. Specifically, at young ages, boys with and without autism had similar scores; however, scores of older boys with FXS/autism diverged increasingly from those of FXS boys without autism.

In a follow-up examination of longitudinal scores on six boys with FXS and autism, Cohen (1995) found that the scores of these children in all four domains did not improve/

increase over periods of time ranging from 1.25 to 7.5 years. Cohen concluded that "the developmental outcome of males with fragile X depends on whether or not they have been diagnosed as having autism" (p. 258). A subsequent comparison of the adaptive skills of the FXS participants with autism to a group of 146 non-FXS males with autism under the age of 22 years revealed no significant differences, suggesting that males with FXS/autism were similar to males with autism of unspecified origin.

Based on earlier work that suggested that males with FXS/autism demonstrated more social avoidance than males with autism alone (Cohen, Vietze, Sudhalter, Jenkins, & Brown, 1989, 1991), Cohen (1995) studied social avoidance in four groups: males with FXS/ no autism, males with FXS/autism, autism, and mental retardation. Dependent measures included the Vineland Adaptive Behavior Scales (Sparrow et al., 1984) and the Autistic Behavior Interview (Cohen et al., 1991). Using principal components analysis and analyses of covariance, Cohen (1995) found that boys with FXS/autism and boys with autism of nonspecific origin performed similarly on social communication scales and measures of repetitive behaviors. Autism rather than FXS was the distinguishing variable in this case, supported by the fact that boys with FXS/no autism performed similarly to a group of IQ-matched controls. However, both autism and FXS seemed to have an additive impact on verbal perseveration; scores were lower for the FXS/autism group, and there was no inter-action between FXS and autism. Autism and FXS had multiplicative effects on aggressive-ness indicated by a significant interaction. According to Cohen (1995), these results suggest that males with FXS/autism were similar to autistic children on social communication and repetitive behaviors; however, they exhibited more verbal perseveration (a marker for high arousal) and more aggression (less tolerance for environmental stimulation) than the other groups. Having both disorders resulted in "greater impairment in functioning in multiple areas" (p. 262) and could account for the lack of progress seen in the six subjects examined longitudinally. Cohen (1995) noted that early diagnosis of autism in individuals with FXS is important because of possible prognostic usefulness.

In studies of language and conversational skills, Paul, Dykens, Leckman, Watson, Breg, and Cohen (1987) found increased echolalia in a group of participants with autism as compared to samples with FXS and mental retardation. Sudhalter, Cohen, Silverman, and Wolf-Schein (1990) found that participants with autism engaged in more deviant repetitive language than children with either FXS or Down syndrome. Males with FXS/autism achieved similar scores on the socialization domain of the Vineland; however, males with autism differed from males with Down syndrome while the FXS participants did not (Sud-halter et al., 1990). Ferrier, Bashir, Meryash, Johnson, and Wolff (1991) found that males with FXS exhibited self-repetition more often in an effort to maintain communication, while males with autism produced more multiply inappropriate responses.

In all of the literature reviewed on FXS and autism, ages varied widely, with very few young children as participants. In most cases, samples were small and there was little consistency in the diagnosis of autism or the measurement of autistic behaviors.

STUDIES BY THE CAROLINA FRAGILE X PROJECT

Early in our longitudinal study of young boys with FXS, clinical observations of autistic behavior in some of the children piqued our interest. As time progressed, it became apparent that children with autistic behaviors did not appear to be doing as well developmentally as children who did not display these behaviors, or who displayed fewer of the behaviors. A review of the literature on FXS and autism suggested some controversy concerning the relationship between FXS and autism, precluding definitive conclusions about this issue. Consequently, we designed a series of three sequential studies to examine the relationship between FXS and autistic behavior. In the first study, we planned to examine the autistic characteristics of subjects in our study and then compare them to reference groups of children with and without autism. After examining the results of that study, it was apparent that a quarter of our sample did have autistic characteristics. To examine their characteristics in more detail, we designed a second study with a matched comparison group of boys with autism that confirmed our earlier findings. Finally, with confirmation of the impact of autistic behavior on development, behavior, and functional status from the second study, we compared the contributions of autistic behavior and FMR protein expression on developmental outcome.

In designing the protocol, we faced several limitations. First, our sample was distributed across a three-state area. Because we assessed children in their homes or schools, substantial time and travel resources were required. Second, our existing comprehensive assessment protocol required considerable time and energy from the parents of the children. Because subject retention has been a primary goal of our longitudinal studies, we did not want to add undue stress to either the parents or children in the study. For these reasons, we selected the Childhood Autism Rating Scale (CARS; Schopler, Reichler, & Renner, 1988) as the most appropriate and feasible measure of autistic behavior for our subjects. In addition, the Battelle Developmental Inventory (BDI; Newborg, Stock, Wnek, Guidubaldi, & Svinicki, 1984) was used across all three studies. Specific details regarding our research protocol can be found in Bailey et al. (1998); Bailey, Hatton, Mesibov, Ament, and Skinner (2000); and Bailey, Hatton, Skinner, and Mesibov (2001).

Autistic Characteristics of Young Males with FXS: Study 1

In a study of 57 boys between the ages of 24 and 133 months, Bailey et al. (1998) used the Childhood Autism Rating Scale (CARS; Schopler et al., 1988) to document autistic behavior in a sample of young boys with full mutation FXS. The profiles of the participants with FXS were then compared to an extant data set of children who had been referred to and evaluated by an agency serving individuals with autism. Two comparison profiles were generated for the autistic reference samples. The profiles of a group of 391 children who were diagnosed with autism and of another 391 children who were evaluated and found not to have autism were compared to those of children with FXS with (FXS/autism) and without autistic behavior.

The CARS scores of 14 (25%) of the children with FXS fell within the autistic range. Twelve fell within the mild to moderate range and two children scored within the severe range. Children who scored high on the CARS tended to have lower developmental scores. When the profile of children with FXS/autism was compared to that of children with autism in the reference sample, no distinguishing features were evident. This was also true for the comparison of profiles of children with FXS without autistic behavior to those of children who were referred for autism evaluation and found not to be autistic. These findings are consistent with those reported by Cohen (1995) when he compared the adaptive behavior ratings of children with FXS/autism to those of a large sample of individuals with autism alone.

Only when profiles of children with FXS/autism were compared to children with FXS and no autistic behavior did differences emerge. The items that children with FXS/autism demonstrated poorer performance on included: relating to people, imitation, object use, verbal communication, and overall impression of autism by examiner. Scores on activity level and intellectual function were virtually identical for children with FXS with and without autistic behavior. These results must be viewed cautiously, however, because the profile of children with FXS/autism was based on scores of 14 children, while the nonautistic FXS profile reflected the scores of 43 children. Seven of the 14 children who scored in the autistic range were nonverbal.

Thus, the findings of our first study of FXS and autistic behavior suggested that:

1. Twenty-five percent of the boys in our sample exhibited autistic behaviors as measured by the CARS.
2. Boys with FXS/autistic behavior had more difficulty than boys with FXS alone in the following: (a) relating to people; (b) imitation; (c) object use; and (d) verbal communication. In addition, examiners gave them higher scores on an overall impression of autism item.
3. The CARS did not distinguish between boys with FXS/autism and those with autism not related to FXS.
4. Boys with high CARS scores tended to have lower developmental quotients.
5. Age was not related to CARS scores.

Developmental, Functional, and Behavioral Status in FXS and Autism: Study 2

After finding that a quarter of our sample of boys with FXS did appear to have autistic characteristics, we designed a comparative study to examine these characteristics in more detail. To examine differences between boys with autism and those with FXS, a sample of 44 boys with full mutation FXS between the ages of 36 and 95 months (mean = 64.1) was matched to a sample of 31 boys with autism on age and ethnicity (Bailey et al., 2000). Then the samples were compared on measures of development, functional status, and behavioral style.

Developmental status was measured using the Battelle Developmental Inventory (BDI; Newborg et al., 1984). An overall age equivalent score and age equivalent scores for the five BDI domains were obtained. Functional status was measured by the ABILITIES Index (Simeonsson & Bailey, 1991), a rating scale that documents the functional status of audition, behavior, intellectual functioning, limbs, intentional communication, tonicity, integrity of physical status, eyes, and structural status. Each dimension was rated by the professional who completed the Battelle on a scale from 1 (normal function) to 6 (extreme limitation in function).

Behavioral style was measured by the Behavioral Style Questionnaire (McDevitt & Carey, 1978–1995). The BSQ examines temperament across the following nine dimensions: activity level, rhythmicity (of physiological functions), approach/withdrawal; adaptability; intensity (of emotional response), mood (positive or negative), persistence/ attention span; distractibility, and threshold (to sensory stimuli—high or low). Parents rate

100 items on a scale of 1 (almost never) to 6 (almost always) that are used to calculate scores on each of the nine dimensions. Finally, the CARS (Schopler et al., 1988) was completed by the same individual who conducted the BDI assessment.

Results were analyzed in two steps based on CARS scores of boys with FXS. Thirty-one of the 44 participants (70%) had scores of <30, indicating that they did not have autistic behavior, while 13 (30%) had scores of >30, representing autistic behavior. The first analysis compared the performance of the FXS boys without autistic behavior to 31 boys with autism of nonspecific origin, matched on chronological age, gender, and ethnicity. In the second analysis, three matched groups were compared: 13 boys with FXS/autistic behavior, 13 with FXS alone, and 13 with autism.

When comparing boys with FXS alone to those with autism, results indicated that the overall developmental level (BDI total score) was similar for boys with FXS and those with autism. Both groups had overall mean age equivalent scores of about 32 months, at a mean chronological age of 63 months. However, when profiles were examined across developmental domains, differences emerged. Boys with FXS showed a relatively flat pattern with similar age equivalent mean scores across the five domains. Boys with autism, however, showed more variability, with lower scores in personal–social development and communication. Boys with autism scored significantly lower on personal–social development than on the other four domains of adaptive, motor, communication, and cognitive development.

Differences in functional development were also noted, with boys with FXS having significantly higher scores (more impairment) on use of limbs, tonicity (more hypotonic), and structural status. However, these scores were only in the suspected range of delay/disability. Boys with autism scored significantly higher on inappropriate behavior, intellectual functioning, and communication, and those scores were in the mild to moderate range of delay/disability.

Both groups were compared to a referent sample of typically developing children on the Behavioral Style Questionnaire (McDevitt & Carey, 1978–1995), designed to measure temperament traits. Boys from both groups differed significantly from the reference sample on adaptability (slower to adapt), persistence (less persistent), and approach/withdrawal (more withdrawing). Boys with FXS were rated as more active than the reference group, while boys with autism were rated as less intense, distractible, and rhythmic, but with a higher sensory threshold. Boys with FXS were significantly more active and intense and had a more negative mood than boys with autism; however, except for activity, they did not differ from the reference sample on those dimensions.

Finally, Bailey et al. (2000) compared three smaller groups of children who were matched on age, gender, and ethnicity. These groups consisted of 13 children with FXS, another 13 with autism, and 13 children with both FXS/autistic behavior. Developmentally, the children with both FXS/autistic behavior showed the lowest scores on the Battelle. Communication, rather than personal social development, however, seemed to be the greatest area of need. On the ABILITIES Index (Simeonsson & Bailey, 1991), boys with both FXS/autistic behavior scored significantly lower than boys with FXS but not boys with autism on intellectual function. Boys with both FXS/autistic behavior had significantly lower tone than boys with autism, and they had significantly more inappropriate behavior and lower communication than boys with FXS. Although temperament trends were similar to those found in the two-way comparison, no significant differences emerged, probably due to the small sample size. These findings supported those of Cohen (1995) who found that autism in addition to FXS resulted in poorer developmental outcome.

Thus, this study demonstrated that boys with FXS and autism have similarities and differences in development, functional abilities, and behavioral style. Although overall levels of developmental function were similar, boys with autism showed more variability across developmental domains, with personal-social development being especially delayed. Boys with FXS were more hypotonic, had more suspected delays in use of limbs, and had more distinct differences in structural status; however, these areas were rated as having suspected delays/differences. Boys with autism exhibited more inappropriate behavior and more impaired intellectual and communication function; these areas were rated as mildly to moderately delayed. Boys with FXS were more active and intense and had a more negative mood than boys with autism; however, they differed from the reference sample of typically developing children only on activity level. Finally, children with both FXS/autistic behavior appeared to have significantly more developmental delays and more impaired functional abilities than the other two groups.

Autistic Behavior, FMR Protein, and Developmental Patterns of Boys with FXS: Study 3

After finding that autistic behavior had a substantial impact on development, behavior, and functional status in Study 2, we wanted to investigate it's relative contribution to outcome when compared to the FMR protein. Because a deficiency in this protein is believed to be responsible for the characteristic symptoms of FXS, we would expect it to influence outcome more than autistic behavior. Consequently, in a third study, we examined the growth curves of a sample of 55 young males with FXS in order to identify variables that affect developmental outcome (Bailey et al., 2001). These 55 boys with a mean age of 46 months (range 24 to 84 months) were assessed on 290 occasions (mean = 5, range = 2–10) using the Battelle Developmental Inventory (Newborg et al., 1984). Independent variables included ethnicity, age, autistic behavior as measured by the CARS (Schopler et al., 1988), maternal education, and the percentage of lymphocytes that expressed FMR protein.

The majority (85%) of boys in the study were from European American families, and all but one mother had finished high school and had some college. Thus, lack of variability in the sample may have accounted for the finding that these factors did not significantly impact developmental outcome.

Approximately 25% of the sample (14 out of 55) obtained CARS scores of 30 or above. Twelve scored between 30 and 36.5, indicating mild to moderate autistic behaviors. Two of the 14 subjects had scores in the severely autistic range (37 or higher).

The effects of FXS are believed to be due to a lack of production of the FMR protein, thought to be necessary for normal brain development. Blood samples were analyzed to determine the percentage of 200 lymphocytes that produced protein. In our sample, the mean percentage of lymphocytes expressing this protein was 8.6 (range 1–40, SD = 8.03). Thus there was little variability in protein expression in our sample.

Initial t-tests were run to test for relationships between CARS scores and FMRP. The sample was divided into two groups—those with (CARS scores ≥30) and those without

(CARS scores <30) autistic behavior. Boys without autistic behavior had slightly higher levels of FMRP; however, the difference was not statistically significant.

Hierarchical linear modeling (HLM: Bryk & Raudenbush, 1987; Burchinal, Bailey, & Snyder, 1994; Willet, 1989) was used to identify variables that significantly affected both the rate and level of growth. This approach produces individual growth curves for each child and uses them to compute estimated population growth curves. Because the age of our participants varied at entry and because of different numbers of observations per child, HLM was the most appropriate analysis technique for our data.

Results of the HLM suggested that autistic behavior significantly affected both the mean level and rate of development of boys with FXS. Specifically, boys whose CARS scores were ≥30, showed slower rates of growth (.26 compared to .53) and lower mean levels of performance (22.7 months versus 33.4 months for overall performance at the centered mean CA of 60 months). Similar patterns were found across all five developmental domains, with greatest differences being in personal–social, language, and adaptive domains. FMR protein expression significantly affected mean levels of performance but not the rate of development.

Thus, autistic behavior as measured by the CARS was related to outcome development more significantly than the amount of FMRP expression. There were no interactions between autistic behavior and FMRP, suggesting that autistic behavior and FMRP expression were not related. However, because the number of boys with autistic behavior was relatively small (*n* = 14) and because there was little variability in the amount of protein expression in our sample, these findings must be viewed cautiously. Nevertheless, our findings and visual inspection of the observed individual trajectories in Figure 6.1 suggest that the development of boys with both FXS and autistic behavior (as measured by the CARS) is quite different from those without autistic behavior. Fragile X syndrome and autistic behavior appear to have an additive influence on developmental outcome. Children

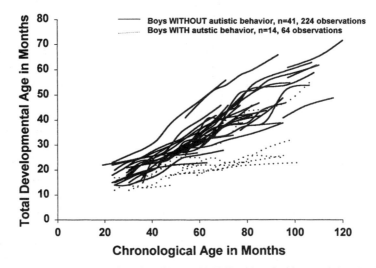

FIGURE 1. Developmental trajectories of boys with FXS with and without autistic behaviors.

with both autism and FXS appear to be at increased risk for developmental delays across domains, again supporting the Cohen's (1995) findings.

IMPLICATIONS FOR INTERVENTION

The results of our three prospective studies of autistic behavior in boys with FXS supports Cohen's (1995) observation that males who meet diagnostic criteria for both disorders do not fare as well developmentally as those with FXS alone. He suggested that early diagnosis of autism was important for early intervention. Currently, however, there is very little research that describes intervention techniques for individuals with FXS/autism. Braden (1996), Scharfenaker, O'Connor, Stackhouse, Braden, Hickman, & Gray (1996), and Spiridigliozzi et al. (1994) provide comprehensive reviews of intervention for individuals with FXS from a clinical perspective.

Throughout the clinical literature, a number of recommendations are made for various types of intervention; however, there is no research literature to support most of those recommendations. Early intervention/special education, speech/language, motor, and sensory integration therapies are routinely recommended, as is a multidisciplinary approach to intervention. In addition, counseling for the individual and family and behavior management/ therapy are also often suggested.

Based on clinical literature and our own experiences, boys with FXS are often prescribed medication at fairly young ages, typically for hyperactivity and/or attention problems. Clinical descriptions of the efficacy of folic acid and of a variety of medications have been reported; however, results seem to be highly variable. To date, however, medication does appear to be one of the most commonly used interventions with individuals with FXS. Hagerman (1996a) provides a useful overview of studies examining the efficacy of folic acid and medications in individuals with FXS.

In a longitudinal study of early intervention services for young boys with FXS, Hatton et al. (2000) found that the average age of entry into early intervention for their sample of 50 boys was 21.6 months. Home visits usually preceded the initiation of physical, speech/ language therapies, and occupational therapists and center-based services. While the amount of early intervention/special education increased over time, the intensity of speech/ language and occupational therapies remained constant, and physical therapy decreased after 5 years of age. Considerable variability was found in the service patterns and amounts of services that were provided. Teachers identified behavior as their primary concern in working with these children; however, they offered a tremendous variety of strategies to deal with behavior. Consequently, the authors concluded that tremendous variability in developmental status, types and amounts of services provided, and teacher recommendations precluded the development of a specific set of recommendations for intervention for children with FXS. Rather, recommendations for intervention must be based on individual needs and circumstances.

As mentioned earlier, several of the children in our longitudinal study of FXS have been served in classes designed for children with autism. Many families have found that their children do well in these settings. Why they do better in such classrooms has not been documented by research. However, we can speculate on the reasons. First, classes designed for children with autism often have a lower student to teacher ratio than other classes. In addition, these classrooms are often structured, well organized, and focused on using visual skills, rather than language, for communication. In addition, children are prepared for transitions and have a consistent routine. Many boys with FXS have language delays at young ages, are easily overwhelmed by sensory overload, and have trouble with transitions. Consequently, they may perform better in a quiet, structured environment compared to a regular classroom and/or a classroom for children with special needs that is less structured.

Hatton et al. (2000) asked teachers, via surveys and interviews, to make recommendations for serving boys with FXS, based on their own experience. Among the recommendations were several that are appropriate for children with autism: have a consistent routine with structured activities; have a structured environment; provide a personal work space; use visual cues and modeling; use picture schedules; break tasks down into manageable steps. In addition, 60% to 70% of the teachers specifically recommended that similarities to autism be considered and that strategies appropriate for autism be used with children with FXS. This recommendation by teachers in the field serves as a concise summary of what is known about intervention for individuals with FXS and FXS/autism. Now that we know more about the characteristics of young children with FXS, in particular that many of them have autistic behaviors, our challenge is to design research that provides an empirical basis for intervention for both groups, children with FXS alone and those with FXS/autism.

SUMMARY AND FUTURE DIRECTIONS

The preliminary studies of FXS and autistic behavior in young boys described in this chapter provide new and unique information to the field. Specifically, these prospective studies focused on young boys within a narrow age range; used one measure of autistic behavior; examined performance across a range of dimensions; and included matched samples of boys with autism, boys with FXS, and boys with FXS/autistic behavior.

Consistent with the literature, we found similarities and differences in boys with FXS and boys with autism. In the process, we discovered that approximately 25% of our sample of boys with FXS exhibited autistic behavior as measured by the CARS. Boys with both FXS/autistic behavior had much lower mean levels and rates of development than boys with FXS alone on longitudinal assessments. Indeed, autistic behavior accounted for more of the variance in developmental outcome than did amount of FMR protein that was expressed.

Boys with FXS alone and boys with autism demonstrated similar levels of development on the Battelle; however, boys with autism showed more variation across developmental domains, scoring significantly lower on personal–social development. These two groups were similar temperamentally on approach/withdrawal (more withdrawing), persistence (less persistent), and adaptability (less adaptable) than the reference sample of typically developing children; however, boys with FXS were more active than boys with autism and the reference sample of typical children.

Because similarities and differences emerged while using global measures of assessment with relatively small samples of children, our findings suggest that more refined measures and larger samples might be useful for future studies. Feinstein and Reiss (1998) eloquently described the benefits of using knowledge gained from the study of FXS and other neurogenetic disorders to inform autism research. They noted that more is known about the pathogenesis from gene to brain to behavior with FXS than with any other disorder. Of particular interest, according to Feinstein and Reiss (1998), is why some individuals with FXS seem to meet full diagnostic criteria for autism while others display a subset of behaviors. By studying behavioral and neurocognitive profiles, genetic characteristics, and brain structure/functioning [via magnetic resonance imaging (MRI) and functional magnetic resonance imaging (fMRI)] in FXS with particular attention to features that are common to autism, we should be able to learn more about autism (Feinstein & Reiss, 1998).

We suggest that even more can be learned by studying individuals and their families longitudinally from very early ages. By employing multiple measures, including psycho-physiological assessments from infancy, we may be able to identify both physiological and environmental factors that contribute to developmental outcome and behavior. In addition, by studying individuals across contexts of home, school/childcare, and community, and by collecting data from multiple sources, we gain a more valid and richer understanding of risk factors and resiliency that will answer the question of why some individuals with FXS have autism, why some have a subset of features, and why others have no features. Not only will this information enhance our ability to promote optimal development and functioning of individuals with FXS through research-based intervention, but it will also further our understanding of autism, and provide the empirical basis required to design much needed treatment studies.

REFERENCES

Bailey, D. B., Hatton, D. H., Mesibov, G., Ament, N., & Skinner, M. (2000). Early development, temperament, and functional impairment in autism and fragile X syndrome. *Journal of Autism and Developmental Disorders, 30*(1), 557–567.

Bailey, D. B., Hatton, D. H., & Skinner, M. (1998). Early developmental trajectories of males with fragile X syndrome. *American Journal on Mental Retardation, 103,* 29–39.

Bailey, D. B., Hatton, D. H., Skinner, M., & Mesibov, G. (2001). Autistic behavior, FMR1 protein, and developmental trajectories in young males with fragile X syndrome. *Journal of Autism and Developmental Disorders, 31,* 165–174.

Bailey, D. B, Hatton, D. H, Tassone, F., Skinner, M., & Taylor, A. K. (2001). FMRP and early development in fragile X syndrome. *American Journal of Mental Retardation, 106,* 16–27.

Bailey, D. B., Skinner, D., Hatton, D. D., & Roberts, J. (2000). Family experiences and factors associated with diagnosis of fragile X syndrome. *Journal of Developmental and Behavioral Pediatrics, 21,* 315–321.

Baumgardner, P. L., Green, K. E., & Reiss, A. L. (1994). A behavioral neurogenetics approach to developmental disabilities: Gene-brain-behavior associations. *Current Opinions in Neurology, 7,* 172–178.

Braden, M. L. (1996). *Fragile Handle with Care: Understanding Fragile X Syndrome.* Chapel Hill, NC: Avanta.

Brown, W. T. (1996). The molecular biology of the fragile X mutation. In R. J. Hagerman, & A. Cronister (Eds.), *Fragile X Syndrome: Diagnosis, Treatment, and Research* (pp. 88–113). Baltimore, MD: Johns Hopkins University Press.

Brown, W. T., Jenkins, E. C., Friedman, E., Brooks, J., Wisniewski, K., Ragathu, S., & French, J. (1982). Autism is associated with the fragile X syndrome. *Journal of Autism & Developmental Disorders. 12*(3), 303–308.

Bryk, A. S., & Raudenbush, S. W. (1987). Application of hierarchical linear models to assessing change. *Psychological Bulletin, 101,* 147–158.

Burchinal, M. R., Bailey, D. B., & Snyder, P. (1994). Using growth curve analysis to evaluate child changes in longitudinal investigations. *Journal of Early Intervention, 18,* 403–423.

Cohen, I. (1995). Behavioral profiles of autistic and nonautistic fragile X males. *Developmental Brain Dysfunction, 8,* 252–269.

Cohen, I., Sudhalter, V., Pfadt, A., Jenkins, E., Brown, W., & Vietze, P. (1991). Why are autism and the fragile X syndrome associated? Conceptual and methodological issues. *American Journal of Human Genetics, 48,* 195–202.

Cohen, I. L., Vietze, P. M., Sudhalter, V., Jenkins, E. C., & Brown, W. T. (1989). Parent-child dyadic gaze patterns in fragile X males and in non-fragile X males with autistic disorder. *Journal of Child Psychology and Psychiatry, 300,* 845–856.

Cohen, I. L., Vietze, P. M., Sudhalter, V., Jenkins, E. C., & Brown, W. T (1991). Effects of age and communication level on eye contact in fragile X males and non-fragile X autistic males. *American Journal of Medical Genetics, 38,* 498–502.

Cook, E., Jr. (1998). Genetics of autism. *Mental Retardation and Developmental Disabilities Research Reviews, 4,* 113–120.

Dykens, E., & Volkmar, F. (1997). Medical conditions associated with autism. In D. Cohen & F. Volkmar (Eds.), *Handbook of Autism and Pervasive Developmental Disorders* (2nd ed., pp. 388–410). New York: John Wiley & Sons.

Feinstein, C., & Reiss, A. (1998). Autism: The point of view from fragile X studies. *Journal of Autism and Developmental Disorders, 28*(5), 393–405.

Ferrier, L., Bashir, A., Meryash, D., Johnson, J., & Wolff, P. (1991). Conversational skills of individuals with fragile X syndrome: A comparison with autism and down syndrome. *Developmental Medicine and Child Neurology, 33,* 776–788.

Fisch, G. S. (1992). Is autism associated with the fragile X syndrome? *American Journal of Medical Genetics, 43,* 47–55.

Fisch, G. S., Cohen, I.. L., Wolf, E. G., Brown, W. T., Jenkins, E. C., & Gross, A. (1986). Autism and the fragile X syndrome. *American Journal of Psychiatry, 143,* 71–73.

Hagerman, R. J. (1996a). Medical follow-up and pharmacotherapy. In R. J. Hagerman, & A. Cronister (Eds.), *Fragile X Syndrome: Diagnosis, Treatment, and Research* (pp. 283–331). Baltimore, MD: Johns Hopkins University Press.

Hagerman, R. J. (1996b). Physical and behavioral phenotype. In R. J. Hagerman, & A. Cronister (Eds.), *Fragile X Syndrome: Diagnosis, Treatment, and Research* (pp. 3–87). Baltimore, MD: Johns Hopkins University Press.

Hatton, D. H., Bailey, D. B., Hargett-Beck, M. Q., Skinner, M., & Clark, R. D. (1999). Behavioral style of young boys with fragile X syndrome. *Developmental Medicine & Child Neurology, 41,* 625–632.

Hatton, D. H., Bailey, D. B., Roberts, J. P., Skinner, M., Mayhew, L., Clark, R. D., Waring, E., & Roberts, J. E. (2000). Early intervention services for young boys with fragile X syndrome. *Journal of Early Intervention, 23,* 235–251.

Mazzocco, M. M. M. (2000). Advances in research on the fragile X syndrome. *Mental Retardation and Developmental Disabilities Research Reviews, 6,* 96–106.

Mazzocco, M., Kates, W., Baumgardner, T., Freund, L., & Reiss, A. (1997). Autistic behaviors among girls with fragile x syndrome. *Journal of Autism and Developmental Disorders, 27*(4), 415–435.

McDevitt, S., & Carey, W. (1978–1995). *Behavioral Style Questionnaire.* Scottsdale, AZ: Behavioral-Developmental Initiatives.

Merenstein, S. A., Sobesky, W. E., Taylor, A. K., Riddle, J. E., Tran, H. X., & Hagerman, R. J. (1996). Molecular-clinical correlations in males with an expanded FMR1 mutation. *American Journal of Medical Genetics, 64,* 388–394.

Newborg, J., Stock, J. R., Wnek, L., Guidubaldi, J., & Svinicki, J. (1984). *The Battelle Developmental Inventory.* Allen, TX: DLM/Teaching Resources.

Paul, R., Dykens, E., Leckman, J., Watson, M., Breg, W., & Cohen, D. (1987). A comparison of language characteristics of mentally retarded adults with fragile X syndrome and those with non-specific mental retardation and autism. *Journal of Autism and Developmental Disorders, 17,* 454–891.

Reiss, A. L. (1996). *Behavioral neurogenetics: Genetic conditions as models for understanding brain development cognition and behavior in children.* Paper presented at the Model for Advancing Research on Developmental Plasticity: Integrating the Behavioral Science and the Neuroscience of Mental Health, Chantilly, VA.

Scharnaker, S., O'Connor, R., Stackhouse, T., Braden, M., Hickman, L., & Gray, K. (1996). An integrated approach to intervention. In R. J. Hagerman & A. Cronister (Eds.), *Fragile X Syndrome: Diagnosis, Treatment, and Research* (pp. 349–411). Baltimore, MD: Johns Hopkins University Press.

Schopler, E., Reichler, R., & Renner, B. (1988). *The Childhood Autism Rating Scale (CARS).* Los Angeles: Western Psychological Services.

Simeonsson, R., & Bailey, D. B. (1991). *The ABILITIES Index.* Chapel Hill, NC: Frank Porter Graham Child Development Center, University of North Carolina.

Small, K., & Warren, S. (1995). Analysis of FMRP, the protein deficient in fragile X syndrome. *Mental Retardation and Developmental Disabilities Research Reviews, 1,* 245–250.

Sparrow, S., Balla, D., & Cicchetti, D. (1984). *Vineland Adaptive Behavior Scales*. Circle Pines, MN: American Guidance Service, Inc.

Spiridigliozzi, G. A., Lachiewicz, A. M., MacMurdo, C. S., Vizoso, A. D., O'Donnell, C. M., McConkie-Rosell, A., & Burgess, D. J. (1994). *Educating Boys with Fragile X Syndrome: A Guide for Parents and Professionals*. (Available from the Gail A . Spiridigliozzi, Child Development Unit, Box 3364, Duke University Medical Center, Durham, NC.

Sudhalter, V., Cohen, I., Silverman, W., & Wolf-Schein, E. (1990). Conversational analyses of males with fragile X, Down syndrome, and autism: Comparison of the emergence of deviant language. *American Journal on Mental Retardation*, *94*(4), 431–41.

Tassone, F., Hagerman, R. J., Ikle, D. N., Dyer, T. N., Lampe, M., Willemsen, R., Oostra, D. A., & Taylor, A. K. (1999). FMRP expression as a potential indicator in fragile X syndrome. *American Journal of Medical Genetics*, 84, 250–261.

Turk, J., & Graham, P. (1997). Fragile X syndrome, autism and autistic features. *Autism*, *1*(2), 175–197.

Weiler, I. J., Irwin, S. A., Klintsoza, A. Y., Spencer, C. M., Brazelton, A. D., Miyashiro, K., Comery, T. A., Patel, B., Eberwine, J., & Greenough, W. T. (1997). Fragile X mental retardation protein is translated near synapses in response to neurotransmitter activation. *Proceedings of the National Academy of the Sciences*, 94, 5395–5400.

Willett, J. B. (1989). Some results on reliability for the longitudinal measurement of change: Implications for the design of studies of individual growth. *Educational and Psychological Measurement*, 49, 587–602.

7

Analysis of Three Coding Region Polymorphisms in Autism

Evidence for an Association with the Serotonin Transporter

Nurit Yirmiya, Tammy Pilowsky, Lubov Nemanov, Shoshana Arbelle, Temira Feinsilver, Iris Fried, and Richard P. Ebstein

THE ORGANIC BASIS OF AUTISM

Autism is a pervasive developmental disorder (*Diagnostic and Statistical Manual of Mental Disorders*, DSM-IV, APA, 1994) characterized by impairments in reciprocal social interaction and verbal and nonverbal communication; and restricted, repetitive, and stereotyped behaviors. Since Kanner's description of autism in 1943, a large body of literature has focused on its nature and etiology. Yet, although autism is a well defined syndrome, and clearly diagnosed by its behavioral characteristics, there is no medical, chemical, or genetic procedure that can confirm the diagnosis, and thus its etiology remains unknown.

Today it is widely accepted that there is an organic basis to autism. Support for this suggestion is based on evidence of neurological impairments and of genetic involvement in autism. Neurologically, there is an elevated rate of epilepsy in individuals with autism, according to which 25% to 30% of the individuals with autism develop epilepsy throughout their lives (Deykin & MacMahon, 1979). Moreover, an elevated rate of soft neurological signs was reported in individuals with autism (DeMyer, Hingtgen, & Jackson, 1981; Jones & Prior, 1985). Further support stems from evidence regarding abnormality in brain func-

NURIT YIRMIYA • Department of Psychology and School of Education, The Hebrew University of Jerusalem, Mount Scopus, Jerusalem, 91905 Israel.   TAMMY PILOWSKY • Department of Psychology, The Hebrew University of Jerusalem, Mount Scopus, Jerusalem, 91905 Israel.   LUBOV NEMANOV, TEMIRA FEINSILVER, and RICHARD P. EBSTEIN • S. Herzog Memorial Hospital, Jerusalem, 91351 Israel.   SHOSHANA ARBELLE and IRIS FRIED • Ben-Gurion University Soroka Medical Center, Beer-Sheeva, 84777 Israel.

The Research Basis for Autism Intervention, edited by Schopler, Yirmiya, Shulman, and Marcus. Kluwer Academic/Plenum Publishers, New York, 2001.

tioning as reflected in abnormalities of EEG (Cantor, Thatcher, Hrybyk, & Kaye, 1986; Coleman, Romano, Laphan, & Simon, 1985), visual and auditory evoked potentials (Verbaten, Roelofs, van Engeland, Kenemans, & Slangen, 1991; Wong & Wong, 1991), and brain imaging (Balottin, Bejor, Cecchini, Martelli, Palazzi, & Lanzi, 1989; Horwitz, Rumsey, Grady, & Rapoport, 1988). In addition, macrocephaly, abnormalities in cerebellar histology, and various brain malformations have been described in autism (Fisher, Van Dyke, Sears, Matzen, Lin-Deyken, & McBrien, 1999). These findings indicate the existence of a neurological impairment in autism, and suggest a strong support for autism as a neurological disorder.

GENETICS AND BEHAVIOR GENETICS OF AUTISM

During the last two decades there has been an increasing interest in the genetic basis of autism. Identification of a genetic component associated with autism may convey vast implications, varying from a possibility of prenatal diagnosis and prevention, to early identification and very early intervention. Support for the genetic hypothesis arrives from the relationship between autism and disorders with a known genetic etiology, and from genetic and behavioral genetic studies.

A relationship between autism and different disorders with a known genetic etiology was described. For example, an elevated rate of autism was found in individuals with fragile X syndrome (Gillberg & Wahlström, 1985), and an elevated rate of tuberous sclerosis was found in individuals with autism (Gillberg, Gillberg, & Ahlsén, 1994; Smalley, Tanguay, & Smith, 1992). A high rate of autistic behavior has been reported in other disorders associated with genetic abnormalities, including Prader–Willi, Klinefelter, and Williams syndromes (Fisher et al., 1999). As suggested by Rutter (2000), these varied findings imply etiological heterogeneity in autism. Yet, these disorders explain only a small percentage of cases of autism.

A more substantial support for the genetic hypothesis is revealed by twin studies. Twin studies in autism consistently reported higher rates of the disorder in monozygotic (identical) twins as compared with dizygotic (fraternal) twins, with the concordance for autism ranging from 36% to 95% in monozygotic twins in comparison with 0% to 24% concordance for autism in dizygotic twins (Bailey et al., 1995; Folstein & Rutter, 1977; Ritvo, Freeman, Mason-Brothers, Mo, & Ritvo, 1985; Steffenburg et al., 1989). Furthermore, twin studies suggest that autism is under a high degree of genetic control and that multiple genes are likely to play a role in conferring a risk for this (Bailey et al., 1995). However, it may be suggested that monozygotic twins also share a common prenatal environment, so that the elevated rate of autism in monozygotic twins may to some degree be attributed to the shared environment. This may emphasize the need for family studies to achieve a more in-depth understanding of the genetic component in autism.

Indeed, family studies provide further support for the genetic hypothesis, in their attempt to determine the rate of autism in relatives of children with autism. Several researchers reported that in comparison to the rate of 0.02% to 0.05% of autism in the general population (DSM-IV, APA, 1994), the risk for autism in siblings of individuals with autism ranges between 2% and 7% (Bolton, Macdonald, Pickles, Rios, & Goode, 1994; Piven et al., 1990; Smalley, Asarnow, & Spence, 1988). Thus, the recurrence risk of autism in siblings is 30 to 100 times in excess of what would be expected based on chance alone (Rutter, 2000). Based on the difference in the risk for autism between monozygotic and dizygotic twins, and between first-degree and second-degree relatives of children with autism, it was suggested that the genetic basis for autism could not involve one gene only, but must involve 2 to 10 genes (Pickles et al., 1995).

Twin and family studies were employed to investigate behavioral phenotypes in autism. This line of research focused on the search for behavioral features characteristic of families of children with autism. In their twin study, Folstein and Rutter (1977) first suggested the existence of a broader autism phenotype, by demonstrating elevated rates of cognitive deficits in the nonautistic monozygotic twins compared to the nonautistic dizygotic twins. The broader phenotype was defined as a milder social and cognitive deficit, typically involving speech or language abnormality, which might be accompanied by circumscribed interest pattern. Other studies supported this notion, by reporting on outcomes in terms of not only an elevated rate of autism, but also of an increased rate of social and communicative impairments in family members (August, Stewart, & Tsai, 1981; Bailey et al., 1995; Bolton, Macdonald, Pickles, Rios, & Goode, 1994; Creak & Ini, 1960; Folstein & Piven, 1991; Folstein & Rutter, 1977; Piven, Palmer, Jacobi, Childress, & Arndt, 1997), implying a potentially broader pattern of difficulties. These studies, using a family history approach, or by directly assessing family members' behavior, showed evidence for aggregation of various difficulties in the families of children with autism, including language difficulties, reading and spelling difficulties, and limited sociability (Piven, 1999). Cognitive abilities were also examined, with conflicting results, indicating the importance of the comparison group employed (Fombonne, Bolton, Prior, Jordan, & Rutter, 1997; Ozonoff, Rogers, Farnham, & Pennington, 1993). In sum, this body of literature on the behavior genetics of autism suggests strong support for a genetic component in autism. It suggests that the liability for autism extends beyond the traditional diagnosis of autism and may cause milder difficulties that resemble the characteristics of autism, and that several genes may be involved (Rutter, 2000). This implies the importance and the need for genetic studies in autism.

As summarized by Rutter (2000), the genetic research in autism faces challenges. Initially, there were no good candidate genes, there was no evidence of the mode for genetic transmission, and the boundaries regarding the phenotype are still unclear. Nevertheless, genetic research in autism has drawn great interest in the last few years. Recently genome wide scans using the affected sib strategy have provisionally located several chromosomal regions harboring possible genes for autism (Barrett et al., 1999; Philippe et al., 1999; Risch et al., 1999). Encouragingly, some overlap of chromosomal regions (2q, 7q, 16p, and 19p) was observed between studies, although in each study unique regions were flagged, suggesting genetic heterogeneity (Risch et al., 1999; Szatmari, 1999). It may be that this genetic heterogeneity reflects the heterogeneity in the phenotype observed in individuals with autism, and it may also reflect an etiological heterogeneity in autism. A similar heterogeneity has been observed in linkage studies of bipolar disorder and schizophrenia.

A number of candidate gene studies have also been carried out in autism (Cook et al., 1997; Herault et al., 1994a,b; Klauck et al., 1997a,b; Limprasert, Zhong, Dobkin, & Brown, 1997; Martineau et al., 1994; Maestrini et al., 1999; McDougle, Epperson, Price, & Gelernter, 1998; Petit et al., 1995; Persico et al., 2000) with conflicting results. It was observed early that autistic children are hyperserotonemic and show high platelet serotonin levels

(Anderson, Horne, Chatterjee, & Cohen, 1990; Cook, Leventhal, Heller, Metz, Wainwright, & Freedman, 1990; de Villard et al., 1986), suggesting the possible involvement of serotonergic genes in this disorder. Serotonin effects mood, aggressive behavior, repetitive behaviors, sleep, memory, pain, anxiety, and neural development (Fisher et al., 1999). Indeed, the serotonin transporter promoter region (5-HTTLPR) polymorphism, first identified by Lesch and his colleagues (Heils et al., 1996; Lesch et al., 1996), has been a focus of interest in autism (Cook et al., 1997; Klauck et al., 1977b; Persico et al., 2000; Maestrini et al., 1999; McDougle, Epperson, Price, & Gelernter, 1998), again with contradictory results.

In the current study, in addition to 5-HTTLPR, we also examined two additional coding region polymorphisms: the dopamine D4 receptor 7 repeat (DRD4) and catechol-O-methyltransferase (COMT). The DRD4 exon III repeat polymorphism has been associated with "novelty seeking" (Ebstein et al., 1996; Benjamin, Li, Patterson, Greenberg, Murphy, & Hamer, 1996) and with attention deficit hyperactivity disorder (Swanson et al., 2000); in both impulsive behavior is prominent, and therefore appeared to be a worthwhile candidate to examine in autism. COMT has been associated with obsessive–compulsive disorder (Alsobrook, Zohar, Leboyer, Chabane, Ebstein, & Paul, in press; Karayiorgou et al., 1997, 1999), heroin addiction (Horowitz, Shufman, Aharoni, Kotler, & Ebstein, in press; Vandenbergh, Rodriguez, Miller, Uhl, & Lachman, 1997), and violence in schizophrenia (Kotler et al., 1999; Lachman, Nolan, Mohr, Saito, & Volavka, 1998).

Therefore, in the current study we examined the role of three functional polymorphisms previously studied in human behavior: the 5-HTTLPR (Heils et al., 1996; Lesch et al., 1996), the DRD4 (Benjamin, Li, Patterson, Greenberg, Murphy, & Hamer, 1996; Ebstein et al., 1996; LaHoste et al., 1996), and COMT (Lachman, Papolos, Saito, Yu, Szumlanski, & Weinshilboum, 1996).

PARTICIPANTS

Thirty-four families participated in the current study. Blood samples were obtained from individuals with autism and from their biological parents. Diagnosis of autism was established using the Autism Diagnostic Interview-Revised (ADI-R; Lord, Rutter, & LeCouteur, 1994). The ADI-R is a standardized, semistructured interview, based on the ICD-10 and the DSM-III-R criteria for autism. It was administered to participants' caregiver(s) by a trained interviewer. The ADI-R relies on a detailed description of behaviors that correspond to developmental deviance rather than developmental delay, and focuses on three areas of functioning: communication and language; reciprocal social interaction; and repetitive, restrictive, and stereotyped behavior. In addition, to receive a diagnosis of autism, evidence of developmental deviance must be present before the age of 36 months. The ADI-R was translated to Hebrew (Yirmiya, Shulman, & Arbelle, 1996) with good interrater reliability (for more details see Pilowsky, Yirmiya, Shulman, & Dover, 1998). All individuals with autism were diagnosed by an independent clinician who was not affiliated with the current study. All 34 participants received the diagnosis of autism according to the ADI-R.

Participants' levels of functioning were assessed using a standard evaluation, according to participants' age and level of functioning. Eleven participants were assessed using the Wechsler Intelligence Scale for Children-Revised (Wechsler, 1974), two participants were assessed with the Leiter International Performance Scale (1948), two participants were assessed with the Measurement of Intelligence of Infants and Young Children-Revised (Cattell, 1960), two participants were assessed with the Mullen Scales of Early Learning (1984), one participant was assessed with the Kaufman Assessment Battery for Children (Kaufman & Kaufman, 1983), and one with the Bayley Scales of Infant Development (Bayley, 1993). For the additional participants who could not be assessed in a direct evaluation, the Vineland Adaptive Behavior Scales (Sparrow, Balla, & Cicchetti, 1984) was administered to their main caregiver(s). Independent professionals not affiliated with the current study collected all developmental information. The participants' chronological ages ranged from 3.6 and 25.5 years (mean = 11.17, SD = 5.85). The participants' level of functioning ranged from mental retardation to a high level of functioning, and their mental ages ranged between 18 months and 13.17 years (mean = 5.85, SD = 3.06).

Each family was seen individually for the blood sample procedure, and participants with autism were seen individually for a developmental assessment. The ADI-R (Lord, Rutter, & LeCouteur, 1994) and the Vineland Adaptive Behavior Scales (Sparrow, Balla, & Cicchetti, 1984) were administered to participants caregiver(s) at a different session.

GENOTYPING

Individuals with autism and their parents were met at their homes for blood sampling. DNA was extracted from frozen blood samples using the phenol procedure. From some individuals, from whom blood sample could not be obtained, DNA was obtained from buccal smears using a MasterPure kit (Epicentre Technologies, Madison WI).

Each individual was genotypes by characterizing the *5-HTTLPR*, the *DRD4*, and *COMT* (for high and low COMT activity).

STATISTICAL METHODS

Data were analyzed using the haplotype relative risk (HRR) and the transmission disequilibrium test (TDT) strategy. The HRR strategy (Falk & Rubenstein, 1987) compares allele and genotype frequency between the proband group and a "virtual" control group constructed from those alleles not transmitted to the proband. This procedure neutralizes the problem of type I errors due to population admixture or stratification that often confounds interpretation of case-control studies. The TDT examines the transmission of alleles from heterozygous parents to the proband. This method controls for stratification biases, and is thought to be more robust than the HRR design (Ewens & Spielman, 1995; Spielman, McGinnis, & Ewans, 1993).

RESULTS AND DISCUSSION

A significant excess (39.4% versus 12.1 %) of the long/long *5-HTTLPR* genotype was observed in the group with autism. Similarly, when allele frequencies were examined, preferential transmission (62.1% versus 40.9%) of the long *5-HTTLPR* allele was observed in the autistic group. We also examined allele transmission from heterozygous parents using the TDT test and found a significant preferential transmission of the long *5-HTTTLPR*. Examination of the high/low enzyme activity *COMT* polymorphism revealed that both genotype and allele frequencies were similar in the group with autism compared to the HRR control group. Similarly when the *DRD4* exon III repeat polymorphism was examined, no significant difference in allele frequency of the various repeats was observed between the autism versus control group. Nor was any difference observed between the various repeats when grouped according to the long versus short classification scheme (Ebstein et al., 1996).

The serotonin transporter gene (*HTT*) is a likely candidate in autistic disorder based on efficacy of potent serotonin transporter inhibitors in reducing rituals and routines (Gilman & Tuchman, 1995; Pigott & Seay, 1999; Todorov, Freeston, & Borgeat, 2000), a core behavioral characteristic of autism. In addition, elevated serotonin levels have been consistently found in 30% to 50% of the patients with autism (Anderson, Horne, Chatterjee, & Cohen, 1990) and may represent a marker for familial autism (Piven, Tsai, Nehme, Coyle, Chase, & Folstein, 1991). Hyperserotoninemia in autism appears to be due to enhanced 5-hydroxytryptamine (5-HT, serotonin) uptake, as free 5-HT levels are normal (Cook, Leventhal, & Freedman, 1988; Katsui, Okuda, Usuda, & Koizumi, 1986). Finally, serotonin also plays a role in brain development, suggesting that subtle changes in serotonin brain levels could contribute to the manifestation of the clinical syndrome (Cases, Vitalis, Seif, De Maeyer, Sotelo, & Gaspar, 1996).

Several studies examined the *5-HTTLPR* polymorphism in autism. The first study by Cook et al. found evidence for preferential transmission of the short allele of this polymorphism in 86 triads (Cook et al., 1997). A second study in a somewhat smaller group of 65 trios also found evidence for preferential transmission, although the preferentially transmitted allele was the long rather than the short allele (Klauck et al., 1997b). Another study (Persico et al., 2000) genotyped 54 singleton families collected in Italy and in 32 singleton and 5 multiplex families collected in the United States, yielding a total sample of 98 trios. Both the Italian and the American samples, either singly or combined, displayed no evidence of linkage/association between *5-HTT* gene promoter alleles and autistic disorder. The IMGSA consortium (Maestrini et al., 1999) examined 90 families and found no evidence for linkage at the *HTTLPR* locus, the *HTT-VNTR* (a *VNTR* in the second intron) locus, or their haplotypes.

In the current study we examined in 34 autistic triads the distribution of the s and l variants of the *5-HTTLPR* gene using the haplotype relative risk and the TDT strategies. Our results, albeit with only a small number of triads, show a significant preferential transmission of the long allele, similar to results observed by Klauck et al., (1997b). It would be tempting to speculate that the excess of the more efficient l/l or l/s genotype in autism could account for the higher 5-HT content observed in autistic platelets. However, in a study of platelets from normal subjects, although the long variant of *5-HTTLPR* was associated with more rapid initial platelet 5-HT uptake (V_{max}), the index of platelet *5-HTT* function most clearly heritable (Greenberg, Tolliver, Huang, Li, Bengel, & Murphy, 1999), the *5-HTTLPR* genotype had no effect on platelet 5-HT content.

In addition to *5-HTTLPR*, we also examined two additional coding region polymorphisms: *DRD4* and *COMT*. The *DRD4* exon III repeat polymorphism has been associated in some studies with the adult personality construct of "novelty seeking" (Ebstein et al., 1996; Benjamin, Li, Patterson, Greenberg, Murphy, & Hamer, 1996) and with attention deficit hyperactivity disorder (Swanson et al., 2000). In both these behaviors impulsive behavior is prominent and this gene therefore appeared a worthwhile candidate to examine in autism. The *COMT* polymorphism *val→met* determines high and low enzyme activity and the *met/met* genotype displays only 20% of the activity of the *val/val* genotype. Serotonin is not a substrate for this enzyme that is involved in the degradation of dopamine and nor-epinephrine. *COMT* has been associated with obsessive–compulsive disorder in two inde-pendent studies (Alsobrook et al., 2000; Karayiorgou et al., 1997, 1999), in heroin addiction (Horowitz et al., 2000; Vandenbergh, Rodriguez, Miller, Uhl, Lachman, 1997) and violence in schizophrenia (Kotler et al., 1999; Lachman et al., 1998). In the current study no association was observed between either of these polymorphisms and autism.

In a genome wide scan of autism (Risch et al., 1999) results were most compatible with a model specifying a large number of loci (perhaps as many as 15). Only modestly positive or negative linkage evidence in candidate regions was identified in other studies. As Risch and his colleagues point out, their results suggest that positional cloning of susceptibility loci by linkage analysis may be a formidable task and that other approaches may be necessary. One such approach was suggested by Risch and Merikangas (1996), who proposed that mapping genes in complex traits might be best accomplished by combining the power of the human genome project with association studies using the TDT. This test has been shown to be immune to confounding due to population stratification (Ewens & Spielman, 1995; Spielman, McGinnis, & Ewans, 1993). Also, in the absence of population stratification, this test has similar power to the usual case-control design (Risch & Teng, 1998; Teng & Risch, 1999). Although several international consortiums are now recruiting affected sib pairs for genome wide scans, the considerations raised by Risch suggest that use of the TDT strategy as currently employed using singleton families is likely to place an increasingly important role in finding genes conferring risk for autism.

CLINICAL IMPLICATIONS

Geneticists and behavioral researchers are currently investigating the genes and the behaviors associated with autism and its broad phenotype. Identification of a specific genetic component associated with autism may will have important clinical implications. It will enable genetic counseling and prenatal genetic diagnosis for families at risk for autism. Based on personal values, parents may decide whether or not to continue a pregnancy at risk for autism or related disorders. This in turn may also eliminate the birth limiting effect now evident in families of children with autism who chose not to have any more children because of the risk of another child with autism.

ACKNOWLEDGMENTS

Nurit Yirmiya's work on this chapter was supported in part by the United States–Israel Binational Science Foundation and by the Israel Science Foundation founded by the Israel Academy of Sciences and Humanities.

REFERENCES

Alsobrook, II J. P., Zohar, A. H., Leboyer, M., Chabane, N., Ebstein, R. P., & Paul, D. L. (in press). Association between the COMT locus and obsessive compulsive disorder in females but not males. *Neuropsychiatric Genetics.*

American Psychiatric Association. (1994). *Diagnostic and Statistical Manual of Mental Disorders,* 4th ed. Washington, DC: American Psychiatric Association.

Anderson, G. M., Horne, W. C., Chatterjee, D., & Cohen, D. J. (1990). The hyperserotonemia of autism. *Annals of the New York Academy of Sciences, 600,* 331–340, discussion 341–2.

August, G. J., Stewart, M. A., & Tsai, L. (1981). The incidence of cognitive disabilities in siblings of autistic children. *British Journal of Psychiatry, 138,* 416–422.

Bailey, A., LeCouteur, A., Gottesman, I., Bolton, P., Simonoff, E., Yuzda, E., & Rutter, M. (1995). Autism as a strongly genetic disorder: Evidence from a British twin study. *Psychological Medicine, 25,* 63–78.

Balottin, U., Bejor, M., Cecchini, A., Martelli, A., Palazzi, S., & Lanzi, G. (1989). Infantile autism and computerized tomography brain-scan findings: Specific versus nonspecific abnormalities. *Journal of Autism and Developmental Disorders, 19,* 109–117.

Barrett, S., Beck, J. C., Bernier, R., Bisson, E., Braun, T. A., Casavant, T. L., et al. (1999). An autosomal genomic screen for autism. *American Journal of Medical Genetics, 88*(6), 609–615.

Bayley, N. (1993). *Bayley Scales of Infant Development,* 2nd ed. The Psychological Corporation. San Antonio: Harcourt Brace.

Benjamin, J., Li, L., Patterson, C., Greenberg, B. D., Murphy, D. L., & Hamer, D. H. (1996). Population and familial association between the D4 dopamine receptor gene and measures of Novelty Seeking. *Nature Genetics, 12*(1), 81–84.

Bolton, P., Macdonald, H., Pickles, A., Rios, P., & Goode, S. (1994). A case-control family history study of autism. *Journal of Child Psychology and Psychiatry, 35*(5), 877–900.

Cantor, D. S., Thatcher, R. W., Hrybyk, M., & Kaye, H. (1986). Computerized EEG analyses of autistic children. *Journal of Autism and Developmental Disorders, 16,* 169–187.

Cases, O., Vitalis, T., Seif, I., De Maeyer, E., Sotelo, C., & Gaspar, P. (1996). Lack of barrels in the somatosensory cortex of monoamine oxidase A-deficient mice: Role of a serotonin excess during the critical period. *Neuron, 16*(2), 297–307.

Cattell, P. (1960). *The Measurement of Intelligence of Infants and Young Children-Revised.* New York: Psychological Corporation.

Coleman, P. D., Romano, J., Laphan, L., & Simon, W. (1985). Cell counts in cerebral cortex of an autistic patient. *Journal of Autism and Developmental Disorders, 15,* 55–76.

Cook, E. H., Jr., Courchesne, R., Lord, C., Cox, N. J., Yan, S., Lincoln, A., et al. (1997). Evidence of linkage between the serotonin transporter and autistic disorder. *Molecular Psychiatry, 2,*(3), 247–250.

Cook, E. H., Jr., Leventhal, B. L., & Freedman, D. X. (1988). Free serotonin in plasma: autistic children and their first-degree relatives. *Biological Psychiatry, 24*(4), 488–491.

Cook, E. H., Jr., Leventhal, B. L., Heller, W., Metz, J., Wainwright, M., & Freedman, D. X. (1990). Autistic children and their first-degree relatives: Relationships between serotonin and norepinephrine levels and intelligence. *Journal of Neuropsychiatry and Clinical Neuroscience, 2*(3), 268–274.

Creak, M., & Ini, S. (1960). Families of psychotic children. *Journal of Child Psychology and Psychiatry, 1,* 156–175.

de Villard, R., Flachaire, E., Thoulon, J. M., Dalery, J., Maillet, J., Chauvin, C., et al. (1986). Platelet serotonin concentrations in autistic children and members of their families. *Encephale, 12*(4), 139–142.

DeMyer, M. K., Hingtgen, J. L., & Jackson, R. K. (1981). Infantile autism reviewed: A decade of research. *Schizophrenia Bulletin, 7,* 390–453.

Deykin, E., & MacMahon, B. (1979). The incidence of seizures among children with autistic symptoms. *American Journal of Psychiatry, 136,* 1310–1312.

Ebstein, R. P., Novick, O., Umansky, R., Priel, B., Osher, Y., Blaine, D., et al. (1996). Dopamine D4 receptor (D4DR) exon III polymorphism associated with the human personality trait of Novelty Seeking. *Nature Genetics, 12*(1), 78–80.

Ewens, W. J., & Spielman, R. S. (1995). The transmission/disequilibrium test: History, subdivision and admixture. *American Journal of Human Genetics, 57,* 455–464.

Falk, C. T., & Rubenstein, P. (1987). Haplotype relative risk: An easy reliable way to construct a proper control sample for risk calculations. *Annals of Human Genetics, 51,* 227–233.

Fisher, E., Van Dyke, D. C., Sears, L., Matzen, J. R. N., Lin-Dyken, D., & McBrien, D. M. (1999). Recent research on the etiologies of autism. *Infants and Young Children, 11*(3), 1–8.

Folstein, S. E., & Piven, J. (1991). Etiology of autism: Genetic influences. *Pediatrics, 87,* 767–773.

Folstein, S. E., & Rutter, M. L. (1977). Infantile autism: A genetic study of 21 twin pairs. *Journal of Child Psychology and Psychiatry, 18,* 297–321.

Fombonne, E., Bolton, P., Prior, J., Jordan, H., & Rutter, M. (1997). A family study of autism: Cognitive patterns and levels in parents and siblings. *Journal of Child Psychology and Psychiatry, 38,* 667–684.

Gillberg, I. C., Gillberg, C., & Ahlsén, G. (1994). Autistic behavior and attention deficits in tuberous sclerosis: A population-based study. *Developmental Medicine and Child Neurology, 36,* 50–56.

Gillberg, C., & Wahlström, J. (1985). Chromosome abnormalities in infantile autism and other childhood psychoses: A population study of 66 cases. *Developmental Medicine and Neurology, 27,* 293–304.

Gilman, J. T., & Tuchman, R. F. (1995). Autism and associated behavioral disorders: Pharmacotherapeutic intervention. *Annals Pharmacotherapeutics, 29*(1), 47–56.

Greenberg, B. D., Tolliver, T. J., Huang, S. J., Li, Q., Bengel, D., & Murphy, D. L. (1999). Genetic variation in the serotonin transporter promoter region affects serotonin uptake in human blood platelets. *American Journal of Medical Genetics, 88*(1), 83–87.

Heils, A., Teufel, A., Petri, S., Stober, G., Riederer, P., Bengel, D., et al. (1996). Allelic variation of human serotonin transporter gene expression. *Journal of Neurochemistry, 66*(6), 2621–2624.

Herault, J., Martineau, J., Petit, E., Perrot, A., Sauvage, D., Barthelemy, C., et al. (1994a). Genetic markers in autism: Association study on short arm of chromosome 11. *Journal of Autism and Developmental Disorders, 24*(2), 233–236.

Herault, J., Petit, E., Buchler, M., Martineau, J., Cherpi, C., Perrot, A., et al. (1994b). Lack of association between three genetic markers of brain growth factors and infantile autism. *Biological Psychiatry, 35*(4), 281–283.

Horwitz, B., Rumsey, J. M., Grady, C. L., & Rapoport, S. I. (1988). The cerebral metabolic landscape in autism: Intercorrelations of regional glucose utilization. *Archives of Neurology, 45,* 749–755.

Horowitz, R., Shufman, A., Aharoni, S., Kotler, M., & Ebstein, R. P. (2000). Confirmation of an excess of the high enzyme activity COMT val allele in heroin addicts in a family-based haplotype relative risk study. *American Journal of Medical Genetics, 96,* 599–603.

Jones, V., & Prior, M. (1985). Motor imitation abilities and neurological signs in autistic children. *Journal of Autism and Developmental Disorders, 15,* 37–46.

Karayiorgou, M., Altemus, M., Galke, B. L., Goldman, D., Murphy, D. L., Ott, J., et al. (1997). Genotype determining low catechol-*O*-methyltransferase activity as a risk factor for obsessive-compulsive disorder. *Proceedings of the National Academy of Sciences USA, 94*(9), 4572–4575.

Karayiorgou, M., Sobin, C., Blundell, M. L., Galke, B. L., Malinova, L., Goldberg, P., et al. (1999). Family-based association studies support a sexually dimorphic effect of COMT and MAOA on genetic susceptibility to obsessive-compulsive disorder. *Biological Psychiatry, 45*(9), 1178–1189.

Katsui, T., Okuda, M., Usuda, S., & Koizumi, T. (1986). Kinetics of 3H-serotonin uptake by platelets in infantile autism and developmental language disorder (including five pairs of twins). *Journal of Autism and Developmental Disorders, 16*(1), 69–76.

Kaufman, A. S., & Kaufman, N. L. (1983). *Kaufman Assessment Battery for Children (K-ABC).* American Guidance Services. Circle Pines, MN: American Guidance Services, Inc.

Klauck, S. M., Munstermann, E., Bieber-Martig, B., Ruhl, D., Lisch, S., Schmotzer, G., et al. (1997a). Molecular genetic analysis of the FMR-1 gene in a large collection of autistic patients. *Human Genetics, 100*(2), 224–229.

Klauck, S. M., Poustka, F., Benner, A., Lesch, K. P., & Poustka, A. (1997b). Serotonin transporter (5-HTT) gene variants associated with autism? *Human Molecular Genetics, 6*(13), 2233–2238.

Kotler, M., Peretz, B., Cohen, H., Averbuch, A. V., Grinshpoon, A., Gritsenko, I., et al. (1999). Homicidal behavior in schizophrenia associated with a genetic polymorphism determining low catechol *O*-methyltransferase (COMT) activity. *American Journal of Medical Genetics (Neuropsychiatric Genetics), 88,* 628–633.

Lachman, H. M., Nolan, K. A., Mohr, P., Saito, T., & Volavka, J. (1998). Association between catechol *O*-methyltransferase genotype and violence in schizophrenia and schizoaffective disorder. *American Journal of Psychiatry, 155*(6), 835–837.

Lachman, H. M., Papolos, D. F., Saito, T., Yu, Y. M., Szumlanski, C. L., & Weinshilboum, R. M. (1996). Human catechol-O-methyltransferase pharmacogenetics: Description of a functional polymorphism and its potential application to neuropsychiatric disorders. *Pharmacogenetics*, 6(3), 243–250.

LaHoste, G. J., Swanson, J. M., Wigal, S. B., Glabe, C., Wigal, T., King, N., et al. (1996). Dopamine D4 receptor gene polymorphism is associated with attention deficit hyperactivity disorder. *Molecular Psychiatry*, 1(2), 121–124.

Leiter International Performance Scale (1948). Chicago: Stoelting Co.

Lesch, K. P., Bengel, D., Heils, A., Sabol, S. Z., Greenberg, B. D., Petri, S., et al. (1996). Association of anxiety-related traits with a polymorphism in the serotonin transporter gene regulatory region. *Science*, 274(5292), 1527–1531.

Limprasert, P., Zhong, N., Dobkin, C., & Brown, W. T. (1997). Polymorphism of FXR1 showing lack of association with autism. *American Journal of Medical Genetics*, 74(4), 453–454.

Lord, C., Rutter, M., & LeCouteur, A. (1994). Autism Diagnostic Interview-Revised: A revised version of a diagnostic interview for caregivers of individuals with possible pervasive developmental disorders. *Journal of Autism and Developmental Disorders*, 24, 659–685.

Maestrini, E., Lai, C., Marlow, A., Matthews, N., Wallace, S., Bailey, A., et al. (1999). Serotonin transporter (5-HTT) and gamma-aminobutyric acid receptor subunit beta3 (GABRB3) gene polymorphisms are not associated with autism in the IMGSA families. *American Journal of Medical Genetics*, 88(5), 492–496.

Martineau, J., Herault, J., Petit, E., Guerin, P., Hameury, L., Perrot, A., et al. (1994). Catecholaminergic metabolism and autism [see comments]. *Developmental Medicine and Child Neurology*, 36(8), 688–697.

McDougle, C. J., Epperson, C. N., Price, L. H., & Gelernter, J. (1998). Evidence for linkage disequilibrium between serotonin transporter protein gene (SLC6A4) and obsessive compulsive disorder. *Molecular Psychiatry*, 3(3), 270–273.

Ozonoff, S., Rogers, S. J., Farnham, J. M., & Pennington, B. F. (1993). Can standard measures identify subclinical markers of autism? *Journal of Autism and Developmental Disorders*, 23(3), 471–478.

Persico, A. M., Militerni, R., Bravaccio, C., Schneider, C., Melmed, R., Conciatori, M., et al. (2000). Lack of association between serotonin transporter gene promoter variants and autistic disorder in two ethnically distinct samples. *American Journal of Medical Genetics*, 96(1), 123–127.

Petit, E., Herault, J., Martineau, J., Perrot, A., Barthelemy, C., Hameury, L., et al. (1995). Association study with two markers of a human homeogene in infantile autism. *Journal of Medical Genetics*, 32(4), 269–274.

Philippe, A., Martinez, M., Guilloud-Bataille, M., Gillberg, C., Rastam, M., Sponheim, E., et al. (1999). Genome-wide scan for autism susceptibility genes. Paris Autism Research International Sibpair Study. *Human Molecular Genetics*, 8(5), 805–812.

Pickles, A., Bolton, P., Macdonald, H., Bailey, A., LeCouteur, A., Sim, L., & Rutter, M. (1995). Latent class analysis of recurrence risk for complex phenotypes with selection and measurement error: A twin and family history study of autism. *American Journal of Human Genetics*, 57, 717–726.

Pilowsky, T., Yirmiya, N., Shulman, C., & Dover, R. (1998). The Autism Diagnostic Interview-Revised and the Childhood Autism Rating Scale: Differences between diagnostic systems and comparison between genders. *Journal of Autism and Developmental Disorders*, 28, 143–151.

Pigott, T. A., & Seay, S. M. (1999). A review of the efficacy of selective serotonin reuptake inhibitors in obsessive-compulsive disorder. *Journal of Clinical Psychiatry*, 60(2), 101–106.

Piven, J. (1999). Genetic liability for autism: The behavioral expression in relatives. *International Review of Psychiatry*, 11, 299–308.

Piven, J., Gayle, J., Chase, J., Fink, B., Landa, R., Wzorek, M. M., & Folstein, S. (1990). A family history of neuropsychiatric disorders in the adult siblings of autistic individuals. *Journal of the American Academy of Child and Adolescent Psychiatry*, 29, 177–183.

Piven, J., Palmer, P., Jacobi, D., Childress, D., & Arndt, S. (1997). Broader autism phenotype: Evidence from a family history study of multiple-incidence autism families. *American Journal of Psychiatry*, 154(2), 185–109.

Piven, J., Tsai, G. C., Nehme, E., Coyle, J. T., Chase, G. A., & Folstein, S. E. (1991). Platelet serotonin, a possible marker for familial autism. *Journal of Autism and Developmental Disorders*, 21(1), 51–59.

Risch, N., & Merikangas, K. (1996). The future of genetic studies of complex human diseases. *Science*, 273, 1516–1517.

Risch, N., Spiker, D., Lotspeich, L., Nouri, N., Hinds, D., Hallmayer, J., et al. (1999). A genomic screen of autism: Evidence for a multilocus etiology. *American Journal of Human Genetics*, 65(2), 493–507.

Risch, N., & Teng, J. (1998). The relative power of family-based and case-control designs for linkage disequilibrium studies of complex human diseases I. DNA pooling. *Genome Research*, 8(12), 1273–1288.

Ritvo, E. R., Freeman, B. J., Mason-Brothers, A., Mo, A., & Ritvo A. M. (1985). Concordance of the syndrome of autism in 40 pairs of afflicted twins. *American Journal of Psychiatry, 142*, 74–77.

Rutter, M. (2000). Genetic studies of autism: From the 1970s into the millennium. *Journal of Abnormal Child Psychology, 28*, 3–14.

Smalley, S., Asarnow, R., & Spence, M. (1988). Autism and genetics: A decade of research. *Archives of General Psychiatry, 45*, 953–961.

Smalley, S., Tanguay, P., & Smith, M. (1992). Autism and tuberous sclerosis. *Journal of autism and Developmental Disorders, 22*, 339–355.

Sparrow, S. S., Balla, D. A., & Cicchetti, D. V. (1984). *Vineland Adaptive Behavior Scales.* Circle Pines, MN: American Guidance Services.

Spielman, R. S., McGinnis, R. E., & Ewans, W. J. (1993). Transmission test for linkage disequilibrium: the insulin gene region and insulin-dependent diabetes mellitus (IDDM). *American Journal of Human Genetics, 52*, 506–516.

Steffenburg, S., Gillberg, C., Hellgren, L., Andersson, L., Gillberg, I. C., Jakobsson, G., & Bohman, M. (1989). A twin study of autism in Denmark, Finland, Iceland, Norway and Sweden. *Journal of Child Psychology and Psychiatry, 30*(3), 405–416.

Swanson, J. M., Flodman, P., Kennedy, J., Spence, M. A., Moyzis, R., Schuck, S., et al. (2000). Dopamine genes and ADHD. *Neuroscience and Biobehavior, 24*, 1, 21–25.

Szatmari, P. (1999). Heterogeneity and the genetics of autism [see comments]. *Journal of Psychiatry and Neuroscience, 24*(2), 159–165.

Teng, J., & Risch, N. (1999). The relative power of family-based and case-control designs for linkage disequilibrium studies of complex human diseases. II. Individual genotyping. *Genome Research, 9*(3), 234–241.

Todorov, C., Freeston, M. H., & Borgeat, F. (2000). On the pharmacotherapy of obsessive-compulsive disorder: Is a consensus possible? *Canadian Journal of Psychiatry, 45*(3), 257–262.

Vandenbergh, D. J., Rodriguez, L. A., Miller, I. T., Uhl, G. R., & Lachman, H. M. (1997). High-activity catechol-*O*-methyltransferase allele is more prevalent in polysubstance abusers. *American Journal of Medical Genetics, 74*(4), 439–442.

Verbaten, M. N., Roelofs, J. W., van Engeland, H., Kenemans, J. L., & Slangen, J. L. (1991). Abnormal visual event-related potentials of autistic children. *Journal of Autism and Developmental Disorders, 21*, 449–470.

Wechsler, D. (1974). *WISC-R Manual: Wechsler Intelligence Scale for Children-Revised.* San Antonio, TX: Psychological Corporation.

Wong, V., & Wong, S. N. (1991). Brainstem auditory evoked potential study in children with autistic disorder. *Journal of Autism and Developmental Disorders, 21*, 329–340.

Yirmiya, N., Shulman, C., & Arbelle, S. (1996). Hebrew version of the Autism Diagnostic Interview-Revised. Available from the authors by request.

8

Autism, Stress, and Chromosome 7 Genes

Michael Shapira, David Glick, John R. Gilbert, and Hermona Soreq

Autism, a disorder affecting 4 out of 10,000 individuals in the general population, is classified as a pervasive developmental disorder. It becomes apparent by the third year of life and its characteristic impairments persist into adulthood. Whereas the inheritance of this disorder does not follow a simple Mendelian pattern, there is compelling evidence for strong genetic basis. This fact places autism in the category of complex genetic traits and predicts difficulties in any attempt to unravel the various genes that contribute to the disorder, genes that may even have different contributions in differen populations. Recently, the rising interest in autism has spawned quite a few multinational efforts aimed at identification of these genes. The projects, taking advantage of experimental approaches designed for the study of complex genetic traits, succeeded in identifying several candidate loci. However, none of these loci was identified with certainty. Among this group of candidate loci, several appear to be more prominent than the rest. The long arm of chromosome 7 (7q) is one of those.

The main characteristics of autism are social and communicative impairments, as well as repetitive and stereotyped behaviors and interests. However, there are also reports of stress response-like behavior in autistic children. Such reports strongly suggest that autism is associated with inherited impairments in stress responses. However, this association has yet to be confirmed. An interesting link that relates impairments in stress responses to autism is found in the chromosome 7 gene *ACHE*, which encodes the enzyme acetylcholinesterase (AChE). The expression of this gene is robustly and persistently up-regulated under stress and was recently found to be affected by a novel mutation in the gene's extended promoter.

This chapter describes the recent advances in the identification of genes or gene loci that contribute to the autistic phenotype, concentrating on what appears to be one of the best candidate loci, 7q. It will further describe the reports that suggest an association between

MICHAEL SHAPIRA, DAVID GLICK, and HERMONA SOREQ • Department of Biological Chemistry, Institute of Life Sciences, The Hebrew University of Jerusalem, Jerusalem, 91904 Israel.   JOHN R. GILBERT • Department of Medicine and Center for Human Genetics, Duke University, Durham, North Carolina 27710.

The Research Basis for Autism Intervention, edited by Schopler, Yirmiya, Shulman, and Marcus. Kluwer Academic/Plenum Publishers, New York, 2001.

autism and impairments in stress responses and will elaborate on putative molecular mechanism(s) that underlie stress responses in conjunction with autism. Finally, to follow the suggested link that connects autism with stress, through the candidate locus 7q, we present in this chapter the results of a survey that determined the frequency of the *ACHE* upstream mutation in affected and nonaffected American families. These results show an extremely low incidence of this mutation, failing to confirm its association with autism in American families. Nonetheless, the results do not rule out a role for this polymorphism in the etiology of autism in the Israeli population, where the mutation is present in a higher frequency.

AUTISM AS A COMPLEX TRAIT, CANDIDATE LOCI, AND GENES

Multigenic diseases differ from monogenic ones in that their occurrence cannot be linked to one specific gene, but is, rather, affected by changes in several genes. They include some of modern medicine's chief concerns, such as risk of cardiac failure, diabetes mellitus, and a plethora of neurologic disorders. Among these, autism is an intriguing disorder both from the aspect of its behavioral symptoms, the scope of which is difficult to define, and because of its complex etiology. The frequency of autism is 4 in 10,000 for the classically defined syndrome (with males affected 4 times more frequently than females (Smalley, Asarnow, & Spence, 1988). Inclusion of the related Pervasive Development Disorders, Not Otherwise Specified (PDD-NOS) and Asperger syndrome increases this incidence to 16 in 10,000 (Rodier, 2000).

It was previously believed that drugs such as the teratogens thalidomide and valproic acid may be risk factors for autism (Rodier, Ingram, Tisdale, Nelson, & Romano, 1996). Although a certain contribution of such environmental factors may exist, it is now known that the main factors for the disorder are genetic (Folstein & Rutter, 1977). The strongest evidence for the contribution of inherited factors to autism comes from studies on twins (Bailey et al., 1995; Folstein & Rutter, 1977; Steffenburg et al., 1989; Wahlstrom, Steffenburg, Hellgren, & Gillberg, 1989). These studies showed a much higher concordance rate (the chance that a child will be diagnosed as autistic when his twin has already been confirmed as autistic) in monozygotic (MZ, identical) twin pairs compared to dizygotic pairs (DZ). The concordance rates found in the largest of these studies (Bailey et al., 1995). were 60% in MZ pairs compared to 0% in DZ pairs. This enabled calculation of the heritability of autism, which was found to be greater than 90%. Moreover, in many of the twin pairs showing a discordance, the nonautistic co-twins presented language impairments in childhood and social deficits that persisted into adulthood (LeCouteur et al., 1996). This supports the understanding of autism as a multigenic and multifactorial disease with a large array of partially overlapping symptoms representing disorders with similar physiological bases. Such similar disorders can be pooled into a related diagnostic group of PDD-NOS. That the concordance rate in MZ twin pairs does not reach the 100% expected for a pure genetic disorder implies that autism, as many other multifactorial diseases, is also affected by environmental factors that are associated with life history. Individual responses to life history, however, are also affected by the genetic makeup of the individual. The assumption is that individuals with genetic susceptibility to adverse responses to certain life events (e.g., a traumatic experience) are more likely to develop autism than others who are similarly exposed, yet do not have the inherited susceptibility. One of the twin studies (Steffenburg et al., 1989) reported that in most of the twin pairs discordant for autism, the autistic twin had more perinatal stress. This possible link of autism with stress is discussed further in the paragraphs that follow.

With the genetic basis of autism well established, the next and more challenging goal is to identify the genes linked to it. So far, no clear-cut linkage has been found between any particular gene or genetic locus and autism. This may be attributed to misdiagnosis of individuals, but probably also stems from the genetic heterogeneity of autism, with affecting genes varying in their contribution within different populations. It is believed that more than 14 loci may be associated with autism (Risch et al., 1999). Table 8-1 presents a summary of the current candidate loci and genes, most of which were determined in recent genome-wide screens. Whereas the majority of these chromosomes are implicated in autism based on a single identification, a few loci came up more than once and are therefore considered more seriously as containing genes that contribute significantly to the etiology of autism. Among these, the most prominent locus is 7q, with most of the markers pointing to the q32–q35 region but with some cytogenetical evidence suggesting q21–q22 as well (Ashley-Koch et al., 1999). Another locus that appears to be a serious candidate for harboring relevant genes based on cytological studies is 15q11–q13 (e.g., see Cook et al., 1997). However, this locus is not favored by results of the genetic screens. The reason for

TABLE 8-1. Candidate Genes and Genetic Loci Associated with Autism[a]

Chromosomal locus[b]	Candidate genes[c]	Reference
1p(13)		Risch et al., 1999
2q(24–31)		IMGSAC, 1998; Philippe et al., 1999
4q(34–35)		Philippe et al., 1999
5p		Philippe et al., 1999
6q(16)	*MACS, GRIK6, GPR6*	Philippe et al., 1999
7q(31–35, 21–22)[d]	*GPR37,[d] SPCH1, PTPRZ1, EPHB6, ACHRM1, PTN, NEDD2/ICH1/ CASP2, GRM8*	IMGSAC, 1998; Barrett et al., 1999; Philippe et al., 1999; Risch et al., 1999
10q(26)		Philippe et al., 1999
13a(21–32)		Risch et al., 1999
15q11–q13		Risch et al., 1999
15q11–q13	*GABR3, UBE3A*	Cook et al., 1998; Martin et al., 2000 but see Barrett et al., 1999; Risch et al., 1999
16p(12–13)		IMGSAC, 1998; Philippe et al., 1999
17a11.1–q12	*HTT, NF1*	Cook et al., 1997; Mbarek et al., 1999
17p	*HOX1A[e]*	Risch et al., 1999
18q(22)		Philippe et al., 1999
19p(13)		IMGSAC, 1998; Philippe et al., 1999
Xp(21–22)		Philippe et al., 1999

[a]Compiled most from four full-genome screens performed in the past 2 years (IMGSAC, 1998; Barret et al., 1999; Philippe et al., 1999; Risch et al., 1999).
[b]Whenver available, the exact location of the linked region is designated. When no exact location has been suggested the position of the markers used for the genetic screening was added (in brackets).
[c]Whenever proposed in the cited papers.
[d]See Ashley-Koch et al. (1999).
[e]See Rodier (2000).

this may be the sampling of individuals for the genetic screens, which excludes those carrying chromosomal abnormalities.

Before further focusing on chromosome 7, a few of the candidate genes believed to contributed to the etiology of autism are worth mentioning. Most of the proposed candidate genes are believed to be causally involved in autism based on their known contribution to neuronal activity or development, combined with linkage analysis of their chromosomal locations. In certain cases, such as with the serotonin transporter (*HTT*). This gene was proposed as a candidate based on a phenotypic abnormality, the high serotonin levels shown by autistic individuals (Cook et al., 1997), a suggestion that was reinforced by genetic association studies (Klauck, Poustka, Benner, Lesch, & Poustka, 1997). Similarly, the neurofibromatosis type 1 gene (*NF1*; Mbarek, Marouillat, Martineau, Barthelemy, Muh, & Andres, 1999) was found be overexpressed in autistic patients. *NF1* is known to regulate the activity of Ras proteins, of which one shows an association with autism (Comings, Wu, Chiu, Muhleman, & Sverd, 1996). A different case involved the γ-aminobutyric acid (GABA) receptor β3-subunit gene (*GABRB3*; Cook et al., 1998). This receptor is activated by GABA, the principal inhibitory neurotransmitter in the brain. Its importance in control of brain excitability, as well as its developmentally regulated expression, indicated possible involvement in the autistic phenotype.

So far, however, genetic screens have failed to unequivocally verify the association of these genes. In most cases, new allelic markers were identified in the gene regions, but not in the same position as the preliminarily associated markers (Martin et al., 2000; Risch et al., 1999). The next two sections point up the stress-related symptoms of autism that have been somewhat neglected in recent years, and which may suggest new candidate genes based on their involvement in such symptoms.

IS AUTISM ASSOCIATED WITH INHERITED IMPAIRMENTS IN STRESS RESPONSES?

Once a genetic basis of autism was established, environmental factors, which had previously been the focus of attention, were pushed aside. However, we now believe that there is reason to consider an interaction of genetic and environmental factors. The correlation of autism with inherited susceptibility to extreme stress responses has been discussed extensively, so far without resolution. Several observations suggest such correlation. First, autistic patients show an exaggerated response to external stimuli that are not stressful in healthy individuals (Bergman & Escalona, 1949; Hutt, Hutt, Lee, & Ounsted, 1964), perhaps suggesting inherited differences in their levels of perceived stress; second, such an exaggerated response to external stimuli may indicate an inherited tendency to impaired control over stress responses (Hutt, Hutt, Lee, & Ounsted, 1965); and third, the long-lasting nature of their repetitive behavior phenotype hints at inherited difficulties in termination of stress responses. Similarly, the impairments in socioemotional reciprocity that are characteristic of autism (Wing & Gould, 1979), the communication impairments and anxiety (Muris, Steerneman, Merckelbach, Holdrinet, & Meesters, 1998), the susceptibility to epileptic seizures (Giovanardi Rossi, Posar, & Parmeggiani, 2000), and the restricted repertoire of activities and interests (Wing & Gould, 1979) may all be associated with inherited defects in the intricate processes that control human responses to stress. In

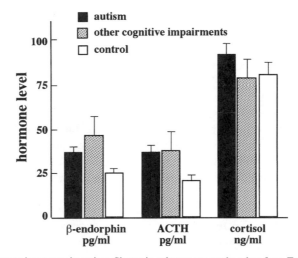

FIGURE 8-1. Plasma stress hormones in autism. Shown in columns are results taken from Tordjman et al. (1997) of data from autistic patients ($n = 46$–48), patients with mental retardation or other cognitive impairments ($n = 15$–16), and normal subjects ($n = 23$–26). Statistics was performed on log-transformed data, as described in the reference.

addition, autism is associated with a mild but reproducible and apparently specific elevation in the stress-related hormones β-endorphin and adrenocorticotropic hormone (ACTH) (Tordjman et al., 1997) (Figure 8-1). All this calls for investigating those nervous system pathways and the corresponding genes that contribute to stress responses. One such pathway involves cholinergic neurotransmission.

Neurons communicating by the neurotransmitter acetylcholine (ACh) are tightly involved in mammalian stress responses. Hyperexcitation of cholinergic neurotransmission has been reported under stress (Kaufer & Soreq, 1999); persistent changes were observed in the expression patterns of the key genes that encode the ACh-synthesizing enzyme choline acetyl transferase, the packaging protein vesicular ACh transporter, and the ACh-hydrolyzing enzyme acetylcholinesterase (AChE) (Kaufer, Friedman, Seidman, & Soreq, 1998), all of which lead to a decrease in cholinergic hyperexcitation and to reestablishment of normal neurotransmission. These stress-induced changes take place primarily in the hippocampus, which has been reported to develop abnormally in autistic individuals (Piven, 1997). The change in AChE expression and its increase under stress conditions is mimicked in AChE-overproducing transgenic mice. These mice display progressive stress-related pathologies, including high density of curled neuronal processes in the somatosensory cortex, accumulation of clustered heat shock protein 70-immunopositive neuronal fragments in the hippocampus, and a high incidence of reactive astrocytes (Sternfeld et al., 2000). They also present progressive impairments in learning, memory, and social behavior (Beeri et al., 1995; Beeri et al., 1997; Cohen, O. et al., personal communication), and appear extremely sensitive to head injury (Shohami et al., 2000) and AChE inhibitors (Shapira et al., 2000b). Moreover, stress was shown to increase the blood–brain barrier permeability (Friedman, Kaufer, Shemer, Hendler, Soreq, & Tur-Kaspa, 1996), thereby allowing potentially harmful xenobiotics to enter the brain. A subset of such xenobiotics, the AChE inhibitors, are commonly used in agriculture and in the household as insecticides. Upon entering the brain, AChE inhibitors may cause the above-mentioned long-lasting increase in AChE expression and persistent excess of this protein may lead to neuropathological changes and to impairment of cognitive and social skills such as those observed in the transgenic mice. Altogether, these data suggest that individuals with an inherited susceptibility to adverse stress responses, itself probably a complex trait, will present exaggerated AChE expression. Similarly, individuals with an inherited abnormal AChE expression may develop a susceptibility to adverse stress responses. The autism-associated symptoms, which appear to indicate increased stress responses, may point to the *ACHE* gene and its transcriptional control as promising ground in which to explore for correlations with the autistic phenotype.

Consider (1) that in everyone, there is a toll in brain neuropathologies to be paid for the daily load of stress, and in experimental animals the appearance of these pathologies seems to exacerbate under AChE overexpression (Sternfeld et al., 2000); (2) this toll may be magnified in individuals with an inherited predisposition to exaggerated responses to stress and to anti-AChE agents, as in some cases hypersensitivity to anti-AChEs was discovered to be associated with a genomic variation that induces constitutive overexpression of AChE (Shapira et al., 2000b); and (3) an additional factor may be a previous exposure to AChE inhibitors, which under stress can cross the blood–brain barrier (Friedman et al., 1996) and induce progressive damage to glia and neurons. Each of these effects, and especially the sum of them, may facilitate the developmental impairments characteristic of autism.

CHROMOSOME 7 AND AUTISM

The long arm of chromosome 7 was marked as a locus of genes that contribute to autism in all of the full genome screens performed so far (IMGSAC, 1998; Barrett et al., 1999; Philippe et al., 1999; Risch et al., 1999) and in a few more restricted screens, for example, by Ashley-Koch et al. (1999). While the linked loci extend from bands q32 to q35, several genes located outside of this region may be equally important. This assumption is based on identified mapping inaccuracies and ambiguities (Hauser, Boehnke, Guo, & Risch, 1996), on the assumption that certain genetic aberrations may involve not only the genetically linked region but also neighboring genes and on potentially relevant functions of the respective gene products, which make them appropriate candidates for association with different aspects of the autistic phenotype. One such candidate gene, *SPCH1*, which fulfills all three criteria, was proposed recently. *SPCH1* is associated with a severe speech and language disorder (Fisher, Vargha-Khadem, Watkins, Monaco, & Pembrey, 1998) and thus may be responsible for the language difficulties observed in autistic children. A family with three affected children, two with autism and one with a language disorder, was recently investigated (Ashley-Koch et al., 1999). Affected members of this family were found to carry an inversion spanning bands 7q21 to 7q34. Further screening of additional families for markers located in the inversion region pointed to part of this inversion region being associated with 25% to 40% of autism cases (Ashley-Koch et al., 1999). However, with the set of chromosome 7 markers included in that screen, the *SPCH1* gene itself was not linked to this syndrome.

We have recently examined the possible involvement of aberrant regulation of another chromosome 7 gene, *ACHE*, located close to *SPCH1*, in the susceptibility to development of the autistic phenotype. Mapped to 7q22, *ACHE* encodes the enzyme AChE which is responsible for hydrolyzing the neurotransmitter ACh and thus for terminating neurotransmission across cholinergic synapses (Massoulie et al., 1998). In addition, *ACHE* is involved in plasticity responses in many more tissues through non-catalytic activities (reviewed in Grisaru, Sternfeld, Eldor, Glick, & Soreq, 1999). Yet more importantly, overproduction of AChE was reported under acute psychological stress (Kaufer et al., 1998). The proximity of the *ACHE* gene to the autism-related 7q32–35 region, its inclusion in the inversion region found in the autism family (reported in Ashley-Koch et al., 1999), and its association with stress responses all make it a plausible candidate. In addition, *ACHE* is expressed in early stages of brain development, long before the formation of functioning synapses (Layer, 1995), which implies that its aberrant regulation can contribute to the developmental defects that are associated with autism. In addition, it should be noted that stress-induced overexpression of 7q22 genes is not limited to *ACHE*; at least one additional gene, *ARS*, which is associated with arsenite resistance, and possibly others at this locus, also appear to be overexpressed (Shapira, Grant, Korner, & Soreq, 2000a).

Although total blockade of ACh hydrolysis is incompatible with life, polymorphisms that modulate the transcriptional control of AChE may cause a milder effect, which is manifested as an inherited susceptibility to changes in cholinergic neurotransmission. Following a search for such polymorphisms (Shapira et al., 2000b), we have recently identified a four-basepair deletion that disrupts one of two binding sites for the transcription factor HNF3β (Kaestner, Hiemisch, Luckow, & Schutz, 1994; Qian, Samadani, Porcella, & Costa, 1995). This deletion is located in a distal enhancer domain, 17 Kb upstream from the transcription start site of *ACHE*, a region dense with binding motifs for other factors, including glucocorticoid hormones (Shapira et al., 2000b) (Figure 8-2). This *ACHE* promoter deletion induces constitutive AChE overproduction, which in turn causes an impaired capacity for up-regulating AChE production under chemical stress insults and results in hypersensitivity to such insults. Because of the molecular mechanisms common to chemical and psychological stress responses, that is, elevated expression of stress-associated transcription factors such as AP1 or HNF3, of AChE (Kaufer & Soreq, 1999) and of heat shock proteins (Sternfeld et

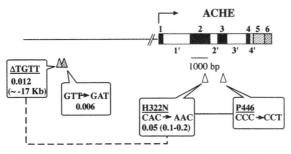

FIGURE 8-2. ACHE polymorphisms. Shown is a drawn-to-scale scheme of the ACHE locus with all known polymorphisms depicted. Exons are depicted as numbered filled boxes, introns as numbered open boxes, and mutations as wedges. A solid line connecting mutations indicates complete linkage between the variants. A broken line represents strong incomplete linkage. Mutation frequencies are taken from Ehrlich et al. (1994) for the coding region mutations (open wedges).

al., 2000), we suspect that carriers of this promoter polymorphism are also hypersensitive to psychological stressors. An extension of this concept implies that autism and susceptibility to stressors share common molecular abnormalities. It may also be that a primary stress event would induce an acquired susceptibility to exaggerated responses to subsequent stress. Under a certain genetic makeup, the risk of developing the full autistic phenotype may also increase. To examine one of the molecular markers associated with such suscep- tibility, we determined the incidence of the transcriptionally activating deletion in the *ACHE* promoter in US families with affected children as compared with screened healthy individuals from Israel and the United States.

In the examined Israeli population, the tested deletion displayed an allele frequency of 0.012 and was strongly linked to the biochemically neutral H322N point mutation in the AChE coding sequence. The H322N mutation, responsible for the rare Ytb blood group, is considerably more frequent in Middle Eastern populations (Ehrlich et al., 1994), much more than in the United States (Giles, Metaxas-Buhler, Romanski, & Metaxas, 1967). Therefore, we predicted that the *ACHE* promoter polymorphism would occur less fre- quently in the US population, regardless of the autistic status. This was, indeed, found to be the case, with 8 heterozygous carriers out of 333 screened Israelis (2.4% incidence) but only 5 carriers in 816 US individuals (0.6%) (Table 8-2). The low incidence of this polymorphism further complicated the data analysis, as it was found in 3 out of 616 normal US individuals (0.5%) as compared with 2 out of 190 affected ones (1.0%). We conclude that if indeed this specific polymorphism is involved in the susceptibility to extreme stress responses in the US survey of autistic patients, its effect is minimal.

PROSPECTS

The current status of this study leaves us with more questions than answers. Because of the rarity of the analyzed promoter polymorphism, we cannot confirm that it is associated with the autistic phenotype in the studied families. The conflicting evidence regarding candidate genes suggests that the genomic basis of autism may differ from one population to another. This is highlighted by the different allelic frequency of the *ACHE* promoter

TABLE 8-2. Screening Autism Families for Δ4 *ACHE* Promoter Polymorphism

Autism	US Families		US Individuals	Carriers	Israeli Individuals	Carriers	Total Individuals	Carriers
Singleton[a]	103	Normal	616	3[c]	333	8	949	11
Multiplex[b]	82	Affected	190	2[d]	—		190	2
Unconfirmed multiplex	18	Unclear status	18	—	—		18	—
Total	203		816	5	333	8	949	13

[a]Nuclear families with an affected child.
[b]Families with at least two affecteds, usually sibs.
[c]Of two families, one female, one male and his grandson.
[d]Two affected males.

polymorphism in the US and Israeli populations that were screened. In addition, the wealth of transcription factor binding motifs in the extended *ACHE* promoter suggests multiple contributions toward its control, both under normal and stress conditions. Therefore, the overall post-transcriptional pattern of *ACHE* gene expression may be more relevant to autism than sequence polymorphisms in particular elements of its promoter.

We do believe, however, that it is worthwhile paying attention to environmental factors, such as stress, that, given a certain genetic makeup, may affect the development of autism. More than identifying affecting environmental factors per se, this approach may offer hints of additional genetic factors, that indirectly contribute to the etiology of autism by processing environmental influences.

ACKNOWLEDGMENTS

This study was supported by a grant from the U.S. Army Medical Research and Material Command (DAMD 17-99-1-9547).

REFERENCES

Ashley-Koch, A., Wolpert, C. M., Menold, M. M., Zaeem, L., Basu, S., Donnelly, S. L., Ravan, S. A., Powell, C. M., Qumsiyeh, M. B., Aylsworth, A. S., Vance, J. M., Gilbert, J. R., Wright, H. H., Abramson, R. K., DeLong, G. R., Cuccaro, M. L., & Pericak-Vance, M. A. (1999). Genetic studies of autistic disorder and chromosome 7. *Genomics, 61*(3), 227–236.

Bailey, A., LeCouteur, A., Gottesman, I., Bolton, P., Simonoff, E., Yuzda, E., & Rutter, M. (1995). Autism as a strongly genetic disorder: Evidence from a British twin study. *Psychological Medicine, 25*(1), 63–77.

Barrett, S., Beck, J. C., Bernier, R., Bisson, E., Braun, T. A.., Casavant, T. L., Childress, D., Folstein, S. E., Garcia, M., Gardiner, M. B., Gilman, S., Haines, J. L., Hopkins, K., Landa, R., Meyer, N. H., Mullane, J. A., Nishimura, D. Y., Palmer, P., Piven, J., Purdy, J., Santangelo, S. L., Searby, C., Sheffield, V., Singleton, J., Slager, S., et al. (1999). An autosomal genomic screen for autism. Collaborative linkage study of autism. *American Journal of Medical Genetics, 88*(6), 609–615.

Beeri, R., Andres, C., Lev Lehman, E., Timberg, R., Huberman, T., Shani, M., & Soreq, H. (1995). Transgenic expression of human acetylcholinesterase induces progress cognitive deterioration in mice. *Current Biology, 5*(9), 1063–1071.

Beeri, R., Le Novere, N., Mervis, R., Huberman, T., Grauer, E., Changeux, J. P., & Soreq, H. (1997). Enhanced hemicholinium binding and attenuated dendrite branching in cognitively impaired acetylcholinesterase-transgenic mice. *Journal of Neurochemistry, 69*(6), 2441–2451.

Bergman, P., & Escalona, S. (1949). Unusual sensitivities in very young children. *Psychoanalytic Study of Children, 34*, 333–352.

Comings, D. E., Wu, S., Chiu, C., Muhleman, D., & Sverd, J. (1996). Studies of the c-Harvey-Ras gene in psychiatric disorders. *Psychiatry Research, 63*(1), 25–32.

Cook. E. H., Jr., Courchesne, R. Y., Cox, N. J., Lord, C., Gonen, D., Guter, S. J., Lincoln, A., Nix, K., Haas, R., Leventhal, B. L., & Courchesne, E. (1998). Linkage-disequilibrium mapping of autistic disorder, with 15q11–13 markers. *American Journal of Human Genetics, 62*(5), 1077–1083.

Cook, E. H., Jr., Lindgren, V., Leventhal, B. L., Courchesne, R., Lincoln, A., Shulman, C., Lord, C., & Courchesne, E. (1997). Autism or atypical autism in maternally but not paternally derived proximal 15q duplication. *American Journal of Human Genetics, 60*(4), 928–934.

Ehrlich, G., Patinkin, D., Ginzberg, D., Zakut, H., Eckstein, F., & Soreq, H. (1994). Use of partially phosphorothioated "antisense" oligodeoxynucleotides for sequence-dependent modulation of hematopoiesis in culture. *Antisense Research Developments, 4*(3), 173–183.

Fisher, S. E., Vargha-Khadem, F., Watkins, K. E., Monaco, A. P., & Pembrey, M. E. (1998). Localisation of a gene implicated in a severe speech and language disorder. *Nature Genetics, 18*(2), 168–170.

Folstein, S., & Rutter, M. (1977). Infantile autism: A genetic study of 21 twin pairs. *Journal of Child Psychology and Psychiatry*, *18*(4), 297–321.

Friedman., A., Kaufer, D., Shemer, J., Hendler, I., Soreq, H., & Tur-Kaspa, I. (1996). Pyridostigmine brain penetration under stress enhances neuronal excitability and induces early immediate transcriptional response. *Nature Medicine*, *2*, 1382–1385.

Giles, C. M., Metaxas-Buhler, M., Romanski, Y., & Metaxas, M. N. (1967). Studies on the Yt blood group system. *Vax Sang*, *13*(2), 171–180.

Giovanardi Rossi, P., Posar, A., & Parmeggiani, A. (2000). Epilepsy in adolescents and young adults with autistic disorder. *Brain Development*, *22*(2), 102–106.

Grisaru, D., Sternfeld, M., Eldor, A., Glick, D., & Soreq, H. (1999). Structural roles of acetylcholinesterase variants in biology and pathology. *European Journal of Biochemistry*, *264*, 672–686.

Hauser, E. R., Boehnke, M., Guo, S. W., & Risch, N. (1996). Affected-sib-pair interval mapping and exclusion for complex genetic traits: Sampling considerations. *Genetic Epidemiology*, *13*(2), 117–137.

Hutt, C., Hutt, S. J., Lee, D., & Ounsted, C. (1964). Arousal and childhood autism. *Nature*, *204*, 908.

Hutt, C., Hutt, S. J., Lee, D., & Ounsted, C. (1965). A behavioural and electroencephalographic study of autistic children. *Journal of Psychiatry Research*, *3*, 181–197.

IMGSAC, International Molecular Genetic Study of Autism Consortium. (1998). A full genome screen for autism with evidence for linkage to a region on chromosome 7q. *Human Molecular Genetics*, *7*(3), 571–578.

Kaester, K. H., Hiemisch, H., Luckow, B., & Schutz, G. (1994). The HNF-3 gene family of transcription factors in mice: Gene structure, cDNA sequence, and mRNA distribution. *Genomics*, *20*(3), 377–385.

Kaufer, D., Friedman, A., Seidman, S., & Soreq, H. (1998). Acute stress facilitates long-lasting changes in cholinergic gene expression. *Nature*, *393*(6683), 373–377.

Kaufer, D., & Soreq, H. (1999). Tracking cholinergic pathways from psychological and chemical stressors to variable neurodeterioration paradigms. *Current Opinions in Neurology*, *12*(6), 739–743.

Klauck, S. M., Poustka, F., Benner, A., Lesch, K. P., & Poustka, A. (1997). Serotonin transporter (5-HTT) gene variants associated with autism? *Human Molecular Genetics*, *6*(13), 2233–2238.

Layer, P. G. (1995). Nonclassical roles of cholinesterases in the embryonic brain and possible links to Alzheimer disease. *Alzheimer's Disease and Associated Disorders*, *9*(Suppl 2), 29–36.

LeCouteur, A., Bailey, A., Goode, S., Pickles, A., Robertson, S., Gottesman, I., & Rutter, M. (1996). A broader phenotype of autism: The clinical spectrum in twins. *Journal of Child Psychology and Psychiatry*, *37*(7), 785–801.

Martin, E. R., Menold, M. M., Wolpert, C. M., Bass, M. P., Donnelly, S. L., Ravan, S. A., Zimmerman, A., Gilbert, J. R., Vance, J. M., Maddox, L. O., Wright, H. H., Abramson, R. K., DeLong, G. R., Cuccaro, M. L., & Pericak-Vance, M. A. (2000). Analysis of linkage disequilibrium in gamma-aminobutyric acid receptor subunit genes in autistic disorder. *American Journal of Medical Genetics*, *96*(1), 43–48.

Massoulie, J., Anselmet, A., Bon, S., Krejci, E., Legay, C., Morel, N., & Simon, S. (1998). Acetylcholinesterase: C-terminal domains, molecular forms and functional localization. *Journal of Physiology* (Paris), *92*(3–4), 183–190.

Mbarek, O., Marouillat, S., Martineau, J., Barthelemy, C., Muh, J. P., & Andres, C. (1999). Association study of the NF1 gene and autistic disorder. *American Journal of Medical Genetics*, *88*(6), 729–732.

Muris, P., Steerneman, P., Merckelbach, H., Holdrinet, I., & Meesters, C. (1998). Comorbid anxiety symptoms in children with pervasive developmental disorders. *Journal of Anxiety Disorders*, *12*(4), 387–393.

Philippe, A., Martinez, M., Guilloud-Bataille, M., Gillberg, C., Rastam, M., Sponheim, E., Coleman, M., Zappella, M., Aschauer, H., Van Maldergem, L., Penet, C., Feingold, J., Brice, A., Leboyer, M., & van Malldergerme, L. (1999). Genome-wide scan for autism susceptibility genes. Paris Autism Research International Sibpair Study. *Human Molecular Genetics*, *8*(5), 805–812.

Piven, J. (1997). The biological basis of autism. *Current Opinions in Neurobiology*, *7*(5), 708–712.

Qian, X., Samadani, U., Porcella., A., & Costa, R. H. (1995). Decreased expression of hepatocyte nuclear factor 3 alpha during the acute-phase response influences transthyretin gene transcription. *Molecular and Cellular Biology*, *15*(3), 1364–1376.

Risch, N., Spiker, D., Lotspeich, L., Nouri, N., Hinds, D., Hallmayer, J., Kalaydjieva, L., McCague, P., Dimiceli, S., Pitts, T., Nguyen, L., Yang, J., Harper, C., Thorpe, D., Vermeer, S., Young, H., Hebert, J., Lin, A., Ferguson, J., Chiotti, C., Wiese-Slater, S., Rogers, T., Salmon, B., Nicholas, P., Myers, R. M., et al. (1999). A genomic screen of autism: Evidence for a multilocus etiology. *American Journal of Human Genetics*, *65*(2), 493–507.

Rodier, P. M. (2000). The early origins of autism. *Scientific American*, *282*(2), 56–63.

Rodier, P. M., Ingram, J. L., Tisdale, B., Nelson, S., & Romano, J. (1996). Embryological origin for autism: Developmental anomalies of the cranial nerve motor nuclei. *Journal of Comparative Neurology, 370*(2), 247–261.

Shapira, M., Grant, A., Korner, M., & Soreq, H. (2000a). Genomic and transcriptional characterization of the human ACHE locus: Complex involvement with acquired and inherited diseases. *Israeli Medical Association Journal, 2*(6), 470–473.

Shapira, M., Tur-Kaspa, I., Bosgraaf, L., Livni, N., Grant, A. D., Grisaru, D., Korner, M., Ebstein, R. P., & Soreq, H. (2000b). A transcription-activating polymorphism in the ACHE promoter associated with acute sensitivity to anti-acetylcholinesterases. *Human Molecular Genetics, 9*(9), 1273–1281.

Shohami, E., Kaufer, D., Chen, Y., Cohen, O., Ginzberg, D., Melamed-Book, N., Seidman, S., Yirmiya, R., & Soreq, H. (2000). Antisense prevention of neuronal damages following head injury in mice. *Journal of Molecular Medicine, 78,* 228–236.

Smalley, S. L, Asarnow, R. R., & Spence, M. A. (1988). Autism and genetics. A decade of research. *Archives of General Psychiatry, 45*(10), 953–961.

Steffenburg, S., Gillberg, C., Hellgren, L., Andersson, L., Gillberg, I. C., Jakobsson, G., & Bohman, M. (1989). A twin study of autism in Denmark, Finland, Iceland, Norway and Sweden. *Journal of Child Psychology and Psychiatry, 30*(3), 405–416.

Sternfeld, M., Shoham, S., Klein, O., Flores-Flores, C., Evron, T., Idelson, G. H., Kitsberg, D., Patrick, J. W., & Soreq, H. (2000). Excess "read-through" acetylcholinesterase attenuates but the "synaptic" variant intensifies neurodeterioration correlates. *Proceedings of the National Academy of Sciences USA, 97*(15), 8647–8652.

Tordjman, S., Anderson, G. M., McBride, P. A., Hertzig, M. E., Snow, M. E., Hall, L. M., Thompson, S. M., Ferrari, P., & Cohen, D. J. (1997). Plasma beta-endorphin, adrenocorticotropin hormone, and cortisol in autism. *Journal of Psychology and Psychiatry, 38*(6), 705–715.

Wahlstrom, J., Steffenburg, S., Hellgren, L., & Gillberg, C. (1989). Chromosome findings in twins with early-onset autistic disorder. *American Journal of Medical Genetics, 32*(1), 19–21.

Wing, L., & Gould, J. (1979). Severe impairments of social interaction and associated abnormalities in children: Epidemiology and classification. *Journal of Autism and Developmental Disorders, 9*(1), 11–29.

III

Communication and Social Issues

9

Communicative Intent in Autism

Cory Shulman, Odette Bukai, and Sigal Tidhar

Autism, a pervasive developmental disorder, is characterized by impairments in communication and social reciprocity and by repetitive behaviors and limited areas of interest
(American Psychiatric Association, 1994). At various times, each of these limitations has
been investigated as a possible primary deficit in autism. In particular, language and
communication deficits have been put forward as possible primary core symptoms that
underlie other essential features of the syndrome (Churchill, 1972; Rutter, 1984). Cognitive
and social skills, areas of deficit in autism, overlap with some language and communication
abilities. For example, language entails the ability to encode and decode symbols and
requires representative thought. Ricks and Wing (1979) linked some of the cognitive
deficits in autism to deficiencies in the ability to encode and decode symbols, such as those
involved in language, while Leslie and Happé (1989) and Sigman (1997) posited that
difficulties in representative thought, which are characteristic of individuals with autism,
may interface with language and communication deficits. Wing (1996) suggested that social
difficulties associated with autism may stem from a failure to participate jointly in social
interaction, which is an integral part of communication.

Attempts to establish the exact nature of the connection between deficits in language
and communication and the other impairments found in autism have been inconclusive.
Moreover, the very investigation of possible primary deficits in autism does not address the
interrelatedness of the linguistic, social, and cognitive deficits found in individuals with
autism (Goodman, 1989). Considering the interplay between the linguistic, cognitive, and
social domains in the development of individuals with autism, it may be futile to interpret
the syndrome primarily as a disorder of any one of these realms. Investigating the interface
between these developmental domains, however, could serve as the basis for a more
cohesive understanding of autism. For this reason, it may be useful to focus on "communicative intent"—which lies at the nexus of language, social, and cognitive development—

CORY SHULMAN • School of Social Work and School of Education, The Hebrew University of Jerusalem,
Mount Scopus, Jerusalem, 91905 Israel.   ODETTE BUKAI and SIGAL TIDHAR • Department of Psychology, The Hebrew University of Jerusalem, Mount Scopus, Jerusalem, 91905 Israel.

The Research Basis for Autism Intervention, edited by Schopler, Yirmiya, Shulman, and Marcus. Kluwer
Academic/Plenum Publishers, New York, 2001.

as a possible construct useful in understanding underlying abilities and disabilities in autism.

In this chapter, we propose that the investigation of communicative intent, a developmental motivational construct, which involves prelinguistic and language skills, as well as social referencing, may have the potential to provide diagnostic clarity and insight into the nature of the social and communicative dysfunction in autism. The chapter begins with a survey of literature that defines communicative intent and its elements, the development of communicative intent in typically developing children, and the development of communicative intent in children with autism. In our attempt to assess the appropriateness of communicative intent in autism, we ran a small pilot study using a systematic series of activities, which encourage communicative overtures. The importance of the development of such an instrument and the methodologies involved in analyzing the information gleaned from the activities are discussed. The applicability of the communicative profiles that emerge from using such a procedure are considered as fundamental information to consider when developing intervention strategies for young children with autism. Some suggestions for directions for further research are raised.

COMMUNICATIVE INTENT: DEFINITION

Bates (1979) defined intentional communication as "signaling behavior in which the sender is aware a priori of the effect that a signal will have in his listener or he persists in that behavior until the effect is obtained or failure is clearly indicated" (p. 36). Communication involves some degree of social engagement; intentional communication requires some notion of social causality and an understanding of other persons as intentional agents, as the signals are aimed at the listener rather than the goal itself. The signal may range from a preverbal gesture, such as pointing or giving, to a grammatically complete sentence. Language symbols are social conventions that gain communicative significance through agreement among the users. A child acquires active use of language for communicative purposes only by agreeing to this social interaction, and by understanding that the desired effect is obtainable through the listener. Examples of such desired effects might include regulating another person's behavior, attracting attention, or directing attention to something (Seibert & Oller, 1981; Wetherby, 1986). These communicative acts are referred to as "social communication" (Bakerman & Adamson, 1984; Carpenter, Nagell, & Tomasello, 1998), as "intentional communication" (Bretherton & Bates, 1979; Camaioni, 1993), and as "communicative intent" (Coggins & Carpenter, 1981; Holdgrafer & Durst, 1990). These communicative acts take place in a social context, with the purpose (intention) of affecting the listener in some predetermined manner.

Not all behavior that is interpreted communicatively is intentional. For example, a young infant's crying may alert the caregiver to the child's feelings of hunger or discomfort, without the infant's planning or intending to do so. Thus, the child's behavior may serve a communicative function without the child's planning or prior understanding of this effect. Consequently, determining intentionality in communication is problematic. Disagreements can be found regarding behavioral criteria for inferring intentionality, and researchers are divided regarding how loose or tight the behavioral criteria for inferring intentionality should be and whether or not there is a precise "moment" in development when a child progresses from preintentional to intentional communication.

COMMUNICATIVE INTENT: DETERMINING INTENTIONALITY

Several approaches have been suggested for determining the intentionality of communicative acts. One approach is defining intentional communication operationally based on the child's behavior (Coggins & Carpenter, 1981; Seibert, Hogan, & Mundy, 1982). Some examples of behavior which presume communicative intent include (1) alternating eye gaze between a goal and the listener, (2) persistent signaling until the goal has been met, (3) changing the quality of the signal until the goal has been met, (4) ritualizing or conventionalizing the form of the signal within specific communicative contexts, (5) awaiting a response from the listener, (6) terminating the signal when the goal is met, and (7) displaying satisfaction when the goal is met and dissatisfaction when it is not met. These behaviors can support the assertion that the child plans and intends to achieve a goal, and is aware that another person can be a means to that end. Although target behaviors associated with communicative intents are identified with this approach, adopting any particular set of behavioral criteria may be somewhat arbitrary and may introduce an artificial discontinuity into the investigation of the development of intentional communication.

An alternative approach to determination of intentionality in communication is based on the premise that developmental changes in communicative behavior may be an index of emerging intentionality (Thal, Bates, Goodman, & Jahn-Samilo, 1997; Wetherby, Cain, Yonclas, & Walker, 1988) and that communicative intent may be inferred by charting these changes. According to this approach, the suggested developmental sequence includes (1) no evidence of an awareness of a goal, (2) evidence of an awareness of a goal, (3) evidence of a simple plan designed to achieve a goal, (4) evidence of a coordinated plan designed to achieve a goal, and (5) evidence of alternative plans designed to achieve a goal. The difficulty inherent in determining intentionality of communicative acts is augmented because of the substantial heterogeneity among individuals with autism. With differing degrees of developmental retardation and severity of the impairment, a qualitative analysis of the communicative intentionality and the social contexts in which these acts occur is essential. As a result of this heterogeneity, the repertoire of behaviors that can be used for communication varies extensively across individuals with autism. Moreover, beyond this interindividual heterogeneity, there is extensive intra-individual heterogeneity across developmental domains within any given child with autism. Thus, the qualitative investigation of communicative intents has broadened researchers' conceptions of what types of behaviors may be considered communicative. Emerging intentional communicative behavior of children with autism initially appears to serve primarily nonsocial and quasi-social functions, such as attempting to obtain objects or directing the behavior of others. This pattern is strikingly different from that of other impaired children who typically express a wide range of intents early in development. In addition, these findings indicate the importance of considering the potential communicative intent underlying aberrant behaviors that are so prevalent in individuals with autism. The investigation of these behaviors and their possible communicative purposes may assist in understanding of the nature of the communication impairment in autism.

ELEMENTS OF COMMUNICATIVE INTENT

Communicative intent is traditionally investigated by quantitatively examining the overall number of communicative acts designated as intentional. In addition to the overall number of communicative acts, quantitative parameters include the frequency, duration, and variety of intentional communicative acts found in a particular communicative profile (Watson, Lord, Schaefer, & Schopler, 1989). The average number, frequency, and duration of communicative acts were not found to differ significantly among different populations of children (Dawson, Hill, Spencer, Galpert, & Watson, 1991; Wetherby, 1986). Analyzing communicative intent qualitatively, as well, is now accepted protocol. The qualitative parameters assessed encompass the evaluation of the function (purpose) of the communicative intent, the means (manner) of expression, as well as the referent (Paul & Shiffer, 1991; Watson et al., 1989). Although no quantitative differences emerged among different groups, the quality of communication, as measured by the function, the manner in which the messages were coordinated among the participants, and the third entity to which both communicative partners referred, are markedly different.

Qualitative analysis for determining the quality of intentionality in communicative acts comprises three dimensions (Prizant & Schuler, 1987; Watson et al., 1989). The first dimension concerns the reason for communicating and is referred to as the communicative purpose or function. Because such types of motivations cannot be observed directly, they must be inferred. These motivations are divided into two categories—imperative and declarative communication. Imperative communication includes requesting (objects, information, activity) and protesting. Declarative communication includes bringing attention (to self, objects, events) and relates to commenting and sharing. The second dimension to be assessed is the means (or form) by which intentions are expressed. These forms are, with some qualifications, developmental. They begin with nonsymbolic communication (e.g., behavior), move to prelinguistic gestures (e.g., pointing) and vocalizations, and continue until symbolic communication (e.g., words) has been attained. Normal communicative development involves the expression of a variety of intents from nonverbal to preverbal with the gradual development of more sophisticated and conventional communicative means to express intentions. The third dimension of intentional communicative behavior involves the analysis of the use of gaze, a social component of communicative intent. The use of alternating gaze reflects the comprehension of differentiation among self and others and the comprehension of people as agents, who can help achieve desired ends (Bakerman & Adamson, 1984; Harding, Stilson, Kromelow, & Weissmann, 1997). Although we analyzed these three elements of communicative intent in our sample, only preliminary data are presented here as future research is still pending.

Previous research reveals that nonverbal children with autism expressed requests, protests, and greeting intentionally, but few gestures of pointing or showing to label or comment were intentional. In addition, all children with autism expressed a limited repertoire of communicative intents. In spite of variability in level of language development and degree of mental retardation, children with autism exhibited a relatively homogeneous profile of communicative intents distinct from that of children without autism. When compared with typically developing children, children with autism communicated more often in an attempt to regulate adult behavior to achieve an environmental end. They seldom attempted to attract and direct adult attention to themselves or objects (Curcio, 1978; Wetherby, 1986).

DEVELOPMENT OF COMMUNICATIVE INTENT IN TYPICALLY DEVELOPING CHILDREN

Normally developing infants appear to begin to communicate intentionally at approximately 9 months of age (Bates, 1979; Carpenter, Nagell, & Tomasello, 1998). A three-stage model for tracing the development of communication has been proposed (Bates, 1979). Infants in the "perlocutionary stage" have a systematic effect on their partners although no intention to do so exists. This preintentional stage commences at birth and is preverbal. At about 9 months, the "illocutionary stage" begins. In this stage, children begin to use preverbal (e.g., gestural, vocal) signals intentionally to affect their listeners. With the emergence of language at approximately 12 to 18 months of age, children begin to communicate intentionally with words and enter the "locutionary stage." This model assumes developmental continuity from preintentional communication through intentional preverbal communication to intentional verbal communication (Sigman, 1997; Zeedyk, 1996). According to the continuum established by this approach, intentional communication emerges from a rudimentary awareness of a goal, through the recognition of a person as a communicative partner, and culminates in the coordination of behaviors to signal a person in the pursuit of a goal. Although this framework may have a solid theoretical base, it lacks operational and systematic definitions; therefore the developmental stages posited are difficult to pinpoint, and the transitions from one stage to another are not defined behaviorally. For example, parallel developments occur in nonsocial, object-oriented acts, and in social, person-oriented acts in typically developing children (Meltzoff, 1995; Zeedyk, 1996). The model proposed by this approach, however, does not provide for the possibility that a child may reach a specific developmental stage in the realm of object-oriented acts at a different time than she or he reaches the same stage in the realm of social acts.

Inasmuch as communicative intent occurs in a social context, shared agreement among the communicators is necessary for successful communication to transpire. The degree to which the meaning of signals is shared or understood by a social community is referred to as "conventionality" in communicative signaling. The conventional meaning in a given message can be analyzed on at least two levels. The first level is pragmatic intent, in which language is used as a social tool (Becker, 1994). From this perspective, the meaning of a communicative act is dependent on the manner in which it is expressed and meaning is closely determined by the intention that underlies or motivates a particular act. If, to accomplish a goal, a person is purposefully "activated" by another, the meaning of the communication is encompassed in the participants' shared understanding of the signals that comprise the communicative act.

The second level of conventional meaning is semantic intent, which refers to referential meaning—the objects, persons, actions, and locations—that particular words denote. Thus, communicative intent has aspects of conventionality and mutuality. For an expression of communicative intent to be successful, it must be interpretable at both the pragmatic and semantic levels. At preverbal levels, referential, semantic meaning is not inherent in the communicative act itself, but is sustained by objects and events in the environment. The listener must decode the referent based on the context, and must derive meaning by looking to environmental objects or events for clues. Nonverbal children use behavioral "signals" in setting up and maintaining social interactions. These signals are predicated on an awareness of the other person as a participant in the interaction, and a desire to initiate an interaction with that person. The child's initiation must then be followed by a response in order for the interaction to proceed. Once children begin to use language, they can communicate successfully on the levels of both pragmatic and semantic intent, and can convey meaning both as a social act and referentially. At this stage, communication of interest on the part of the child is still necessary to establish an interactive social exchange, but referential meaning can be conveyed explicitly by utterances, without the need for contextual support.

COMMUNICATIVE INTENT AND AUTISM

Difficulties in communication and social relationships have been identified as the major symptoms of the autistic syndrome, with severe repercussions for the development of autistic individuals (Volkmar & Klin, 1994). One of the first identifiable and measurable parameters of communication and social relatedness is communicative intent, which develops at around 9 months in typically developing children. Communicative intent in autism has been studied over the years, but, unfortunately, variability in the definition of this construct and the differing methodologies used to study it complicate the interpretation and applicability of the findings in this important field.

Hermelin and O'Connor (1985) made a distinction between nonintentional (spontaneous or unlearned) and intentional (voluntary) communication in their analyses of communication abilities in autism. According to their definition, nonintentional communication refers to information that is transmitted without deliberate or conscious awareness. Nonintentional productions are spontaneous and presumably unlearned, and they generally reflect emotional states. Some examples of nonintentional communication include the startle response, and a smile in response to a pleasant stimulus or to the voice intonation of a tense and anxious speaker. In contrast, intentional communication refers to a deliberate and voluntary attempt to convey information. Asking for food, pointing to a desired toy, or pushing away undesired work are examples of intentional communication.

In typically developing children, nonintentional communicative overtures are usually consistent with information conveyed intentionally. For example, a typically developing child who approaches a peer and says, "Want to play?" may establish eye contact, increase proximity to the other child, extend a toy, and perhaps smile. Although the request may be deliberate, other components of social communicative interaction (e.g., eye contact, smiling) are likely produced automatically and nonintentionally. In many children with autism, however, discrepancies between what is communicated nonintentionally and intentionally are common. For example, voice intonation may not match the contact of that which is said. In addition, nonverbal body language may have little to do with how the child with autism actually feels in a particular situation; for instance, the child's body may be turned away from the person with whom he or she is interacting. For these children, unlearned, innate behaviors may simply not be part of their internal wiring. Rather than reflecting some sort of negative attitude to the situation or indicating a negative affect toward the other person, these behaviors may simply be a manifestation of the basic lack of social skills of many children with autism. One social implication that arises from this problem in communication is that children with autism may be misunderstood by their peers, because nonintentionally transmitted information may be given more credence than information that is produced intentionally.

Bates' developmental model has been employed in the study of communication development of children with autism (Prizant, 1984; Wetherby, 1986), but because of the fundamental communication impairments in autism, the use of the model was problematic, particularly in determining the underlying communicative intent of children with autism. Both pragmatic intent, which entails the use of language as a social tool, and semantic intent, which encompasses referential communication, may be obscure in the communicative attempts of autistic children. For example, the communicative attempts of nonverbal children with autism, who communicate through gestures and vocalization, may not be understood, because the gestures and vocalization may be indirect, aberrant, or unclear. These expressions are often unconventional, idiosyncratic, or tied to particular events or situations not shared with the listener. Determining communicative intent in children with autism who communicate verbally is likewise problematic. Whereas the normal child's use of speech almost always implies intentionality, as the child is using a conventional symbolic code that reflects an intention to communicate (Bates, 1979; Nagel & Fontaine, 1989), this is often a false assumption regarding children with autism. In practice, the challenge lies in determining whether unconventional and idiosyncratic behavior is an expression of communicative intent.

The focus on communicative intent of children with autism provides important insights into the nature of the social communication impairments characteristics of autism. In comparative studies, children with autism display as many communicative acts as typically developing children matched for language level (Prizant & Schuler, 1997). However, children with autism express a more limited repertoire of communicative intents (e.g., fewer communicative functions and means). These limitations in communicative intent displayed by children with autism may be related to their social dysfunction (van Engeland, Bodnar, & Bolhuis, 1986).

Cross-sectional comparisons of communicative behaviors of children with autism at various language levels indicate predictability in the order by which communicative intents emerge. Wetherby (1986) presented a model of the ontogency of communicative intentionality in autism, in which communication for nonsocial, quasisocial, and social goals was delineated. Communication for nonsocial ends include attempts to regulate another's behavior to achieve environmental ends, such as requesting an object or an action, and protesting. Communication for quasi-social ends, which are focused on self or self needs, include attempts to attract another's attention to one's self, such as requesting a social routine, greeting, calling, requesting permission, or showing and showing off. Communication for social ends that are focused on interaction/sharing include directing another's attention to an object or event, such as naming an interactive label, commenting, and requesting information.

Whereas typically developing children develop a solid communicative foundation before the emergence of words, it may be possible that children with autism progress from relatively primitive means for achieving environmental ends to more sophisticated ones before expressing intentions for more social purposes. In addition, in contrast to the synchronous development of social and nonsocial communicative intents in normal and other developmentally delayed and language impaired children, it may be possible that children with autism may acquire communicative intents one at a time (Wetherby, 1986). The investigation of communicative intents addresses both cross-sectional descriptions, as well as longitudinal studies of the characteristic sequence of the development of communicative intents.

Around the same time that communicative intent emerges in the developing child, joint attention appears. Joint attention, which involves the child, the adult, and some third entity, which the participants both reference, has been found to be deficient in children with autism (Mundy, Sigman, & Kasari, 1994). Moving from dyadic (involving two people) to triadic interaction (involving two people and a third entity) is particularly difficult for children with autism. Hobson (1993) asserts that this difficulty comes from an innate difficulty in comprehending people's emotional signals, whereas Leslie and Happé (1989) believe that difficulties in triadic interactions stem from difficulties in processing more than one signal at a time, which is necessary for successful triadic interaction. As intentional communication implies the comprehension of people as agents who can act upon an object or event in the environment, in a predetermined manner, triadic interaction is intrinsic for intentional communication. Consequently, intentional communication may be a particularly salient construct in the study of autism as it cosigns communication, social interrelatedness, and cognitive processing of the social and nonsocial environment.

PURPOSE OF THE CURRENT STUDY: IMPORTANCE OF SYSTEMATIC PROCEDURES

The current study was designed to describe and characterize communicative acts, designated as intentional, in young children with autism. These communicative behaviors between young children with autism and adults were observed systematically, during semistructured, interactive activities, which encourage communication. The first purpose of this research was to formulate a short battery of activities that would encourage intentional communicative behavior in young children with autism. These activities which were to occur in a social context would be nonthreatening, enjoyable exercises, which could be used when first meeting a young child with a suspicion of autism or related communication deficits. Wetherby (1986) proposed a similar protocol for screening young children with a possible communication disorder. This diagnostic clarity is equally important after establishing a diagnosis of autism, for many intra-individual differences exist among the individuals with this diagnosis. To assess the intentionality of communicative behavior, we developed a series of eight semistructured activities in which to observe and code behavior designated as intentional, which were coded according to communicative function, expressive means, and the use of gaze.

Describing communicative and social anomalies associated with autism based upon data obtained from direct behavioral observation, such as suggested here, is accepted practice (Lord, Rutter, & diLavore, personal communication, 1998; Schopler, Reichler, & Renner, 1988; Stone & Caro-Martinez, 1990; Tardif, Plumet, Beaudichon, Waller, Bouvard, & Leboyer, 1995; Volkmar & Klin, 1994). Behavioral descriptions obtained through direct observation are analyzed according to two methodologies. One methodology codes unitary behaviors on a behavioral grid, on a second-by-second basis (Buitelaar, van Engeland, deKogel, deVries & van Hoof, 1991; van Engeland et al., 1985). This approach is limited, however, in that coding systems differs with regard to which behaviors are included in the behavioral coding grids. The descriptions mostly focus on the behavior of the child with autism and pay less attention to the partner's behavior. A second methodology has a more global approach, wherein social behavior in fairly complex and large units is coded, according to predefined, coding categories, devised by the experimenter. These categories examine behaviors according to the specific questions raised by the research. For example, McHale, Simeonsson, Marcus, and Olley (1980) coded the symbolic and social levels of interactive behaviors, comparing situations involving the presence or absence of an adult. Mundy, Sigman, Ungerer, and Sherman (1986, 1987) devised hierarchical scales of social behavior in the areas of social interaction, joint attention, and behavioral regulation. Each coded item was delineated according to a predefined combination of the child and partner's behavior (e.g., gazes, gestures). In other studies, observed interactions between children with autism and their mothers were coded qualitatively, focusing on such measures as level of involvement (Dawson et al., 1991; Howlin & Rutter, 1989). We adopted the second methodology, as our classifications were globally defined and based on the results of previous research, which identified function, means, and use of gaze as particularly salient elements in intentional communication.

The quality of communicative interactions between children with autism and a partner have been found to be affected by the amount of structure, the type of partner, and the type of activity. Children with autism manifest more interactive behaviors in structured situations than in unstructured situations (Clark & Rutter, 1981). Their behaviors are also less stereotyped when they are with adults than when they are with other children with autism (McHale et al., 1980). A familiar, nonautistic, adult partner appears to be the most conducive partner for establishing rich interactions. Objects seem to facilitate interactions by serving as exchange mediators (Charman, Swetenhan, Baron-Cohen, Cox, Baird, & Drew, 1997; Tiegerman & Primavera, 1981). Because the quality of the communicative exchanges of children with autism and their partners is influenced by these parameters, the activities we chose to include in the battery involved objects, actions, and routines, some familiar and some unfamiliar. The eight interactive communicative activities consist of a free play period, a peek-a-boo game, requesting candy after it was placed in a visible but unobtainable place, balloon play, reading a familiar book, attempting to activate a broken remote control car, responding to recorded laughter, and reaction to a laser beam close to the child.

PARTICIPANTS

The participants included 30 children with a diagnosis of autism, aged 3 to 5 years, the age when diagnosis of autism can be reliably ascertained. Inclusion criteria included minimum score on the communication domain of the Vineland Adaptive Behavior Scales (VABS: Sparrow, Balla, & Cicchetti, 1984) of 9 months, the age at which intentional communication begins to emerge in typically developing children and a minimum overall composite score on the VABS of 18 months, the age at which communicative, social, and cognitive abilities develop. An autism diagnosis was established by meeting the criteria of autism on the Autism Diagnostic Interview-Revised (ADI-R: Lord, Rutter, & LeCouteur, 1994) and the Childhood Autism Rating Scale (CARS; Schopler et al., 1988). All children were Israeli born and native Hebrew speakers, living with their biological parents.

The children were referred from child development centers and early childhood, special education programs throughout Israel. After referral, contact with parents was established to explain the research. One parent was interviewed using the ADI-R and the Vineland. The child was evaluated during approximately two sessions, which included the use of the eight interactive situations, which were videotaped for validation of the instrument. The administration of various diagnostic, psychological, adaptive, and language measures was also accomplished during the two sessions with the child, according to each child's level of abilities and attention span.

QUANTITATIVE ASPECTS OF COMMUNICATIVE INTENT

The examiner spent up to 2 hours interacting with each child. This allowed the children to familiarize themselves with the examiner prior to their interaction in the eight experimental situations. Each interaction was videotaped and then coded for communicative intents. In addition to coding the overall number of overtures made by each child in each situation, the means of expression (motor response, vocalization, gesture, or word), the function (requesting/refusing or commenting/sharing), and the direction of gaze (undirected, to object, to person, alternating) were coded. The overall number of communicative intents that were expressed in each situation as well as the number of children who expressed themselves intentionally in each situation are presented in Table 9-1.

The attempt to reactivate a remote control car, which had previously worked and then did not, and requesting food that was placed on a high shelf, encouraged the most overtures. The children's interest was caught and their expectations were not met in both situations. First, the batteries were removed from the car when the children were otherwise occupied and they did not see their removal, so they expected the car to move when they activated it. Similarly, after enjoying eating the food, the child was usually still interested in it, although

TABLE 9-1. Distribution of Number of Communicative Overtures and Number of Children Expressing Themselves in Each Situation

Situations	Number of children ($n = 30$)	Number of intents
Warm up play	27	156
Peek-a-boo	23	84
Unobtainable food	29	164
Balloon play	25	118
Reading a book	23	138
Activating broken remote car	29	171
Hearing recorded laughter	13	17
Seeing beamed laser light	18	38

the examiner placed it out of reach. In this situation, the child actually followed the examiner's actions when she placed the food on the shelf. In contrast, the audio recording of laughter stimulated the least number of communicative responses from the smallest number of children. Likewise, there were fewer responses from fewer children in response to beaming a laser light on the table where the child was sitting. The children were not directly engaged during these two situations, but rather responded to stimulation. As Howlin and Rutter (1989) noted activities involving physical contact trigger the most responses from children with autism. In the car activity, the children activated the car themselves while in the laser activity they did not even see the source of the light beam. It is also possible that laughter does not stimulate the same response in children with autism than in typically developing children because of issues with reading and understanding expressions of emotions (Hobson, 1993).

QUALITATIVE ASPECTS OF COMMUNICATIVE INTENT

Before discussing the significance of communicative intent for the study of autism, it is important to emphasize that the results presented here portray a very small sample of 30 young children with autism and represent only a preliminary attempt to understand and treat communication and social limitations manifest in autism. Despite the small number of participants, our findings supported previously reported results, with the children in this study expressing communicative intent with relative high frequency, despite their diagnosis of autism. Intentional communication, which requires the awareness of people as agents of change, was investigated as a possible construct through which autism can be better understood.

The operational definition of communicative intent involves three basic elements: means, function and use of gaze. First, the function or purpose of the communicative overture were assessed. In our sample, both imperative (requests/protests) and declarative (sharing/commenting) intentions were recorded, but the communication of nonverbal children was limited to requests/protests only. Declarative functions, such as sharing and commenting, depend on reciprocity, which is impaired in children with autism (Rutter, 1984). It is even possible that some of their "commenting," assumed to be declarative, may actually fulfill imperative functions, as children with autism often express themselves indirectly (Tager-Flusberg & Sullivan, 1994). For example, when a child said, "The candy is up high," he may not have been commenting on the placement of the candy, but rather he may have been requesting that we get it for him.

The method by which children expressed their intentions was coded according to the following generally hierarchical categories of increasing complexity: motor responses, vocalizations, gestures, and words (Watson et al., 1989). Prizant and Schuler (1987) postulated that when typically developing children reach a more complex means of communication, the complex expressions supersede the primitive means of expression and more primitive levels are no longer used. In our sample, words, the most complex means of communication, surpassed other more basic means of expressing communicative intent. However, only one child used words exclusively to communicate intent; all the other children continued to communicate using words accompanied by other more primitive, less complex means (motor behavior, gestures, and vocalizations). Words were used in combination with other forms as if the children were not sure of the efficacy of passing on a message through words alone. Perhaps children with autism do not realize that if one word does not sufficiently express their intentions, an alternative word can be substituted; rather, they return to more developmentally immature, less complex methods of communication. Normally, when children adopt a manner of communication, they use that method in parallel contexts, which did not occur in our sample. However, in our sample, the children used different means of communication in the eight different situations, without establishing a set mode of expression. This phenomenon may be explained by the findings of Jarrold, Boucher, and Smith (1996) that children have difficulty generalizing from one context to another or by Sigman's (1997) finding that children with autism have inherent deficits in symbolic representation. An additional explanation for the specificity of the means used by children with autism to express their intentions communicatively that takes into account the problems in generalizations and in symbolic representations involves the general inflexibility, which characterizes so many children with autism. It is possible that expressions of general inflexibility in understanding and dealing with the world may also manifest themselves in expressions of pragmatic and semantic intention.

The third element of intentional behavior in communication that was investigated in this research was direction of gaze. Gaze is one of the factors that helps determine intentionality in typically developing children. Because impairments in the use of gaze (Baron-Cohen, Baldwin, & Crowson, 1997; Hobson, 1993) have been documented in autism, it was particularly difficult for us to code the use of gaze during the interactions. Some overtures from our sample were coded as intentional, despite the absence of accompanying gaze, usually because the children persisted until the goal was achieved. Use of gaze in communicative exchanges is distinguished from the purpose and the means of the communicative overture in that it is dependent on the social context, independent of the purpose for communicating and the chosen method of communication. Gaze deals with the referent involved in the communicative interchange.

While children with autism may fail to gaze alternatively at the partner with whom they are interacting and at the desired objects (i.e., joint attention), their communicative behavior may be judged as intentional when behaviors, such as persistence, associated with intention are observed. Deficits in joint attention are most notable in young children with autism (Lewy & Dawson, 1992; Mundy et al., 1994). Before any true verbal language exists, children with typical development use their gaze as a means of sharing their affective experiences, which becomes the social context of communication with another person. Because children with autism lack crucial joint attention skills, their ability to engage others and forge social and communicative relations is greatly diminished.

SUMMARY

After discussing the definition of communicative intent and the importance of its qualitative analysis, it is our hope that the developmental construct of communicative intent will contribute to the understanding of autism and will enhance our ability to identify and meet the needs of children with autism. The use of semistructured situations for the assessment of communicative intent is a significant contribution of this research, because previously semistructured assessments have been employed for basically diagnostic purposes. For example, both the Autism Diagnostic Observation Schedule (ADOS: Lord, Rutter, DiLavore, & Risi, 2001) and the Childhood Autism Rating Scale (CARS: Schopler et al., 1988) result in a diagnostic decision, based on methodical observation and interaction with children. The eight semistructured play situations presented here can be employed to achieve three distinct but related objectives. First, the examiner can use these activities to establish an initial relationship with the child, based on interacting with the child, at his or her own pace, according to his or her own interests. These pleasant and nonthreatening interactions allow the examiner to focus on the child, and not on whether the child passes or fails a particular item. Second, the examiner can use these activities to obtain a communication sample in a systematic manner, focusing on identifying those situations in which the child initiates communication. This type of communicative sample can be a base for subsequent intervention programming. By analyzing the purposes for which the child initiates the contact, the manner in which the communicative overture is expressed, and how gaze is incorporated in the interaction, critical information about incentives for communicative contact of an individual child is obtained. Third, the use of a defined set of interactions, which has been designed to encourage communicative interactions, can serve as a technique for evaluating changes resulting from intervention programs. The instrument presented here can serve as an evaluative marker, by obtaining a communicative sample before an intervention procedure that can be compared to one obtained subsequent to the intervention.

POSSIBLE SUBTYPING ACCORDING TO COMMUNICATIVE INTENT

Communicative intent has emerged as a pivotal issue in the study of autism. In addition to having implications for intervention, communicative intent may provide a standard of reference from which children with autism can be differentiated from one another. Because of the variability among individuals with autism, several systems of grouping children with autism into subcategories have been found to be useful in service provision (Wing & Attwood, 1987). Typologies have been suggested based on aspects of the triad of impairments associated with the autistic spectrum. Wing and Gould (1979) suggested that the social impairment should be at the base of a system of subclassification, and proposed dividing individuals with autism into three types: aloof, passive, and active but odd. They claim that each group tends to be associated with particular clinical pictures and with specific intervention priorities and needs. Those who support classifying on the basis of intellectual function feel that high functioning individuals with autism have different educational and social needs than low functioning individuals with autism (e.g., Tsai, 1992). Indeed, supporting the salience of these two systems of classification, Prior et al. (1998) found that differences in children with autism were explained by the degrees of social and cognitive impairments. Diagnosing autism with the Childhood Autism Rating Scale (Schopler et al., 1988) results in a rating of severity of autism, classifying individuals as having mild to moderate autism or severe autism. Proponents of subclassifying on the basis of severity of symptoms maintain that the supports and intervention these two groups need vary according to the behavioral impairment, although treatment is based on the same intervention principles. We propose that communicative intent may be a particularly salient construct for subclassifying individuals with autism, as it lies at the interface of language and social and cognitive development, the identified areas of impairments in autism. It is clear that these impairments have significant impact on communicative behavior itself, as well as the manner in which communication affects social functioning. Intervention can be individualized, based on profiles of intentional communication. While the existence of discrete groupings of individuals with autism according to their communicative and intentional abilities has not been established, we feel that the grouping of individuals with autism in this fashion may provide a useful framework for conceptualizing communication in individuals with autism.

IMPLICATIONS FOR INTERVENTION

These interactive activities result in a profile of communicative intent, which can be helpful in deciding on intervention strategies, based on the child's strengths and interests. In addition, the interpretation of the communicative profile can help set up priorities for intervention. First, a comprehensive understanding of the particular child's communicative abilities and efforts is attained, thus providing the baseline for appropriate, individualized intervention goals. The child's range of communicative intentions should be considered when setting treatment goals. Enhancement must begin at the child's present level of communication. Identifying the purposes for which a child communicates may provide the transitional links to other communicative functions. By underscoring pragmatic intent, children with autism are reminded that communication is a powerful tool through which it is possible to influence the world around them. For example, if behavior regulation already appears in a child's communicative profile, once gains in behavior regulation are made, greater emphasis can then be placed on communicating for more social purposes, such as sharing.

According to Fogel (1993), social communication is best understood as a process of co-regulation based on continuous adaptation to both the present and the anticipated behavior of another person. Thus, communication is only partly planned and is an open process subject to modification and adaptation. Such joint processes, which are dependent on the understanding of intention and social causality, are particularly challenging for children with autism, who often rely on routines and structure to understand and communicate in social situations.

The importance of providing systematic settings in which children with autism interact and communicate cannot be minimized. The influence on a skill exerted by the context in which communication occurs has profound implications for potential behavioral change. Numerous intervention studies have demonstrated that providing opportunities to initiate communication and then responding contingently results in meaningful gains in eye gaze and communicative behavior (Dawson & Adams, 1984; Klinger & Dawson, 1992; Mirenda & Donnellan, 1986; Peck, 1985). Similarly, Stone and Caro-Martinez (1990) report that in "ritualized" contexts, such as turn taking activities, children with autism reveal more social commenting behavior than in other contexts. By identifying the behavioral characteristics related to communicative intent and analyzing each behavior as it occurs, it may be possible to target environments in which specific behaviors occur and thus induce their occurrence. This approach, which is based on profiles of communicative intent, can aid in motivating children to respond to social and environmental stimulation, by building on existing skills, by identifying referents, and by generalizing between familiar and novel situations. Although it is only one piece of the very complex clinical picture in autism, communicative intent involves overlapping areas of development. As such, it promises to offer important prospects for the understanding and treatment of autism.

REFERENCES

American Psychiatric Association. (1994). *Diagnostic and statistical manual of mental disorders, (DSM-IV)*, 4th edit. Washington DC: American Psychiatric Association.

Bakerman, R., & Adamson, L. B. (1984). Coordinating attention to people and objects in mother–infant and peer–infant interaction. *Child Development, 55*, 1278–1289.

Baron-Cohen, S., Baldwin, D. A., & Crowson, M. (1997). Do children with autism use the speaker's direction of gaze strategy to crack the code of language? *Child Development, 68*, 48–57.

Bates, E. (1979). *The Emergence of Symbols*. New York: Academic Press.

Becker, J. (1994). Pragmatic socialization: Parental input to preschoolers. *Discourse Processes, 17*, 131–148.

Bretherton, I., & Bates, E. (1979). The emergence of intentional communication. *New Directions for Child Development, 4*, 81–100.

Buitelaar, J. K., van Engelander, H., deKogel, K., deVries, H., & van Hoof (1991). Differences in the structure of social behavior of autistic children and non-autistic retarded controls. *Journal of Child Psychology and Psychiatry, 32*, 995–1015.

Camaioni, L. (1993). The development of intentional communication—A reanalysis. In: J. Nadel & L. Camaioni (Eds.), *New Perspectives in Early Communicative Development* (pp. 82–96). London: Routledge.

Carpenter, M., Nagell, K., & Tomasello, M. (1998). Social cognition, joint attention, and communicative competence from 9 to 15 months of age. *Monographs of the Society for Research in Child Development, 63*.

Charman, T., Swettenham, J., Baron-Cohen, S., Cox, A., Baird, G., & Drew, A. (1997). Infants with autism: An investigation of empathy, pretend play, joint attention and imitation. *Developmental Psychology, 33*, 781–789.

Churchill, D. (1972). The relation of infantile autism and early childhood schizophrenia to developmental language disorders of childhood. *Journal of Autism and Childhood Schizophrenia, 2*, 182–197.

Clark, P., & Rutter, M. (1981). Autistic children's responses to structure and to interpersonal demands. *Journal of Autism and Developmental Disorders, 11*, 201–217.

Coggins, T. E., & Carpenter, R. L. (1981). The communicative intention inventory: A system for observing and coding children's early intentional communication. *Applied Psycholinguistics, 2*, 235–251.

Curcio, F. (1978). Sensorimotor functioning and communication in mute autistic children. *Journal of Autism and Childhood Schizophrenia, 8*, 281–292.

Dawson, G., & Adams, A. (1984). Imitation and social responsiveness in autistic children. *Journal of Abnormal Child Psychology, 12*, 209–225.

Dawson, G., Hill, D., Spencer, A., Galpert, L., & Watson, L. (1991). Affective exchanges between young autistic children and their mothers. *Journal of Abnormal Child Psychology, 19*, 115.

Fogel, A. (1993). *Developing Through Relationships*. Chicago: The University of Chicago Press.

Goodman, R. (1989). Infantile autism: A syndrome of multiple primary deficits? *Journal of Autism and Developmental Disorders, 19*, 409–424.

Harding, C. G., Stilson, S. R., Kromelow, S., & Weissmann, L. (1997). Shared minds: How mothers and infants co-construct early patterns of choice within intentional communication partnerships. *Infant Mental Health Journal, 18*, 24–39.

Hermelin, B., & O'Connor, N. (1985). The logico-affective disorder in autism. In E. Schopler & G. B. Mesibov (Eds.), *Communication Problems in Autism*. New York: Plenum.

Hobson, P. R. (1993). *Autism and the development of mind*. Trowbridge: Erlbaum.

Holdgrafer, G. E., & Durst, C. (1990). Use of low structured observation for assessing communicative intent in young children. *First Language, 10*, 103–124.

Howlin, P., & Rutter, M. (1989). Mothers' speech to autistic children: A preliminary causal analysis. *Journal of Child Psychology and Psychiatry, 30*, 819–843.

Jarrold, C., Boucher, J., & Smith, P. K. (1996). Generativity deficits in pretend play in autism. *British Journal of Developmental Psychological Society, 14,* 275–300.

Klinger, L., & Dawson, G. (1992). Facilitating early social and communicative development in children with autism. In S. F. Warren (Ed.), *Causes and Effects in Communication and Language Intervention* (pp. 157–186). Baltimore, MD: Paul Brookes.

Leslie, A., & Happé, F. (1989). Autism and ostensive communication: The relevance of metarepresentation. *Development and Psychopathology. 1,* 205–212.

Lewy, A., & Dawson, G. (1992). Social stimulation and joint attention in young autistic children. *Journal of Abnormal Child Psychology, 20,* 555–566.

Lord, C., Rutter, M., DiLavore, P., & Risi, S. (2001). Autism Diagnostic Observation Schedule. Los Angeles: Western Psychological Services.

Lord, C., Rutter, M., & LeCouteur, A. (1994). Autism diagnostic interview-revised: A revised version of a diagnostic interview for caregivers of individuals with possible pervasive developmental disorders. *Journal of Autism and Developmental Disorders, 24,* 659–685.

McHale, M., Simeonsson, R., Marcus, L., & Olley, J. G. (1980). The social and symbolic quality of autistic children's communication. *Journal of Autism and Developmental Disorders, 10,* 299–310.

Meltzoff, A. N. (1995). Understanding the intentions of others: Re-enactment of intended acts by 18-month-old children. *Developmental Psychology, 31,* 838–850.

Mirenda, P., & Donnellan, A. (1986). Effects of adult interaction style on conversational behavior in students with severe communication problems. *Language, Speech and Hearing Services in Schools, 17,* 126–141.

Mundy, P., Sigman, M., & Kasari, C. (1994). Joint attention, developmental level, and symptom presentation in autism. *Development and Psychopathology, 6,* 394–401.

Mundy, P., Sigman, M., Ungerer, J., & Sherman, T. (1986). Defining the social deficits of autism: The contribution of non-verbal communication measures. *Journal of Child Psychology and Psychiatry, 27,* 657–669.

Mundy, P., Sigman, M., Ungerer, J., & Sherman, T. (1987). Nonverbal communication and play correlates of language development in autistic children. *Journal of Autism and Developmental Disorders, 17,* 349–364.

Nagel, J., & Fontaine, A. (1989). Communicating by imitation: A developmental and comparative approach to transitory social competence. In B. H. Schneider (Ed.), *Social Competence in Developmental Perspective.* (pp. 131–144). Dordrecht, Netherlands: Kluwer.

Paul, R., & Shiffer, M. (1991). Communicative initiations in normal and late-talking toddlers. *Applied Psycholinguistics, 12,* 419–431.

Peck, C. (1985). Increasing opportunities for social control by children with autism and severe handicaps: Effects on student behavior and perceived classroom climate. *Journal of the Association for Persons with Severe Handicaps, 10,* 183–193.

Phillips, W., Baron-Cohen, S., & Rutter, M. (1992). The role of eye contact in goal detection: Evidence from normal infants and children with autism or mental handicap. *Development and Psychopathology, 4,* 375–383.

Prior, M., Eisenmajer, R., Leekam, S., Wing, L., Gould, J., Ong, B., & Dowe, D. (1998). Are there subgroups within the autistic spectrum? A cluster analysis of a group of children with autistic spectrum disorders. *Journal of Child Psychology and Psychiatry, 39,* 893–902.

Prizant, B. M. (1984). Assessment and intervention of communicative problems in children with autism. *Communicative Disorders, 9,* 127–142.

Prizant, B. M., & Schuler, A. (1997). Facilitating communication: Language approaches. In D. J. Cohen & A. M. Donnellan, (Eds.), *Handbook of Autism and Developmental Disorders.* (pp. 316–332). New York: John Wiley & Sons.

Prizant, B., & Wetherby, A. (1987). Communicative intent: A framework for understanding social-communicative behavior in autism. *Journal of the American Academy of Child and Adolescent Psychiatry, 26*(4), 472–479.

Ricks, D. M., & Wing, L. (1975). Language, communication, and the use of symbols in normal and autistic children. *Journal of Autism and Childhood Schizophrenia, 5,* 191–220.

Rutter, M. (1984). Cognitive deficits in the pathogenesis of autism. *Annual Progress in Child Psychiatry and Child Development,* 321–345.

Schopler, E., Reichler, R. J., & Renner, B. R. (1988). *The Childhood Autism Rating Scale (CARS) for Diagnostic Screening and Classification of Autism.* New York: Irvington Press.

Seibert, J. M., Hogan, A. E., & Mundy, P. C. (1982). Assessing interactional competencies: The early social-communication scales. *Infant Mental Health Journal, 3,* 244–258.

Seibert, J. M., & Oller, D. K. (1981). Linguistic pragmatics and language intervention strategies. *Journal of Autism and Developmental Disorders, 11,* 75–88.

Sigman, M. (1997). *Children with Autism: A Developmental Perspective.* Cambridge, MA: Harvard University Press.

Sparrow, S., Balla, D., & Cicchetti, D. V. (1984). *Vineland Adaptive Behavior Scales.* Circle Pines, MN: American Guidance Service.

Stone, W., & Caro-Martinez, L. (1990). Naturalistic observations of spontaneous communication in autistic children. *Journal of Autism and Developmental Disorders, 20,* 437-453.

Tager-Flusberg, H., & Sullivan, K. (1994). A second look at second order belief attribution in autism. *Applied Psycholinguistics, 16,* 241–256.

Tardif, C., Plument, M. H., Beaudichon, J., Waller, D., Bouvard, M., & Leboyer, M. (1995). Micro-analysis of social interactions between autistic children and normal adults in semi-structured play situation. *International Journal of Behavioral Development, 18,* 727–747.

Thal, D., Bates, E., Goodman, J., & Jahn-Samilo, J. (1997). Continuity of language abilities: An exploratory study of late and early talking toddlers. *Developmental Neuropsychology, 13,* 239–273.

Tiegerman, E., & Primavera, L. (1981). Object manipulation: An interactional strategy with autistic children. *Journal of Autism and Developmental Disorders, 11,* 27–38.

Tsai, L. (1992). Diagnostic issues of high functioning autism. In: E. Schopler & G. Mesibov (Eds.), *High Functioning Individuals with Autism,* (pp. 11–40). New York: Plenum.

van Engeland, H., Bodnar, F. A., & Bolhuis, G. (1986). Some qualitative aspects of the social behavior of autistic children: An ethological approach. *Journal of Child Psychology and Psychiatry, 26,* 879–893.

Volkmar, F., & Klin, A. (1994). Social development in autism: Historical and clinical perspectives. In S. Baron-Cohen, H. Tager-Flusberg, & D. J. Cohen (Eds.), *Understanding Other Minds—Perspectives from Autism.* (pp. 40–55). New York: Oxford University Press.

Watson, L., Lord, C., Schaffer, B., & Schopler, E. (1989). *Teaching Spontaneous Communication to Autistic and Developmentally Handicapped Children.* New York: Irvington.

Wetherby, A. (1986). Ontogeny of communicative functions in autism. *Journal of Autism and Developmental Disorders, 16,* 295–316.

Wetherby, A., Cain, D. H., Yonclas, D. G., & Walker, V. G. (1988) Analysis of intentional communication of normal children from the prelinguistic to the multiword stage. *Journal of Speech and Hearing Research, 31,* 240–252.

Wing, L. (1996). *The Autistic Spectrum.* London: Constable.

Wing, L., & Attwood, A. (1987). Syndromes of autism and atypical development. In D. J. Cohen & A. M. Donnellan (Eds.), *Handbook of Autism and Pervasive Developmental Disorders* (pp. 3–19). New York: John Wiley & Sons.

Wing, L., & Gould, J. (1979). Severe impairments of social interaction and associated abnormalities in children: Epidemiology and classification. *Journal of Autism and Developmental Disorders, 9,* 11–29.

Zeedyk, M. S. (1996). Developmental accounts of intentionality: Toward integration. *Developmental Review, 16,* 416–461.

10

Issues in Early Comprehension Development of Children with Autism

Linda R. Watson

The diagnostic criteria for autism (e.g., American Psychiatric Association, 1994) include qualitative impairments in communication. The specific diagnostic features, however, are described in terms of impairments of expressive communication, both verbal and nonverbal. Although not a criterial diagnostic feature, impairments in the *comprehension* of nonverbal and verbal communication are universally associated with autism. Evidence suggests that individuals with autism comprehend language more poorly than their peers with specific language impairments or cognitive impairment not associated with autism, even after matching on mental age (Fein et al., 1996; Paul & Cohen, 1984).

Although there has been considerable research on language comprehension in typically developing children, we continue to lack a comprehensive theoretical model to account for the development of language comprehension skills. Nevertheless, for the purposes of this chapter, we will juxtapose several areas of development and processing that are generally accepted as having importance for the development of language comprehension. First, the ability to comprehend spoken language entails an ability to appropriately perceive, discriminate, and categorize the sounds of the particular language being heard, as well as the intonational patterns that carry meaning in the language. Second, comprehension of language requires an ability to understand that it is part of a communicative process through which people can share ideas and emotions, and attempt to impact the behavior of communicative partners. Third, language comprehension entails symbolic processing abilities that enable a person to relate spoken words to the objects, action, people, and ideas they represent. The identification of these three components of language comprehension is not offered here as a complete account of the processes involved in language comprehension, but rather these areas are regarded as essential components that have special relevance for

LINDA R. WATSON • Division of Speech and Hearing, University of North Carolina at Chapel Hill, Chapel Hill, North Carolina 27599-7190.

The Research Basis for Autism Intervention, edited by Schopler, Yirmiya, Shulman, and Marcus. Kluwer Academic/Plenum Publishers, New York, 2001.

considering how language comprehension may develop during the first 24 months in typically developing children, and why language comprehension may be so problematic for children with autism.

There has been limited attention in research to comprehension of language by individuals with autism. Lord (1985) provided a detailed review of the literature 15 years ago, and there have been few studies since that time that have explicitly examined the development of language comprehension in this population (see Lord & Paul, 1997 for a recent review). There has been, on the other hand, considerable research examining some of the nonverbal interactive behaviors that may help us understand the developmental origins or nature of these comprehension impairments. This chapter examines literature related to the normal development of communicative comprehension during the first 2 years of life and the available literature on young children with autism. The premise of this chapter is that many of the foundational abilities and interactions leading to the development of comprehension in other children are the very areas in which children with autism show their earliest impairments. Intervention aimed at producing dramatic improvements in functional outcomes for individuals with autism needs to address the foundations of comprehension early and intensively. The three major areas we consider correspond to the components of language comprehension identified in the preceding paragraph, and are considered under the topics of speech perception, construction of meaning in social interactions, and symbol formation.

SPEECH PERCEPTION IN INFANTS

Newborns show remarkable abilities in speech perception that appear to be well adapted to acquiring language (Jusczyk, 1997; Kuhl, 1998). They are able to perceive speech sounds categorically and to discriminate between different consonant sounds. In the newborn period, the perceptual boundaries for speech sounds are the same across infants born into different language environments. Kuhl proposes that the infant's initial discrimination of speech sound boundaries is based on innate auditory processing mechanisms demonstrated to be shared by nonhuman animals. In addition to discriminating between speech sounds, neonates show preferences for listening to the mother's voice as opposed to other speakers, and also preferences for listening to the native language as opposed to a strongly contrasting nonnative language. These latter pieces of evidence indicate that even newborns have been influenced by their experiences of in utero exposure to their mother's voice and to the "mother tongue."

Kuhl (1998) describes a process through which, with development and exposure to the native language, speech perception is altered by "warping the underlying acoustic space" (p. 300). This results in an increase in infants' discrimination of speech sounds according to the categorical boundaries of the native language and a decrease in sensitivity to nonnative boundaries. Kuhl emphasizes that infants' speech representations involve not just auditory properties, but also visual and proprioceptive properties, and are thus "polymodal." The process of developing these perceptual maps results in the infant sharing perceptions with adults who are part of their culture. According to Kuhl, these shared perceptions assist not only in the later development of language, but also in the infant's understanding of others outside of the domain of language.

Recent research on infant speech perception has begun to tie infants' early abilities to the development of language comprehension. Some of the important developments include sensitivity to prosodic markers of syntactic units such as clauses and phrases at ages as young as 4½ months; sensitivity to the phonotactic constraints (i.e., constraints on allowable sequences of sounds) of the native language by 9 months; and an ability to segment word units from within a stream of fluent speech by 11 months (see Jusczyk, 1997).

SPEECH PERCEPTION IN AUTISM

It has long been recognized that a typical cognitive profile of individuals with autism shows relative strengths in visual–perceptual tasks and weaknesses in tasks requiring auditory–verbal processing (Rapin, 1994). This has led to the exploration of hypotheses that there are specific auditory and/or speech perception deficits in children with autism (e.g., Courchesne, 1987; Dawson, Finley, Phillips, & Lewy, 1989), which could account for or at least contribute to difficulties in language comprehension. There is currently no published research on the speech perception skills of young children with autism that is comparable to the aforementioned work with typically developing infants, although Kuhl (personal communication, September 6, 1999) is currently investigating speech processing in children with autism. The results of studies examining auditory brainstem responses (ABRs) have conflicted to some extent, but the weight of evidence suggests there are no differences in the ABRs of children with autism compared to comparison groups (Minshew, Sweeney, & Bauman, 1997), suggesting that subcortical differences in auditory processing are not present in most children with autism. In studies examining auditory evoked potentials (AEPs), there appear to be some differences in later waves, which presumably reflect a cortical level of participation in the processing of the auditory stimuli. It is not clear, however, how these differences correspond to psychological levels of organization. The differences may reflect problems with auditory processing at a general level, problems with speech sound processing specifically, or problems with more complex language processing that are exerting a downward effect on the speech processing. (See Minshew et al., 1997 for a review of this research.)

Several reports have suggested that young children with autism fail to attend to speech or fail to show the same attentional preferences as other children. For example, Klin (1991) found that whereas children developing typically and children with mental retardation preferred listening to their mother's voice over listening to the noise from a busy canteen, young children with autism either preferred the sounds of the busy canteen or showed no preference. Several retrospective videotape studies of young children later diagnosed with autism have indicated that these children differ from their peers with typical development or other developmental disabilities as early as 9 to 12 months of age in terms of more limited responses to the child's own name (e.g., Baranek, 1999; Osterling & Dawson, 1996).

Minshew et al. (1997) have presented cogent arguments against hypotheses positing domain-specific processing disorders in autism, and argued instead that there are deficits in complex information processing across domains. If neonatal speech sound discrimination abilities are based on general innate auditory processing mechanisms, then we could extrapolate the arguments of Minshew et al. (1997) to predict that children with autism would demonstrate the same universal speech processing abilities demonstrated by neonates. Further, if social interactive experiences play a role in the infant's development of shared perception with other members of the culture (Kuhl, 1998), and children with autism have deficits in their abilities to engage in these early social interactions, then we would predict that children with autism would be very slow in making the transition to culturally shared speech perception. It is therefore important to consider that speech differs from many other types of auditory stimuli in that it is social in nature. Recent work by Dawson and colleagues (Dawson, Meltzoff, Osterling, Rinaldi, & Brown, 1998) found that children with autism were less responsive to social than to nonsocial stimuli that included auditory components. Therefore, any speech perception difficulties in young children with autism may be attributable more to the social nature of speech stimuli than to their auditory nature. In a subsequent section, we examine the possibility that social impairments of children with autism affect their earliest experiences critical to language comprehension.

CONSTRUCTING MEANING IN SOCIAL INTERACTIONS

As mentioned earlier, there is no consensus on the developmental process through which infants who are typically developing come to understand the language and communicative acts of their culture. One theoretical perspective that seems especially applicable to the consideration of comprehension deficits in children with autism is that meaning is constructed in social interactions and mapped onto the linguistic symbols embedded in those social interactions (e.g., Nelson, 1985). Some would argue that this process of constructing meaning begins with the interactions between adults and very young infants during the period of what Trevarthan (1979) has called "primary intersubjectivity." Meltzoff and Moore (1998) point out that inferring intersubjectivity requires evidence that an infant takes "into account the *psychological* aspects of the other, not solely the physics of the other" (p. 48). Observations of young infants show that in face-to-face interactions, infants participate in affective exchanges involving facial gestures and vocalizations, long before the ability to derive meaning from the language symbols is present. Reddy and colleagues (Reddy, Hay, Murray, & Trevarthan, 1997) summarized research supporting the proposition that interactions in the early months of life reflect mutual regulation by the infant and caregiver rather than unilateral adjustments of the caregiver. By 6 to 8 weeks of age, infants demonstrate strategies for both initiating and avoiding interaction. Protoconversational turntaking, reflecting complementary affect and vocalizations, is also apparent by this age. These intersubjective interactions may help establish the infant's recognition that "language is special" in regulating the interactions between humans.

Meltzoff and others have investigated the imitation of infants during this period of primary intersubjectivity (see Meltzoff & Moore, 1998). There have now been numerous replications of the findings that even newborns demonstrate an ability to imitate such movements as tongue protrusion and mouth opening and closing. Meltzoff and Moore argued that this demonstrates some knowledge on the part of the infant as being "like" the other person, enabling the infant to replicate a movement that she or he can see but not feel by producing a movement she or he can feel but not see. Although the ability to imitate behaviors based on cross-modal perceptions is present from birth, the infant's knowledge of "self" and "other" is elaborated through further engagement in mutual imitation activities with caregivers. Neonatal imitation appears to be linked to later imitation by infants.

Research by Kugiumutzakis (1999) has indicated that the ability to imitate is stable in infants studied longitudinally through the first 6 months of life, although what the infant is most likely to imitate undergoes changes with age. In addition to changes in the content of the imitations, there are also changes in the rapidity and control with which an infant imitates, as seen in comparisons of neonatal imitation to the same movements imitated at 3 months of age (Heimann, 1998). Individual differences in neonatal imitation have been found to predict individual differences at 3 weeks and 3 months of age, but not at 12 months of age; however, imitation at 3 months of age is predictive of imitation at 12 months of age (Heimann, 1998).

From these dyadic interactions between the young infant and another person, infants progress to "secondary intersubjectivity" (Trevarthan & Hubley, 1978), in which there is a focus outside of the face-to-face interactions between infant and partner. The early emergence of an ability to share a joint focus of attention with another is seen in the infant's ability to follow the direction of gaze of another person. As described by Messer (1994), a typical developmental sequence would involve being able to follow a partner's gaze toward the correct side of the room at age 6 months, but with limited proficiency in locating the correct target; being able to localize the correct target even with distracters at the age of 12 months; and being able by 18 months to follow gaze directed at objects further away and separated by less distance from distracters, as well as learning to look behind oneself to locate a target when none are in the visual field in front of the infant.

Between 9 and 12 months, typically developing infants show an increasing awareness of the act of sharing another person's focus of attention, and will look from person to object back to person, or from object to person and back to object, thus participating in what have been called triadic interactions. A related phenomenon has been reported in studies of social referencing, in which infants of 8 to 12 months of age are observed to visually check a parent's reaction in ambiguous situations (such as the activation of a novel mechanical toy), and then to respond affectively to the situation in accordance with the parental affect (see Baldwin, 1995).

Triadic interactions can occur in conveying both protoimperative (behavior regulation, including requesting) and protodeclarative (joint attention) intents. By 12 months of age, many infants have begun to actively direct others' attention to objects or events by pointing for protodeclarative purposes. Mundy, Sigman, and Kasari (1993) have argued that this development of joint attention is one of the important early steps toward acquiring a "theory of mind" (Baron-Cohen, 1993). They suggest that joint attention behaviors may emerge out of the earlier dyadic affective interactions of the infant and caregiver, and that joint attention behaviors (in contrast to requesting behaviors) involve conveying an affective attitude toward the shared experience or object.

EARLY STRATEGIES FOR THE SOCIAL CONSTRUCTION OF MEANING

Chapman (1978) described the ways in which an infant of 8 to 12 months of age applies the array of the nonlinguistic developmental abilities described earlier to the task of responding to linguistic input. In other words, before the child has much ability to comprehend linguistic symbols, she or he uses these nonlinguistic skills to interpret linguistic messages. This implies that the infant has made considerable progress in understanding the communicative process that underlies the exchange of linguistic messages, and is an active participant in using cues from the environmental and social context to construct a possible meaning for those messages. Specifically, at 8 to 12 months, Chapman suggested that infants' nonlinguistic response strategies to linguistic input include the following:

- Look at objects the adult looks at.
- Act on objects noticed.
- Imitate ongoing action .

It is important to examine the evidence for the relationship between these proposed nonlinguistic response strategies and the development of language comprehension skills. There is accumulated evidence for a causal relationship between the use of a "follow-in" strategy in adult–child interaction and the child's early receptive vocabulary development (e.g., Ahktar, Dunham, & Dunham, 1991; Tomasello & Farrar, 1986). A "follow-in" strategy entails the adult observing the child's focus of attention and providing the linguistic input that relates to what the child is looking at or doing. For example, if the child's attention is attracted by an airplane flying overhead, the adult may say, "There's an airplane!" This suggests that even though children are developing their ability to follow another's gaze as early as 6 months on, they still benefit in the earliest stages of language acquisition from being able to map language onto their own current focus of attention, rather than having to follow an adult's line of regard to discover the visual and linguistic target. This type of interactive support from adults appears to be especially related to promoting the acquisition of object labels (see Akhtar & Tomasello, 1998). Baldwin (1995) has reviewed the literature on joint attention and the development of language comprehension, and concludes that typically developing children resist errors in mapping meaning onto symbols by the age of 18 months owing to their proficiency in attending to the speaker's direction of gaze. Prior to that, infants may rely more on the supportive scaffold provided when adults use a follow-in strategy in talking to children. On the other hand, there is also evidence that infants who are better early on at gaze-following will later demonstrate better vocabulary comprehension. Individual differences in gaze-following proficiency at 6 and 16 months of age have been found to correlate with receptive vocabulary at 12 and 20 months of age, respectively (Morales, Mundy & Rojas, 1998; Mundy, & Gomes, 1998).

Research has also demonstrated that imitation skills are related to the development of comprehension, although the exact nature of the relationship has not been established. Several studies have found a correlation between both vocal and gestural imitation and concurrent receptive language level for young, typically developing children as well as children in clinical groups (see Smith & Bryson, 1994).

DEFICITS IN EARLY SOCIAL CONSTRUCTION OF MEANING BY CHILDREN WITH AUTISM

If meaning is indeed constructed through the ontogenetic course of the early social interactions described above, the infant with autism comes to the task of learning communicative comprehension with considerable disadvantages. There has been almost no opportunity to date to directly study the intersubjective interactions of infants with autism below the age of 12 months. In retrospective reports, parents of children with autism have been more likely than parents of children with other developmental disabilities to report their child as "having an expressionless face" as an infant or toddler (Hoshino, Kumashiro, Yashima, Tachibana, Watanabe, & Furukawa, 1982), and retrospective videotape research has suggested a lack of social smiling in infants later diagnosed with autism (Adrien et al., 1993). Hobson (1993) has theorized that deficits in intersubjective processes are at the core of the deficits seen in children with autism, and his studies as well as others of older children with autism have confirmed difficulties with such skills as "reading" facial expressions, matching facial expressions to the appropriate verbally expressed messages, and comprehending emotion-laden words. There is also behavioral and physiological evidence that children with autism may be limited in their empathetic responses. Charman et al. (1997) demonstrated this with respect to 20-month-old children with autism, in terms of the likelihood of looking at and showing facial concern for an experimenter expressing distress. Similarly, Corona and colleagues (Corona, Dissanayake, Arbelle, Willington, & Sigman, 1998) found that 3- to 5-year-olds with autism were less likely to look at a distressed experimenter than children with mental retardation, and did not show increases in heart rate in response to another's distress as shown by the children with mental retardation.

If intersubjective deficits originate in infancy in children with autism, then there could be a wide-ranging cascade of effects on the development of comprehension skills. One impact may be a lack of learning that "language is special" in regulating human interactions. Suggestive evidence that young children with autism may lack such an awareness comes from a study by Lord (1995), who reported that 2-year-olds with autism differed from 2-year-olds with other developmental disabilities in their relative failure to attend to voice. Other evidence supporting this lack of attention to or preference for speech among children with autism was discussed in a previous section.

Motor imitation deficits have also been widely documented in children with autism (see Smith & Bryson, 1994; Stone, 1997 for reviews). We do not know how early imitation deficits are apparent in children with autism. Rogers and Pennington (1991) hypothesized that infants who later exhibit autism would not have the ability to engage in neonatal imitation owing to an innate impairment of this important social ability. Imitation deficits are evident in the youngest children with confirmed diagnoses of autism. Charman and colleagues (1997) have reported that 20-month-old children with autism show less proficiency in procedural imitation of actions on objects than children who are typically developing or those with other developmental delays. Results of work by Stone, Ousley, and Littleford (1997) with 2-year-olds with autism suggests that children with autism have the same developmental patterns as other children with respect to the order of difficulty of motor imitation, but that children with autism show less proficiency overall.

Moving from primary intersubjective interactions to secondary intersubjectivity, the accumulated evidence for deficits in young children with autism is especially strong. Children with autism have deficits in responding to bids for joint attention, such as following another person's gaze and/or point (Sigman & Kasari, 1995). In addition, young children with autism are less likely than children with other developmental disabilities to initiate joint attention through nonverbal communicative acts in which they are attempting to share attention/interest with another person. The same differences are not apparent in the use of requesting behaviors (see Mundy, 1995 for a review). Children with autism also rarely use social referencing (Sigman & Kasari, 1995).

Phillips and colleagues (Phillips, Gómez, Baron-Cohen, Laá, & Rivière, 1995) suggested that the critical element is not so much the communicative function involved, but rather the element of recognizing the other person as having attentional mental states separate from those of the child. They examined the strategies used by children with autism when confronted with a problem-solving task involving obtaining an out-of-reach object. Fewer than half of the children with autism used "person-as-perceiving-subject" strategies, compared to more than 80% of the children in the two control groups. These entailed any strategies through which the child attempted to enlist the adult's assistance to obtain the object *combined with* eye contact with the adult.

In contrast, Mundy et al. (1993) argued that joint attention behaviors are specifically impaired in children with autism relative to requesting behaviors owing to the importance of affective sharing in joint attention as well as the higher level representational skills involved in recognizing other persons as "agents of contemplation" rather than merely as "agents of action" (p. 188).

As pointed out by Lord (1985), the early nonlinguistic response strategies postulated to help typically developing infants interpret and respond to language messages (Chapman, 1978) are strategies that the child with autism is ill equipped to employ. Thus the child with autism may be quite disadvantaged in bootstrapping him/herself into linguistic comprehension via these nonlinguistic strategies.

One possibility is that the transactional effects of interacting with a child with autism might result in less optimal input from the child's caregivers. Using groups matched for children's language comprehension level, Watson (1998) compared the interaction of mothers with their preschool children with autism to that of mothers with their typically developing children. Results indicated that mothers of children with autism used "follow-in" strategies as frequently as did mothers of children developing typically. Thus, the young children with autism did not have fewer of these early, more optimal opportunities to map language onto the objects and events in their focus of attention.

On the other hand, there is evidence that children with autism are less proficient in using the strategy "look at objects the adult looks at." Leekam and colleagues (Leekam, Baron-Cohen, Perrett, Milders, & Brown, 1997; Leekam, Hunnisett, & Moore, 1998) demonstrated that children with autism were poor at spontaneously monitoring the gaze direction of a communicative partner, and unlike a comparison group of children with Down syndrome, they did not show an increase in spontaneous gaze monitoring with an increase in mental age. On a more encouraging note, improvements in performance in gaze monitoring occurred in response to more salient cues, such as the partner's body orientation, pointing, and possibly accompanying language (Leekam et al., 1998).

The examination of the relationship between the early nonlinguistic response strategies proposed by Chapman (1978) and comprehension in children with autism has not been widely studied. In a study of acquisition of receptive labels, Baron-Cohen, Baldwin, and Crowson (1997) found that children with autism were more likely than children with other developmental disabilities to make mapping errors. These errors occurred when the children with autism erroneously assigned a verbal label to an object at which they were looking when a speaker used the label, rather than to the object at which the speaker was looking. This study is consistent with the findings of longitudinal work by Sigman (1998), who reported a prospective correlation between joint attention skills in children with autism at 2 to 5 years and gains in language level 8 to 9 years later.

LATER STRATEGIES FOR CONSTRUCTING MEANING IN SOCIAL INTERACTIONS

Chapman (1978) summarized the ways in which children's response strategies to linguistic communication change in accordance with their increasing developmental sophistication. In the 12- to 18-month period, children are beginning to comprehend some words, particularly those labeling objects in the environment. Thus the first response strategy at 12 to 18 months involves the child using the comprehended object labels to guide his or her focus of attention. Chapman outlined the response strategies in this age range as follows:

- Attend to objects mentioned.
- Give evidence of notice.
- Do what you usually do with objects at hand (e.g., carry out an action routine with the object, or use it in a conventional way).

These strategies assume that the child has begun to successfully engage in some sound to symbol mapping, and also that the child has learned to use objects conventionally. As in the early response strategies, imitation skills are important at 12 to 18 months, although at this stage the infant's ability to engage in delayed imitation via mental images of the "usual" actions on objects is implicated.

According to Chapman (1978), response strategies at 18 to 24 months of age are very similar to ones of the previous 6 months, but now the child has an ability to comprehend words in the absence of the mentioned object, and will search for an object that is not present. Also, the child is developing a comprehension of other words in sentences, such as those describing actions. Thus, the strategies Chapman outlines at this stage are:

- Locate the objects mentioned.
- Do what you usually do.
- Act on objects in the way mentioned.

Children are still largely constrained to comprehension at the lexical level at this stage rather than understanding syntactical cues to meaning. They use contextual cues and their own past experiences to supplement their lexical comprehension, and assume that they themselves will be the agent of any mentioned action. For example, if a child at this age is instructed to "Make the alligator kiss the cow," a probable response is for the child to pick up the alligator and/or the cow and kiss it.

In their acquisition of lexical meaning, typically developing toddlers of 18 months of age are able to apply strategies for the acquisition of novel labels that do not entail having to observe a direct correspondence between the word and the referent (Akhtar & Tomasello, 1998). For instance, 18-month-olds are able to apply a novel label to an absent referent that has been previously associated with a specific location, but is not actually visible in the location when the child first hears the novel word (e.g., the experimenter says, "Now let's find the TOMA!" and tries unsuccessfully to open the barn in which an object has been habitually placed). In addition, 2-year-olds are able to associate a novel label with an object based on the target object being new to the discourse context for the adult providing the label, even when it is not new to the context for the child. This ability entails taking the psychological perspective of the other person into account.

CASCADING DEFICITS IN CONSTRUCTION OF MEANING BY CHILDREN WITH AUTISM

For the child with autism, using the nonlinguistic response strategies proposed by Chapman (1978) as important for 12- to 18-month-olds is initially hampered by the impairments in skills required for the earlier response strategies upon which these later strategies are founded. If the child's deficits in gaze monitoring have resulted in mapping errors, as suggested by Baron-Cohen et al. (1997), then at this stage the child with autism may apply the first strategy and attend to the wrong object. Even if the young child with autism succeeds with the first strategy and consequently attends to the same object as the communicative partner, she or he is likely to encounter problems with the second strategy, "Give evidence of notice." This strategy requires that the child engage in joint attention behaviors to communicate she or he is focusing on the object mentioned, a behavior young children with autism are unlikely to initiate (Mundy, 1995). The child with autism will also be likely to encounter difficulties with the third strategy, "Do what you usually do with objects at hand." For the child with autism, the usual action on a particular object may bear little relationship to the conventional use of the object, and therefore may not correspond well to the language used by the partner in talking about expected actions on the object. Mundy et al. (1993) have summarized evidence that children with autism at early developmental stages show deficits in functional play, which involves socially conventional use of objects, although Charman et al. (1997) did not confirm functional play deficits in their 20-month-old children with autism.

Chapman (1978) described children at 18 to 24 months as adding the strategy "Act on objects in the way mentioned." Bearing on this strategy, Menyuk and Quill (1985) hypothesized that children with autism have particular difficulty with the acquisition of relational words (including verbs) compared to their acquisition of concrete words (such as object labels). This hypothesis has not been thoroughly explored, although Watson and Fox (1988) found preliminary evidence supporting it. If this is the case, children with autism will be particularly delayed in their ability to "act on objects in the way mentioned" even after they develop the ability to "locate object mentioned."

SYMBOL FORMATION AND AUTISM

The emphasis in the previous sections has been on the possible social–cognitive foundations for the construction of meaning. It is possible, however, that the child with autism experiences problems in acquiring language comprehension owing to difficulties in symbol formation beyond the difficulties stemming from poor intersubjectivity, joint attention, and imitation. There is ample evidence and longstanding evidence that young children with autism are deficient in symbolic play skills in comparison to groups of children with developmental disabilities and typically developing children at similar mental age levels, and that symbolic play skills are correlated with children's language skills, including comprehension (e.g., Sigman & Ungerer, 1984; Ungerer & Sigman, 1981). In research with very young children, Charman et al. (1997) found that spontaneous symbolic play (object substitution) was uncommon among 20-month-old children with autism as well as among children with developmental delay; in contrast, more than half of the children in a typically developing control group engaged in these behaviors. It is more intriguing, however, to consider these findings in comparison to the results in a structured play task. With scaffolding (open-ended cues, specific suggestions, models of behavior), all the children with developmental delay produced play acts involving object substitution, but none of the children with autism did so. It is difficult to know, however, whether the symbolic deficits are a result of cascading effects of earlier social–cognitive deficits, or whether there is a specific additional difficulty with symbol formation that is not a direct outgrowth of the deficits in intersubjectivity, imitation, and joint attention.

Another possibility is that children with autism make different assumptions regarding the way meaning is mapped onto symbols. For instance, Messer (1997) proposed that in early linguistic mapping for typically developing children, there is a bias in favor of the "whole-object" assumption, that is, that a word refers to a whole object rather than to a part of the object. In the literature on individuals with autism, however, there are clinical descriptions and some research evidence pointing toward a tendency to attend to parts rather than to integrate the parts into a whole. Happé (1997) has described the problem as one of "weak central coherence." To the extent this model accounts for a cognitive style typical of children with autism, it implies that children with autism have mapping difficulties that involve nonsocial aspects of cognition as much as social–cognitive aspects. In a similar vein, Smith and Bryson (1994) hypothesized that the difficulties children with autism experience with both imitation and symbol formation result from nonsocial deficits in cross-modal integration of information. Cross-modal representation has been previously discussed both in reference to imitation skills (Meltzoff & Moore, 1998) and speech perception skills (Kuhl, 1998); thus, problems in this area could have implications for the foundations of comprehension emerging prior to symbol formation. At this point, however, there is limited research examining cross-modal integration in children with autism.

IMPLICATIONS FOR INTERVENTION

Current research does not support intervention to improve language comprehension skills in children with autism via bottom-up efforts to improve the speech perception skills. Nevertheless, there are therapy programs used with children with autism that are directed to improving auditory processing and/or speech perception, including auditory integration training (Rimland & Edelson, 1994), and more recently the Fast ForWord program (Tallal, Saunders, Miller, Jenkins, Protopapas, & Merzenich, 1997). The evidence to date regarding the efficacy of auditory integration training has been unconvincing (American Academy of Pediatrics, 1998). There are limited data available on Fast ForWord for children with autism. The development of the Fast ForWord program was based on research indicating that children with specific language impairment have difficulties in processing rapidly changing acoustic input, such as that characterizing the formant transitions from consonants to vowels in speech. In this program, children engage in computerized exercises that include work on discriminating speech sounds via graded changes in the formant transitions of synthetic speech stimuli. Research by Tallal et al. indicated that children in the autism spectrum made significant gains on standardized language measures (including comprehension) following participation in Fast ForWord. More research is needed on which children with autism may benefit from this program, and what aspects of the program may be beneficial for them.

In comparison to our relative lack of knowledge regarding speech perception skills of children with autism, there is substantial evidence that the posited social–cognitive foundations for the construction of meaning are early deficits of the disorder. To various degrees, there have been efforts to address these deficits in early intervention programs. In their review of early intervention programs for children with autism, Dawson and Osterling (1997) identify a number of common elements of successful programs. Two common curricular elements pertinent to the present discussion are a focus on improving attention to aspects of the environment essential for learning, *including attention to people*, and improving imitation skills. Klinger and Dawson (1992) and Rollins and colleagues (Rollins, Wambacq, Dowell, Mathews & Reese, 1998) have described strategies for promoting attention to other people, imitation, and joint attention in children with autism. To the extent that a model involving the construction of meaning in social interactions is a valid account, we can expect that successfully promoting these abilities in intervention programs for young children with autism will be associated with improvements in the comprehension of verbal and nonverbal communication.

In communication intervention programs for very young or very language-impaired children with autism, there is often an initial emphasis on improving functional communication skills through nonsymbolic means (e.g., Schuler, Prizant & Wetherby, 1997; Watson, Lord, Schaffer, & Schopler, 1989). In most cases, children progress to a point at which the emphasis shifts to facilitating symbolic communication. For children who do not readily verbalize, alternative symbolic systems are helpful, such as sign language or picture communication systems (Watson et al., 1989). Children with autism have demonstrated an ability to learn to use such symbols in communicating (e.g., Bondy & Frost, 1995; Bonvillian, Nelson, & Rhyne, 1981; Layton, 1988), and studies are also suggestive that learning to use these alternative symbol systems does not inhibit and may even facilitate the subsequent development of verbal communication. One early study addressed issues particularly pertinent to the issue of comprehension. Findings suggested that teaching the expressive use of signs prior to their receptive use facilitated learning the receptive use of the signs, but that teaching the receptive use of signs first interfered with learning expressive use (Watters, Wheeler, & Watters, 1981).

SUMMARY

Three components widely viewed as important in the development of language comprehension are speech perception skills, construction of meaning in social situations, and symbol formation. The premise of this chapter is that each of these areas is potentially important for explaining the language comprehension deficits of young children with autism and developing effective intervention strategies.

One severe limitation to our knowledge of whether and to what extent speech perception processes may affect the development of language comprehension in children with autism is the dearth of speech perception research with this population. Research examining speech perception skills in children with autism would have relevance for both theory (e.g., through determining whether deficits are exhibited at the level of "universal" auditory perceptions or only at the level of culturally shared perceptions, or neither) and for intervention planning.

In considering specifically the ontogeny of early comprehension development, a question posed by Nelson (1985) continues to be relevant: "Do words mean or do people mean?" As Nelson pointed out, language is understood on the basis of not only the meaning and organization of the words, but also on the broad context of the utterance. In studying the emergence of language comprehension of children with autism, there is a need to examine their experiences and ongoing adaptations in the social–communicative contexts in which linguistic messages are embedded prior to the time the child demonstrates an ability to comprehend the linguistic components of these messages. Thus, a second research need is for prospective, longitudinal research of prelinguistic children with or at risk for autism, to examine the various social–cognitive processes out of which comprehension may evolve, and the extent to which facilitating development of intersubjective exchanges, imitation, gaze-following, and joint attention impacts the development of language comprehension.

Symbol formation is clearly an essential component of language comprehension, and there is considerable evidence for deficits in the symbolic functioning of young children with autism in both the language and play domains. Several theoretical positions imply that problems in symbol formation may be attributable to deficits in autism that are not inherently social, such as weak central coherence or deficits in cross-modal integration. Research clarifying the processes and barriers to efficient symbol formation for young children with autism could have important implications for communication intervention planning. Whereas the current approaches to early language intervention for children with autism emphasize social approaches, it may be that symbol formation would facilitated more efficaciously with a combination of the types of social–communicative strategies discussed in the preceding and nonsocial strategies aimed at improving processes such as central coherence and cross-modal integration.

There is no consensus on an adequate theoretical account for the evolution of language comprehension in children developing typically. An improved understanding of the comprehension deficits in children with autism will undoubtedly benefit from the development and testing of models to account for typical development. On the other hand, the study of children with autism has the potential for contributing to such models as we define the specific deficits in children with autism and examine their impact on the emergence of comprehension skills.

REFERENCES

Adrien, J. L., Pascal, L., Martineau, J., Perrot, A., Hameury, L., Larmande, C., & Sauvage, D. (1993). Blind ratings of early symptoms of autism based upon family home movies. *Journal of the American Academy of Child and Adolescent Psychiatry*, *32*, 617–626.

Ahktar, N., Dunham, F., & Dunham, P. J. (1991). Directive interactions and early vocabulary development: The role of joint attentional focus. *Journal of Child Language*, *18*, 41–49.

Ahktar, N., & Tomasello, M. (1998). Intersubjectivity in early language learning and use. In S. Bråten (Ed.), *Intersubjective Communication and Emotion in Early Ontogeny* (pp. 316–335). Cambridge: Cambridge University Press.

American Academy of Pediatrics (1998). Auditory integration training and facilitated communication for autism. *Pediatrics, 102*, 431–433.

American Psychiatric Association (1994). *Diagnostic and Statistical Manual of Mental Disorders*, (4th ed.). Washington, DC: Author.

Baldwin, D. A. (1995). Understanding the link between joint attention and language. In C. Moore & P. J. Dunham (Eds.), *Joint Attention: Its Origins and Role in Development* (pp. 131–158). Hillsdale, NJ: Erlbaum.

Baranek, G. T. (1999). Autism during infancy: A retrospective video analysis of sensory-motor and social behaviors at 9–12 months of age. *Journal of Autism and Developmental Disorders, 29*, 213–224.

Baron-Cohen, S. (1993). From attention-goal psychology to belief-desire psychology: The development of a theory of mind and its dysfunction. In S. Baron-Cohen, H. Tager-Flusberg, & D. Cohen (Eds.), *Understanding Other Minds: Perspectives from Autism* (pp. 59–82). Oxford: Oxford University Press.

Baron-Cohen, S., Baldwin, D., & Crowson, M. (1997). Do children with autism use the speaker's direction of gaze strategy to crack the code of language? *Child Development, 68*, 48–57.

Bondy, A. S., & Frost, L. A. (1995). Educational approaches in preschool: Behavior techniques in a public school setting. In E. Schopler & G. B. Mesibov (Eds.), *Learning and Cognition in Autism* (pp. 311–333). New York: Plenum.

Bonvillian, J. D., Nelson, K. E., & Rhyne, J. M. (1981). Sign language and autism. *Journal of Autism and Developmental Disorders, 11*, 125–137.

Chapman, R. (1978). Comprehension strategies in children. In J. F. Kavanaugh & W. Strange (Eds.), *Language and Speech in the Laboratory, School, and Clinic* (pp. 309–327). Cambridge, MA: The MIT Press.

Charman, T., Swettenham, J., Baron-Cohen, S., Cox, A., Baird, G., & Drew, A. (1997). Infants with autism: An investigation of empathy, pretend play, joint attention, and imitation. *Developmental Psychology, 33*, 781–789.

Corona, R., Dissanayake, C., Arbelle, S., Willington, P., & Sigman, M. (1998). Is affect aversive to young children with autism? Behavioral and cardiac responses to experimenter distress. *Child Development, 69*, 1494–1502.

Courchesne, E. (1987). A neurophysiological view of autism. In E. Schopler & G. Mesibov (Eds.), *Neurobiological Issues in Autism* (pp. 285–324). New York: Plenum.

Dawson, G., Meltzoff, A., Osterling, J., Rinaldi, J., & Brown, E. (1998). Children with autism fail to orient to naturally occurring social stimuli. *Journal of Autism and Developmental Disorders, 28*, 479–485.

Dawson, G., Finley, C., Phillips, S., & Lewy, A. (1989). A comparison of hemispheric asymmetries in speech-related brain potentials of autistic and dysphasic children. *Brain and Language, 37*, 26–41.

Dawson, G., & Osterling, J. (1997). Early intervention in autism. In M. Guralnick (Ed.), *The Effectiveness of Early Intervention* (pp. 307–326). Baltimore: Brookes.

Fein, D., Dunn, M., Allen, D. A., Aram, D. M., Hall, N., Morris, R., & Wilson, B. C. (1996). Language and neuropsychological findings. In I. Rapin (Ed.), *Preschool Children with Inadequate Communication* (pp. 123–154). London: Mac Keith.

Happé, F. G. E. (1997). Central coherence and theory of mind in autism: Reading homographs in context. *British Journal of Developmental Psychology, 15* (Pt. 1), 1–12.

Heimann, M. (1998). Imitation in neonates, in older infants, and in children with autism: Feedback to theory. In S. Bråten (Ed.), *Intersubjective Communication and Emotion in Early Ontogeny* (pp. 89–104). Cambridge: Cambridge University Press.

Hobson, P. (1993). Understanding persons: The role of affect. In S. Baron-Cohen, H. Tager-Flusberg, & D. J. Cohen (Eds.), *Understanding Other Minds: Perspectives from Autism* (pp. 204–227). Oxford: Oxford University Press.

Hoshino, Y., Kumashiro, H., Yashima, Y., Tachibana, R., Watanabe, M., & Furukawa, H. (1982). Early symptoms of autistic children and its diagnostic significance. *Folia Psychiatrica et Neurologica Japonica, 36*, 367–374.

Jusczyk, P. W. (1997). *The Discovery of Spoken Language*. Cambridge, MA: The MIT Press.

Klin, A. (1991). Young autistic children's listening preferences in regard to speech: A possible characterization of the symptom of social withdrawal. *Journal of Autism and Developmental Disabilities, 21*, 29–42.

Klinger, L., & Dawson , G. (1992). Facilitating early social and communicative development in children with autism. In S. Warren & J. Reichle (Eds.), *Causes and Effects in Communication and Language Intervention* (pp. 157–186). Baltimore: Brookes.

Kugiumutzakis, G. (1999). Genesis and development of early infant mimesis to facial and vocal models. In J. Nadel & G. Butterworth (Eds.), *Imitation in Infancy* (pp. 36–59). Cambridge: Cambridge University Press.

Kuhl, P. K. (1998). Language, culture and intersubjectivity: the creation of shared perception. In S. Bråten (Ed.), *Intersubjective Communication and Emotion in Early Ontogeny* (pp. 297-315). Cambridge: Cambridge University Press.

Layton, T. L. (1988). Language training with autistic children using four different modes of presentation. *Journal of Communication Disorders, 21,* 333–350.

Leekam, S., Baron-Cohen, S., Perrett, D., Milders, M., & Brown, S. (1997). Eye-direction detection: A dissociation between geometric and joint attention skills in autism. *British Journal of Developmental Psychology, 15,* 77–95.

Leekam, S. R., Hunnisett, E., & Moore, C. (1998). Targets and cues: Gaze-following in children with autism. *Journal of Child Psychology and Psychiatry, 39,* 951–962.

Lord, C. (1985). Language comprehension and cognitive disorder in autism. In L. S. Siegel & F. J. Morrison (Eds.), *Cognitive Development in Atypical Children* (pp. 67–81). New York: Springer-Verlag.

Lord, C. (1995). Follow-up of two-year-olds referred for possible autism. *Journal of Child Psychology and Psychiatry, 38,* 1365–1382.

Lord, C., & Paul, R. (1997). Language and communication in autism. In D. J. Cohen & F. R. Volkmar (Eds.), *Handbook of Autism and Pervasive Developmental Disorders* (pp. 195–225). New York: John Wiley & Sons.

Meltzoff, A. N., & Moore, M. K. (1998). Infant intersubjectivity: broadening the dialogue to include imitation, identity and intention. In S. Bråten (Ed.). *Intersubjective Communication and Emotion in Early Ontogeny* (pp. 47–62). Cambridge: Cambridge University Press.

Menyuk, P., & Quill, K. (1985). Semantic problems in autistic children. In E. Schopler & G. B. Mesibov (Eds.), *Communication Problems in Autism* (pp. 127–145). New York: Plenum.

Messer, D. J. (1994). *The Development of Communication: From Social Interaction to Language.* Chichester: John Wiley & Sons.

Messer, D. J. (1997). Referential communication: Making sense of the social and physical worlds. In G. Bremmer, A. Slater, & G. Butterworth (Eds.), *Infant Development: Recent Advances.* East Sussex: Psychology Press.

Minshew, N. J., Sweeney, J. A., & Bauman, M. L. (1997). Neurological aspects of autism. In D. J. Cohen & F. R. Volkmar (Eds.), *Handbook of Autism and Pervasive Developmental Disorders* (pp. 344–369). New York: John Wiley & Sons.

Morales, M., Mundy, P., & Rojas, J. (1998). Following the direction of gaze and language development in 6-month-olds. *Infant Behavior and Development, 21,* 373–377.

Mundy, P. (1995). Joint attention and social-emotional approach behavior in children with autism. *Development and Psychopathology, 7,* 63–82.

Mundy, P., & Gomes, A. (1998). Individual differences in joint attention skill development in the second year. *Infant Behavior and Development, 21,* 469–482.

Mundy, P., Sigman, M., & Kasari, C. (1993). The theory of mind and joint-attention deficits in autism. In S. Baron-Cohen, H. Tager-Flusberg, & D. Cohen (Eds.), *Understanding Other Minds: Perspectives from Autism* (pp. 181–203). Oxford: Oxford University Press.

Nelson, K. (1985). *Making Sense: The Acquisition of Shared Meaning.* New York: Academic Press.

Osterling, J., & Dawson, G. (1996). Early recognition of children with autism: A study of first birthday home videotapes. *Journal of Autism and Developmental Disorders, 10,* 433–443.

Paul, R., & Cohen, D. J. (1984). Outcomes of severe disorders of language acquisition. *Journal of Autism and Developmental Disorders, 14,* 405–422.

Phillips, W., Gómez, J. C., Baron-Cohen, S., Laá, V., & Riviére, A. (1995). Treating people as objects, agents, or "subjects": How young children with and without autism make requests. *Journal of Child Psychology and Psychiatry, 36,* 1383–1398.

Rapin, I. (1994). Introduction and overview. In M. L. Bauman & T. L. Kemper (Eds.), *The Neurobiology of Autism* (pp. 1–17). Baltimore: Johns Hopkins.

Reddy, V., Hay, D., Murray, L., & Trevarthen, C. (1997). Communication in infancy: Mutual regulation of affect and attention. In G. Bremmer, A. Slater, & G. Butterworth (Eds.), *Infant Development: Recent Advances* (pp. 247–273). East Sussex: Psychology Press.

Rimland, B., & Edelson, S. M. (1994). The effects of auditory integration training on autism. *American Journal of Speech-Language Pathology, 3,* 41–51.

Rogers, S. J., & Pennington, B. F. (1991). A theoretical approach to the deficits in infantile autism. *Development and Psychopathology, 3,* 137–162.

Rollins, P. R., Wambacq, I., Dowell, D., Mathews, L., & Reese, P. B. (1998). Joint attention as a intervention technique for children with autistic spectrum disorders. *Journal of Communication Disorders, 31,* 1–13.

Schuler, A. L., Prizant, B. M., & Wetherby, A. M. (1997). Enhancing language and communication development: Prelinguistic approaches. In D. J. Cohen & F. R. Volkmar (Eds.), *Handbook of Autism and Pervasive Developmental Disorders* (pp. 539–571). New York: John Wiley & Sons.

Sigman, M. (1998). Joint attention as a predictor of language skills and peer engagement in children with autism. *Infant Behavior & Development, 21,* 144. (Special International Conference on Infant Studies Issue).

Sigman, M., & Kasari, C. (1995). Joint attention across contexts in normal and autistic children. In C. Moore & P. J. Dunham (Eds.), *Joint Attention: Its Origins and Role in Development* (pp. 189–203). Hillsdale, NJ: Erlbaum.

Sigman, M., & Ungerer, J. A. (1984). Cognitive and language skills in autistic, mentally retarded and normal children. *Developmental Psychology, 20,* 293–302.

Smith, I., & Bryson, S. E. (1994). Imitation and action in autism: A critical review. *Psychological Bulletin, 116,* 259–273.

Stone, W. L. (1997). Autism in infancy and early childhood. In D. J. Cohen & F. R. Volkmar (Eds.), *Handbook of Autism and Pervasive Developmental Disorders* (pp. 266-282). New York: John Wiley & Sons.

Stone, W. L., Ousley, O. Y., & Littleford, C. D. (1997). Motor imitation in young children with autism: What's the object? *Journal of Abnormal Child Psychology, 25,* 475–485.

Tallal, P. Saunders, G. H., Miller, S., Jenkins, W. M., Protopapas, A., & Merzenich, M. M. (1997). *Rapid training-driven improvement in language ability in autistic and PDD-NOS children.* Berkeley, CA: Scientific Learning Corporation. Retrieved January 29, 2000 from the World Wide Web: http://www.scilearn.com/html/pro/sciposter7.html. Portions of the article presented at the October, 1997 Annual Meeting of the Society for Neuroscience, New Orleans, LA.

Tomasello, M., & Farrar, M. J. (1986). Joint attention and early language. *Child Development, 57,* 1454–1463.

Trevarthan, C. (1979). Communication and cooperation in early infancy: A description of primary intersubjectivity. In M. Bullowa (Ed.), *Before speech* (pp. 321–347). New York: Cambridge University Press.

Trevarthan, C., & Hubley, P. (1978). Secondary intersubjectivity: Confidence, confiding and acts of meaning in the first year. In A. Lock (Ed.), *Action, Gesture and Symbol: The Emergence of Language* (pp. 183–229). London: Academic Press.

Ungerer, J. A., & Sigman, M. (1981). Symbolic play and language comprehension in autistic children. *Journal of the American Academy of Child Psychiatry, 20,* 318–337.

Watson, L. R. (1998). Following the child's lead: Mothers' interactions with children with autism. *Journal of Autism and Developmental Disorders, 28,* 51–59.

Watson, L. R., & Fox, M. (1988). Autistic children's understanding of concrete versus relational words. Unpublished manuscript, University of North Carolina at Chapel Hill.

Watson, L. R., Lord, C., Schaffer, B., & Schopler, E. (1989). *Teaching Spontaneous Communication to Autistic and Developmentally Handicapped Children.* Austin: Pro-Ed.

Watters, R. G., Wheeler, L. J., & Watters, W. E. (1981). The relative efficiency of two orders of training autistic children in the expressive and receptive use of manual signs. *Journal of Communication Disorders, 14,* 273–285.

11

The Experience of Loneliness and Friendship in Autism

Theoretical and Practical Issues

Nirit Bauminger and Connie Kasari

Loneliness is a negative complex social emotion that is assumed to have strong social, cognitive, and emotional components (Perlman & Peplau, 1982; Weiss, 1973). A full understanding of loneliness incorporates social (e.g., a direct reflection of the desire to have friends), cognitive (e.g., an understanding of the gap between an actual and desired social status), and emotional (e.g., a lack of affective bonding) capabilities. Loneliness and social relationships are closely related; in fact, loneliness arises in the absence of social relationships (Asher, Parkhurst, Hymel, & Williams, 1990; Weiss, 1973). A lack of affective bonding as manifested in an absence of close friends and low social status are predictors of loneliness in typically developing children (Parker, Saxon, Asher, & Kovacs, 1999).

Despite the fact that friendships are generally deficient in autistic children *Diagnostic and Statistical Manual of Mental Disorders* (DSM-IV); American Psychiatric Association, 1994), loneliness and friendship in this population are both overlooked issues in many studies. The present chapter examines the ability of children with autism to experience and understand loneliness and to develop friendships with peers. The chapter begins by presenting theories of loneliness and continues with the study of loneliness in autism. The major focus of this chapter is a discussion of the feasibility of friendship in autism.

NIRIT BAUMINGER • Department of Special Education, School of Education, Bar-Ilan University, Ramat-Gan, 52900 Israel.   CONNIE KASARI • Graduate School of Education and Information Studies, University of California at Los Angeles, Los Angeles, California 90095.

The Research Basis for Autism Intervention, edited by Schopler, Yirmiya, Shulman, and Marcus. Kluwer Academic/Plenum Publishers, New York, 2001.

LONELINESS IN TYPICAL DEVELOPMENT: CONCEPTUAL BASIS

The social need theory (e.g., Bowlby, 1973; Sullivan, 1953; Weiss, 1973) and the cognitive theory (e.g., Perlman & Peplau, 1982) are two conceptual approaches that contribute to the understanding of loneliness. The social need theory is a psychodynamic approach that emphasizes the inherent human needs for intimacy: "The human being is born with the need for contact and tenderness" (Fromm-Reichmann, 1980, p. 342). According to this view, loneliness is caused not by being alone, but by being without some valued close interpersonal relationship (Sullivan, 1953; Weiss, 1973). Alternatively, the cognitive approach focuses on cognitions (e.g., perceptions, comparisons, and evaluations of social relationships) as mediating factors between deficits in sociability and the experience of loneliness (Perlman & Peplau, 1982). Loneliness results from perceived dissatisfaction with one's social relationships—that is, a discrepancy between one's desired and achieved level of social contact (Terrell-Deutsch, 1999).

These two different approaches to loneliness can be combined within the two forms of loneliness identified by Weiss (1973): emotional loneliness and social loneliness. Emotional loneliness emphasizes the affective or feelings aspect of loneliness. It represents subjective responses to the lack of truly intimate ties, "the absence of a close emotional relationship in which one feels accepted, secure, cared about, and understood" (Terrell-Deutsch, 1999, p. 12). According to Weiss, the symptoms of emotional loneliness (sadness, fear, restlessness, emptiness, etc.) stem from the young child's fear of being abandoned by the parents; thus, the formation of a secure attachment may be a precursor to later development of emotional loneliness (Cassidy & Berlin, 1999).

The second form of loneliness, social loneliness (Weiss, 1973), arises when children do not have accessible social networks or peer groups, or when they perceive their social relationships as unsatisfactory. According to Weiss, social loneliness is based on cognitive processes such as self-evaluation, self-perception, and social comparison; it induces feelings of exclusion, meaninglessness, marginality, and boredom rather than the sadness, depression, or emptiness aroused by emotional loneliness. Altogether, irrespective of whether the nature of loneliness is social–cognitive or affective, loneliness is a subjective response to a relational difficulty.

LONELINESS IN AUTISM

In 1943, Kanner described a group of children who were content to play for hours with objects, had few relationships with others, and who were observed to move among other children "like strange beings, as if moving between the pieces of furniture" (p. 241). Kanner suggested "a powerful desire for aloneness" (p. 249) in these children. Since the time of Kanner's observation, the study of loneliness in autism has been a subject of speculation in clinical reports but has not been empirically investigated. The lack of empirical attention may be attributable to the diagnostic criteria for autism, which specify an inability to form satisfactory social relationships (American Psychiatric Association, 1994; *International Classification of Diseases*, World Health Organization, 1990). Thus, almost by definition, children with autism are considered lonely; yet the implications of these diagnostic criteria are unclear. Are children with autism satisfied with their aloneness, lacking a social desire to be involved with their peers, and thus they do not feel lonely? Or do these children in fact have a social desire for relationships but are unable to form them satisfactorily, and thus they feel lonely?

Loneliness is always associated with undesired isolation and with unpleasant and negative feelings, thereby reflecting the child's subjective perception of his or her social isolation (Margalit, 1994). For children to feel lonely, however, it appears that several cognitive abilities are critical. These include an understanding of the self as a distinct entity, and an ability to compare one's accomplishments in social relationships to normative standards (i.e., to peers' social accomplishments). Difficulties have been reported among autistic children in understanding the self vis-á-vis others (e.g., Baron-Cohen & Swettenham, 1997), and in understanding other complex social emotions such as pride, embarrassment, and guilt (e.g., Capps, Yirmiya, & Sigman, 1992; Kasari, Chamberlain, Paparella, & Bauminger, 1999; Kasari, Paparella, & Bauminger, 1999). Thus, one might expect that these children also have difficulty in understanding complex emotions such as loneliness.

In a recent study, we examined the feelings and understanding of loneliness in 22 high functioning children with autism and a comparison group of typically developing peers (Bauminger & Kasari, 2000). Children's understanding of loneliness was examined through direct interview, in which children were asked to describe: "What does being lonely mean?" Following Cassidy and Asher's (1992) procedure, children's answers were coded along two dimensions: (1) whether the child indicated that loneliness included affective involvement such as being sad, afraid, or depressed (corresponding to emotional loneliness); and (2) whether the child indicated that loneliness involved unfulfilled relationships, exclusion, or dissatisfaction with social relationships (corresponding with social–cognitive loneliness).

Similar to typically developing children, the children with autism identified social–cognitive dimensions of loneliness—that is, they described being alone, or having no one to play with or "do stuff with." Unlike typically developing children, however, the autistic children rarely identified feelings associated with emotional loneliness such as sadness or depression. The manifestation of only the social–cognitive aspect in children with autism suggests their tendency to conceive a more cognitive interpretation of loneliness (Bauminger & Kasari, 2000). It may be that these children use their "knowledge of loneliness" rather than their emotional experience of loneliness (Hobson, 1993; Kanner, 1943).

Despite the differences in their understanding of loneliness, the autistic children in our study reported greater loneliness compared with typically developing children on the Illinois Loneliness Questionnaire (Asher, Hymel, & Renshaw, 1984). This questionnaire provides a global score of loneliness that encompasses both the social and emotional aspects of loneliness. As a result, it is difficult to know whether the nature of the loneliness reported by the autistic children in our sample was of the emotional or the social–cognitive form. On the other hand, this recent exploration of loneliness in high functioning children with autism adds a unique contribution to our understanding. High functioning children with autism as a group reported that they *experienced* loneliness more intensively and more frequently compared with typically developing children, even though their *understanding* of loneliness was less comprehensive and less coherent. Considering that loneliness is seen as one of the most significant social drives or motivations for children to take part in social relationships (Weiss, 1973), the implication of this finding is that perhaps high functioning children with autism do have the social desire to be involved in social relationships and that they are well aware of their social isolation. However, because we examined older high functioning children with autism (i.e., preadolescents and adolescents), questions remain regarding the chronology of the development of social desire in autism and its universality to the disorder. Future studies might examine whether more severely developmentally delayed children with autism similarly experience and understand loneliness. Further research would also do well to explore the onset of loneliness experiences among low and high functioning subgroups of this population.

Loneliness and friendship are basic constructs for the development of social relationships. By reporting on being lonely, the child expresses a *desire* to be affectively involved in relationships. Friendship is a direct reflection of the child's *ability* to form an affective tie. Friendship and loneliness are related in such a way that the understanding and experience of the former are critical for the development of the latter. Thus, the exploration of friendship in autism can expand our knowledge regarding the emotional nature of these children's loneliness in terms of their lack of affective ties and closeness. The remainder of this chapter discusses issues regarding the feasibility of friendship in autism.

FRIENDSHIP IN AUTISM

Even if friendships with peers are an uncommon social experience and a major area of difficulty for the child with autism (American Psychiatric Association, 1994), recent data have shown that high functioning children with autism perceive themselves as having friends (Bauminger & Kasari, 2000). Despite this recent evidence, the question of whether children with autism are actually able to develop friendships remains a theoretical dilemma in the understanding of the disorder. Why might that be? There are likely several possible explanations.

According to Bronfenbrenner's (1979, 1992) ecological model, the child's social development is affected by continuous transactions (interactions over time) among the child's unique characteristics on the one hand and a broad array of contextual variables that operate at various levels in the child's social environment on the other hand (e.g., school or home environments; cultural assumptions based on research and clinical perceptions) (Bronfenbrenner, 1979; Cairns, McGuire, & Gariepy, 1993; Sontag, 1996). The major factors that affect our thinking about the likelihood of friendship in autism can be conceived within this ecological perspective.

First, at the broadest level of analysis (cultural beliefs according to Bronfenbrenner's model), theoretical assumptions may be critically examined regarding the perception of friendship as an unattainable social experience for the child with autism. Second, at the narrowest level of analysis (the child himself or herself, according to Bronfenbrenner), characteristics of the child with autism may be identified that might predict the development of friendship in autism. Third, the ecological view emphasizes the significance of the child's social environment in enhancing social functioning, thus calling for an examination of the role that teachers, parents, and peers—the child's immediate social environment—might play in the formation of friendship in autism.

Conceptual Assumptions

Peer interaction and friendship are considered in the literature as two different social experiences for typically developing children (Asher, Parker, & Walker, 1996; Parker,

Rubin, Price, & DeRosier, 1995). The one criterion that clearly differentiates friendship from peer interaction is that friendship alone contains a close, intimate affective tie between children (Howes, 1996). Thus, the ability to form affective bonding is a prerequisite for the development of friendship. Likewise, according to Howes, the ability to develop social skills is necessary for the formation of friendship. The following comprise two basic assumptions that might constrain our thinking about the development of friendship in autism:

1. Friendship is not possible in autism owing to the child's limited abilities to form affective bonding with significant others.
2. Friendship is a complex social experience that may be notably difficult for the child with autism to engage in, owing to his or her poor social skills; therefore, enhancement of the child's social skills will result in the development of friendship.

Assumption 1: Deficits in Affective Bonding Lead to a Lack of Friendship in Autism

As emphasized in the preceding, one of the core deficits of the autistic syndrome is abnormality in interpersonal relationships (American Psychiatric Association, 1994; Waterhouse & Fein, 1997). The social impairments of children with autism range from a lack of awareness of others (among those with the most severe social impairments) to abnormalities in peer relationships (among those who are less impaired). Even very high functioning individuals with autism across different ages have difficulties in interpersonal relationships (Bemporad, 1979; Kanner, Rodriguez, & Ashenden, 1972; Volkmar & Cohen, 1985). The affective explanation for this social deficit focuses on the autistic child's inability to establish an affective bond or to develop social relationships based on emotions (Hobson, 1993; Kanner, 1943). According to Kanner, autistic children "come into the world with innate inability to form the usual, biologically provided affective contact with people" (p. 250). This perspective, focusing on affective deficiencies, will predict major difficulties in the formation of friendship in autism.

Studies of attachment in children with autism are of interest when debating the likelihood of friendship attributable to affective factors. If the child with autism is capable of forming a secure attachment, he or she should be able to establish affective contacts with significant others and, by definition, to form selective affective bonding with a peer (e.g., friendships) at least to some extent. A closer look at findings from studies on attachment reveals that, despite a low frequency of prosocial behaviors in children with autism compared with their typically developing counterparts, children with autism were able to: differentiate between their mother and a stranger, react to their mother's departure, direct more social behaviors to a caregiver than to a stranger, and (among the majority) increase proximity behaviors toward their caregiver after separation (Dissanayake & Crossley, 1996; Shapiro, Sherman, Calamari, & Koch, 1987; Sigman & Mundy, 1989; Sigman & Ungerer, 1984). Also, a significant percentage of children with autism (40%) have been described as forming a secure attachment with their mothers (Capps, Sigman, & Mundy, 1994; Rogers, Ozonoff, & Masline-Cole, 1991, 1993; Shapiro et al., 1987).

On the whole, empirical results have demonstrated that subgroups of children with autism were able to establish secure attachments with their caregivers. Therefore, studies on attachment have moved from the question of whether the child with autism is able to form affective bonding—attachment with significant others—to two other questions: (1) identifying which characteristics are unique to those children with autism who are capable of establishing attachment; and (2) elucidating the different manifestations and qualities of attachment behaviors in autism. With regard to their unique characteristics, the ability to form an attachment in children with autism has been positively linked with the child's various developmental variables. Such variables include receptive language level (Capps et al., 1994), mental age (Rogers et al., 1993), representational abilities (joint attention and symbolic play), and affective expressiveness (Capps et al., 1994; Shapiro et al., 1987; Sigman & Ungerer, 1984). However, autistic children's ability to form an attachment was not correlated with the severity of the disorder (Rogers et al., 1993; Shapiro et al., 1987).

    With regard to variance in manifestations of attachment, researchers have noted that attachment behaviors in autism appear to differ from those of typically developing children. Rogers et al. (1993) developed a customized rating scale to tap the attachment behaviors of autistic children in her sample, in response to the fact that these children's behaviors were too subtle to fit the classic ABC classification (e.g., Ainsworth, Blehar, Waters, & Wall, 1978). Similarly, Capps et al. (1994) were able to classify securely attached children using only a secondary classification; in their first classification, the majority of children were classified as disorganized/disoriented. The inability to use typical classification systems attests to differences in autistic children's expression of relationships.

    Attachment and friendship are both forms of affective bonding that children develop throughout their lives (Hartup & Sancilio, 1986). Howes (1996) devised a model for understanding early friendships among typically developing toddlers and preschoolers. She argued that the child is able to construct internal representations of relationships with caregivers through attachment and with peers through friendship, on the condition that the child has ongoing opportunities for familiarity and interaction with caregivers and peers. Based on this model and in view of the aforementioned studies of attachment in children with autism, it might be speculated that at least some of the children with autism should be able to establish friendships with a familiar peer, although their relationships will probably differ in quality compared with those of typically developing children. Owing to the paucity of studies investigating the link between attachment and friendship in autism, it is difficult to predict working models on how attachment may develop or transfer into friendship relationships with peers. Thus, the quality of peer friendship in autism is still unclear. It might be that, for some children with autism, attachment relationships do not transfer into highly evolved friendships based on intimacy, but rather into friendships based on companionship.

    Indeed, Hobson (1993) argued that to know what persons are, one needs to experience and understand the kinds of relationships that can exist between oneself and others—specifically, reciprocal relationships based on feelings. Hobson suggested that the child with autism "stands outside social relationships and merely watches behaviors" (p. 5). In addition, he stressed that it is the lack of intersubjective sharing with others that leads to the incomprehension of what it means to have or to be a "friend," a conceptual deficit that stands in contrast to the understanding of other sophisticated concepts. Without emotional experience of appropriate kinds of interpersonal relationships, the individual with autism will have largely impersonal relationships with others. Hobson proposed that basically children with autism—owing to their emotional deficit in forming affective bonding—might be able to form a more superficial friendship—friendship that differs in quality compared with typically developing children. They would, at best, perceive a friend as a "companion" and would rarely achieve intimacy or express affection in their relationships.

As mentioned previously, friendship is an overlooked field of inquiry in autism, and some of the data to be presented here are still preliminary. In Bauminger and Kasari's (2000) study, all 22 high functioning preadolescents and adolescents with autism could identify at least one friend; however, their understanding of friendship as well as its quality differed in comparison with typically developing children. Among children with autism, quality of friendship diverged on the dimensions of help, intimacy/trust, and companionship, but not on the dimension of closeness. Also, in accordance with Hobson's (1993) hypothesis, these children tended to describe a friend as a companion with whom to carry out activities and games rather than as a close and intimate friend with whom to share feelings.

In an ongoing project, Bauminger and Shulman (2001) have been particularly interested in investigating if high functioning preadolescents and adolescents with autism would relate to issues such as reciprocity, closeness, and intimacy in their perception of a friend. The preliminary data suggest that the majority of children: (1) could explain correctly what a friend is but, similarly to Bauminger and Kasari's (2000) results, tended to perceive a friend as a companion for various activities (e.g., board and card games, football, movies), rather than as an intimate or close figure; (2) described a friend as someone either with whom you play or who plays with you, but not as someone with whom to play *together*; and (3) tended to describe the physical details of pictures depicting two friends sharing secrets together (e.g., the color of the children's clothing, a description of the tree), rather than describing the children in the picture as intimate and close friends.

It is important to note, however, that despite the more·impersonal rather than personal perception of a friend revealed for the majority of children in both of these recent studies, a substantial minority (almost one third) of the children were able to identify the intimate, reciprocal nature of friendship. This subgroup of children with autism could relate to aspects such as trust and intimacy (e.g., "someone you can rely on and trust, tell him problems at school or at home"); could pinpoint the affective relatedness and reciprocity (e.g., "someone who loves you and cares about you, you *also* love him," or "it is like two children who joined together"); and could describe the children in the friendship picture as "*soul* friends—friends for life," or as "two kids who started a friendship" (Bauminger & Kasari, 2000; Bauminger & Shulman, 2001). In sum, recent preliminary research findings have yielded a significant subgroup of children with autism who, similar to the data on attachment, demonstrate a more personal and affective perception of relationships. An important direction for future inquiry would be to determine if these children also experience emotional loneliness, which is the reflection of the absence of an emotional tie. Next, the assumption regarding the connection between social skills and the ability to form friendships is examined.

Assumption 2: The Link between the Formation of Friendship and Social Skills

The development of friendship requires social skills (e.g., sharing, negotiating, compromising); yet at the same time, the very experience of friendship helps in developing these skills (Newcomb & Bagwell, 1995). We might say, then, that the autistic child is caught in a vicious circle. He or she does not develop friendship owing to a lack of social skills, yet is unable to develop those social skills that can be gained via peer friendships owing to that very lack of participation in such relationships (Sigman & Ruskin, 1999).

Regardless of their well documented deficiencies in social skills (American Psychiatric Association, 1994), children with autism have been found to respond consistently to certain social stimuli. Specifically, they show higher levels of social engagement in contexts containing structured social stimuli and in predictable social environments (e.g., Bacon, Fein, Morris, Waterhouse, & Allen, 1998; Ungerer, 1989), when compared with unstructured social situations such as school recess (e.g., Sigman & Ruskin, 1999). In addition, children with autism can cooperate more easily with one particular child than with a group of peers, and it is easier for them to interact with a familiar than an unfamiliar peer (Hauck, Fein, Waterhouse, & Feinstein, 1995; Lord, 1984). Therefore, it can be argued that friendship is a social framework advantageous for the enhancement of social skills among children with autism.

Friendship offers a one-on-one social experience with a familiar peer. Its benefits include continuity over time and greater predictability as children learn to know one another's interests and to develop shared play routines (Grenot-Scheyer, Staub, Peck, & Schwartz, 1998). Studies on typical and atypical friendship have demonstrated that children become more similar during the course of a friendship in response to mutual influences. Also, children grow in their awareness of others' needs and base their relationships on complex attributions and shared characteristics and areas of interest, rather than on proximity and shared material (Berndt, 1982; Grenot-Scheyer et al., 1998). Thus, in friendship relationships, the child with autism can develop and practice social skills (e.g., cooperation, social initiations, play skills, taking other person perspectives, sharing activities and feelings) within an ongoing, secure social experience.

Another common belief regarding the association between social skills and friendship is that a focus on social skills training will enhance the integral social functioning of the child with autism and will result in development of friendship. We would like to argue that social skills comprise only one part of a more integral social competency in children. The need for a multidimensional definition of social competence finds support within the conceptual framework of friendship termed the social relationship approach (Hinde, 1976, 1979). In this approach, individual social behaviors and skills or the interaction of skills are not as important as the social relationships constructed between two people over longer periods (Dunn, 1993; Parker & Gottman, 1989). The development of friendship reflects the "wholeness and order" principle taken from the general systems theory. Wholes are considered to be more than the sum of their parts; likewise, relationships are developed in a way that cannot be attributed to their single elements (Sameroff, 1983). Social skill training focuses on the parts with the aim of generalizing to the whole; however, the teaching of social behaviors alone will not result in the development of friendship (Hurley-Geffner, 1995).

Furthermore, friendship is but one component of the child's social competency. If children are socially competent with peers, they can form friendships and vice versa. However, friendship is independent of social competence with peers because children with friends are not always competent with peers (e.g., a rejected child who has a best friend), and those competent with peers do not always have friends (Furman & Bierman, 1983). Indeed, Farmer, Pearl, and Van Acker (1996), in an extensive review on social competence in children with different diagnoses (learning disabilities, mental retardation, and emotional behavioral disorders) revealed large within-group variation in social status for each etiology. These findings indicated that some students with disabilities are viewed favorably by their peers and do have friends. Evans, Salisbury, Palombaro, Berryman, and Hollowood (1992) and Grenot-Scheyer et al. (1998) reported similar findings regarding children with severe developmental disabilities.

Thus, a multidimensional approach toward social competence should be taken into consideration when considering the formation of friendship in autism. Such an approach—a cognitive–behavioral view of social competence—assumes reciprocity between the ways an individual thinks, feels, and behaves in social situations. Social functioning is "reciprocally determined"—cognitions, emotions, and behaviors are functionally related, and changing one can change the other. Thus, the child's internal cognitive processes and feelings and his or her external behavioral variables should constitute the relevant units of analysis for treatment programs (Hart & Morgan, 1993; Kendall & Panichelli-Mindel, 1995).

Although it seems important to adapt a more comprehensive view of social competence, social skills training programs form the core of most interventions with autistic children (Sigman & Capps, 1997). A review of the literature reveals that many intervention programs have treated social skills by decreasing problematic behaviors such as aggressiveness and echolalic responses that interfere with the child's ability to engage in appropriate social behaviors (e.g., Russo & Koegel, 1977). Other interventions have aimed to teach new behaviors such as appropriate eye contact, greeting responses, play skills, recognizing other people's needs, and initiating and responding to interaction with peers (Belchic & Harris, 1994; Gaylord-Ross, Haring, Breen, & Pitts-Conway, 1984; Harris & Handleman, 1997; Koegel & Frea, 1993; Koegel, Koegel, Hurley, & Frea, 1992; McGee, Krantz, & McClannahan, 1984; Niemtimp & Cole, 1992; Oke & Schreibman, 1990).

Children who have participated in these programs demonstrated improved functioning; however, several issues remain unresolved. First, these programs generally limit themselves to addressing some facet of the child's overall social difficulty, a strategy that results in difficulties when attempting to integrate these behaviors into the integral social competency that will allow the child to develop social relationships and friendships with peers (Hurley-Geffner, 1995). Second, although children have been shown to improve their skills at initiating social behaviors with peers, friendship requires the development of relationships over time. Hence, the maintenance of the relationships is still an issue for children with autism. Third, these programs emphasize different aspects of social behaviors and social interaction, whereas friendship is also dependent on emotional abilities such as the capacity to express and recognize emotions in the self and in others, an ability posing major difficulties even for high functioning children with autism (Borman-Kischkel, Vilsmeier, & Baude, 1995; Celani, Battacchi, & Arcidiacono, 1999; Jaedicke, Storoschuk, & Lord, 1994; Sigman & Ruskin, 1999). According to Hobson (1993), these children exhibit an interplay between their restricted social and emotional experience, and their poor social and emotional understanding. The latter has rarely been the focus of social skills interventions.

The fourth issue concerns the agent of intervention. Teachers and/or typical peers have been the major agents in most social skills training programs to date (e.g., Odom & Strain, 1986; Odom & Watts, 1991; Roeyers, 1996). However, friendships occur in the child's home as well as at school; consequently, parents, teachers, and peers should contribute together to the development and maintenance of friendship in autism.

Altogether, intervention programs to facilitate friendship in autism should adapt a more multidimensional cognitive–behavioral definition of social competence (i.e., they should attempt to enhance the ability for social and emotional understanding as well as specific social behaviors) and should utilize an ecological concept of intervention (i.e., including parents, teachers, and typical as well as atypical peers). In terms of social–cognitive targets of intervention, training should aim to enhance the child's: (1) theory of mind abilities—the child's ability to understand people in terms of their internal states such as their beliefs, desires, and emotions; (2) understanding of social norms and rules; and (3) social problem abilities. The facilitation of the child's ability to read verbal and nonverbal social cues in different social situations would help the child make correct social interpretations in different social situations, expand the child's repertoire of behavioral alternatives, and enhance the child's ability to consider the anticipated results of the various social alternatives. Also, issues such as what a friend is, why friends are important, why it is important to listen to a friend, how we listen to a friend, and what we can do with friends should be topics for discussion and instruction in classes for children with autism

In terms of the emotional targets of intervention, training should focus on expanding the child's affective repertoire (e.g., teaching complex emotions for the high functioning child with autism); fostering the child's recognition of emotions in the self and others; and helping the child to associate a given social situation with the emotion it elicits. In general, interventions that combine cognitive, emotional, and behavioral abilities seem more apt to lead to the development of friendship in autism, at least for high functioning children with autism. This subgroup of children are seen as compensating for their social–emotional deficiencies by utilizing their relatively high cognitive abilities (Capps et al., 1992; Hermelin & O'Connor, 1985; Yirmiya, Sigman, Kasari, & Mundy, 1992). Yet it might be that high functioning children with autism are unable to construct friendships spontaneously owing not only to their social–emotional deficits, but also to their restricted social opportunities and limited environmental mediators (e.g., teachers or parents). Consequently, interventions may be most effective if they incorporate a real social experience in which the child can practice and rehearse newly learned cognitive and emotional skills in an actual ongoing social situation. If given the opportunity to share time with one particular familiar peer in a supportive friendship-oriented environment, these children might be able to better generate friendships (Grenot-Scheyer et al., 1998).

In addition to its potential benefits, friendship also appears to be a need, at least for high functioning children with autism, who were found to express loneliness and to long for a friend (Bauminger & Kasari, 2000; Wing, 1992). Wing reported that the awareness of these high functioning individuals to their social isolation made them more vulnerable to feelings of rejection and depression. Among typically developing children, having friends helps reduce loneliness, but there do not seem to be particular benefits of having a greater number of friends (Parker & Seal, 1996). Likewise, even one friend can lessen the severity of loneliness among high functioning children with autism who long for a friend.

On the whole, similarly to the research trends described previously for attachment, several main implications for the study of friendship in autism might be drawn from the present discussion. First, instead of asking if friendships are possible in autism, the focus of researchers and practitioners needs to shift to the task of identifying the characteristics of those children with autism who are able to establish friendships. Another major implication is that friendship in autism may manifest itself differently (e.g., more shared activities rather than shared emotions) compared with friendship among their typically developing counterparts. Hence, future studies should examine the unique manifestations of friendship behaviors and qualities in children with autism. In terms of implications for intervention, efforts should be made to work on enhancing the child's social cognitive abilities and emotional understanding simultaneously with the child's social behaviors. To this end, the child's environment (peers, teachers, parents) plays a crucial role in the enhancement of friendship. In line with Bronfenbrenner's (1979, 1992) emphasis on the child's unique characteristics and on his or her social–environmental milieu, the remainder of this chapter will elaborate on these issues.

Child Characteristics in the Formation of Friendship in Autism

Owing to the paucity of empirical data, we can only speculate about which characteristics might predict the formation of friendship in children with autism. Our speculations are based on three main sources of evidence. First, in studies on normative populations, formation of friendship has been shown to be related to other domains of development such as symbolic thinking, emotional understanding and expressiveness, cognitive and linguistic abilities, and representational abilities (Dunn, 1993; Hartup & Sancilio, 1986; Howes, 1992; Parker & Gottman, 1989). Second, research on disabled children who do have friends highlighted a pattern of characteristics. The more functional the disabled child was in terms of social skills and overall developmental level, especially cognitive–linguistic abilities (e.g., more extroverted, more assertive, more expressive, more verbal, higher IQ scores)— the greater was the child's likelihood of having friendships with handicapped or nonhandicapped peers (Buysse, 1993; Field, 1984; Siperstein & Bak, 1989; Strain, 1984). Third, several factors have been correlated with the autistic child's ability to engage in peer interactions, including cognitive abilities (Hauck et al., 1995; Sigman & Ruskin, 1999) and emotional understanding (Hauck et al., 1995). Language abilities, prosocial behaviors, and emotional responsiveness were likewise correlated with a high level of social play and a high frequency of initiations (Sigman & Ruskin, 1999). Taking all of these research findings into consideration, we might predict that high functioning children with autism who display good communicative, verbal, affective, and representational (symbolic play) abilities will be more likely to develop friendships.

A related major issue is the child's interest in being involved with peers. Children with autism show more social interest as adolescence approaches (American Psychiatric Association, 1994; Mesibov & Handlan, 1997). Therefore, we might expect to find more friendships or a greater desire for a friend at the onset of adolescence. Findings from studies of attachment in autism have demonstrated that the severity of the child's disorder was not associated with his or her ability to form a secure attachment (e.g., Rogers et al., 1993). On the other hand, although their interrelations remain unclear, it seems that IQ or mental age and linguistic competence are important factors in friendship formation. However, we have inadequate knowledge on the extent to which a child's speech, language, thinking, and play abilities may be impaired and yet he or she still succeeds in having friends. What competence levels are sufficient to allow the autistic child to form friendships? These issues call for further study.

The Role of Peers, Parents, and Teachers

According to the ecological view, the child's social environment (e.g., school and home) plays a significant role in helping the child with autism to establish and maintain friendships with peers (Bronfenbrenner, 1979, 1992). The following section examines the role that the child's peers, parents, and teachers have in the implementation of friendship in autism.

Peers' Role in Friendship

Parents' reports concerning high functioning preadolescents and adolescents with autism who did succeed in maintaining friendships demonstrated large variations in the characteristics of those friends (Bauminger & Shulman, 2001). Their friendships differed regarding their peers' age (younger, older, same age) and developmental status (e.g., high functioning peers with autism, peers with mental retardation, typically developing peers). Thus, the ability to predict specific peer characteristics that enhance friendship in autism remains problematic. However, based on the study of friendship in severely handicapped children (Grenot-Scheyer et al., 1998) some issues call for attention in planning interventions that facilitate friendship with peers: (1) common areas of interest and hobbies seem to be important for the initiation and the maintenance of friendship; (2) friendship should be significant, pleasant, and beneficial for both children; (3) teachers and parents need to support both children in the process of becoming friends; (4) reciprocity should be emphasized; and (5) children need to operate in a safe, accepting environment—implying, for example, that a typically developing child should have access to help when dealing with difficult autistic behaviors.

Grenot-Scheyer et al. (1998) revealed that some typically developing children were able to develop caring, affectionate, and secure relationships with severely handicapped children. These researchers described several important outcomes for typically developing children who have a severely handicapped child as a friend. They were found to reveal growth in their social cognitions and self-concept; to increase their tolerance and patience; to expand their awareness, understanding, and reactions to the needs of the child with disabilities; and to become more committed to personal and ethical principals. Future studies might focus more specifically on the benefits of having a child with autism as a friend.

Parents' Role in Friendship

The significant role of parents in promoting positive peer relationships has been recognized for typically developing children (Rotenberg, 1999). More specifically, parents (especially mothers) can increase their children's success in peer relationships by arranging their children's contacts with peers, and by facilitating children's cooperation and synchrony within peer relationships. Rotenberg suggested that children can also increase their social skills as a result of parental guidance and support in the process of friendship. Likewise, parents of children with autism reported that they had a significant role in providing opportunities for their child to meet with other children, and in supporting the ongoing process by physically bringing the friend, by "being nice to their child's friend," or by helping the two children find shared activities (Bauminger & Shulman, 2001). Thus, parents' ongoing support in their autistic children's friendships seems crucial.

Teachers' Role in Friendship

Although the classroom teacher is an important element in the child's support system within the school environment (e.g., Furman & Buhrmester, 1985), few studies have examined how the quality of teacher–child relationships is associated with children's affective experiences (e.g., friendship) in the school. Certain aspects of teacher–child interaction were found to be related with typically developing children's loneliness, including the level of conflict, closeness, and dependency experienced in those relationships (Burgess, Ladd, Kochenderfer, Lambert, & Birch, 1999). Closeness reflects warmth, affective ties, and security in relationships with significant adults. With teachers, closeness reflects whether children feel sufficiently secure to approach the teacher on personal matters and whether they use the teacher as a source of support. As a result, closeness seems important for any child's well being at school. In contrast, according to Burgess et al. (1999), conflictual teacher–child interactions and overly dependent relationships may result in a child's negative affective state, which may involve loneliness.

In autism, teachers have a greater role. They can: (1) identify potential pairs in class; (2) arrange common activities for the "identified pair" to experience, such as working together on shared projects; (3) incorporate conversations on friendship (e.g., what a friend is, how we choose friends, what we can do with friends) within the didactic program; (4) teach skills that facilitate the child's social competence and social understanding; and (5) inform parents about the potential friendships that have been identified in class.

Inter-Agent Collaboration

According to the ecological model, all of the aforementioned social agents—peers, parents, and teachers—operate in a shared environment and are thus interrelated. Some of the potential interrelationships between different settings appear to be particularly important for the formation of friendship in autism. Cooperation, shared efforts, and open communication between school and home seem critical. For example, a teacher may identify potential pairs but, by notifying the parents, these friendships will find another important source of nurturing and encouragement. When the parents of a typically developing child express concern regarding their child's friendship with a child with autism, open channels of communication with the school, support from the teacher, and contact with the other set of parents may enhance the former set of parents' understanding and cooperation. Other potential important interrelations would include open cooperation between different professionals at school (e.g., educational counselors who support the teacher). These sets of interrelations might directly and indirectly influence the formation of friendship in autism, and should be taken into consideration in intervention planning.

SUMMARY AND CONCLUSIONS

Loneliness and friendship have been presented in this chapter as two forms of social engagement. While the former, loneliness, reflects the lack of social engagement, the latter, friendship, reflects its presence. We have shown that the desire to have social relationships seems to be present at least among high functioning children with autism, but these youngsters possess less knowledge regarding how to create such relationships.

The formation of friendship with peers was perceived in the present chapter as having significant benefits to the enhancement of social skills for children with autism owing to the fact that it provides a predictable, familiar, and secure social framework. Issues that affect the formation of friendship in autism were discussed from an ecological perspective, an approach that emphasizes transactional influences between the child's characteristics and his or her social environment. On the whole, although friendship is a developing area for study in autism, findings do suggest that, for some children with autism, friendship is a concrete experience, while, for others, longing for a friend is a key source of personal frustration. Parents, teachers, and peers were identified as fundamental agents contributing to the formation of friendship, with an emphasis on their interrelations, such as open school–home communication.

The results of the examination of theoretical assumptions regarding friendship suggested that future studies should focus on the following issues to help the child with autism establish and maintain friendships with peers: (1) identifying subgroups of children with autism who are able to form friendships; (2) examining the unique manifestations of friendship in autism; (3) adapting a more cognitive–behavioral definition of social competence, together with an ecological model of intervention; and (4) examining the correlation between autistic children's ability to form a secure attachment and their ability to form friendships with peers.

In addition, further research would do well to examine the effectiveness of several avenues of intervention within a multidimensional, cognitive–behavioral approach toward social competence and friendship in autism. These may include: (1) direct training in specific social and behavioral skills, which may be helpful even for individuals who do not acquire the holistic, more meaningful friendship traits; (2) interventions targeting those indirect friendship qualities necessary for more highly evolved relations, that is, social and emotional understanding; and (3) supportive interventions that bolster the formation and maintenance of friendships. Using these three categories, attempts might be made to individualize intervention according to developmental level and in terms of the subgroups identified within the population on indices of attachment and social impairment.

ACKNOWLEDGMENTS

The authors would like to express their appreciation to Dee B. Ankonina for her editorial contribution.

REFERENCES

Ainsworth, M. D. S., Blehar, M. C., Waters, E., & Wall, S. (1978). *Patterns of Attachment: A Psychological Study of the Strange Situation*. Hillsdale, NJ: Erlbaum.
American Psychiatric Association. (1994). *Diagnostic and Statistical Manual of Mental Disorders* (4th ed.). Washington, DC: Author.
Asher, S. R., Hymel, S., & Renshaw, P. D. (1984). Loneliness in children. *Child Development, 55*, 1456–1464.

Asher, S. R., Parker, J. G., & Walker, D. L. (1996). Distinguishing friendship from acceptance: Implications for intervention and assessment. In W. M. Bukowski, A. F. Newcomb, & W. W. Hartup (Eds.), *The Company They Make: Friendships in Childhood and Adolescence* (pp. 366–406). Cambridge: Cambridge University Press.

Asher, S. R., Parkhurst, J. T., Hymel, S., & Williams, G. A. (1990). Peer rejection and loneliness in childhood. In S. R. Asher, & J. D. Coie (Eds.), *Peer Rejection in Childhood* (pp. 253–273). New York: Cambridge University Press.

Bacon, A. L., Fein, D., Morris, R., Waterhouse, L., & Allen, D. (1998). The responses of autistic children to the distress of others. *Journal of Autism and Developmental Disorders, 28,* 129–142.

Baron-Cohen, S., & Swettenham, J. (1997). Theory of mind in autism: Its relations to executive function and central coherence. In D. J. Cohen & F. R. Volkmar (Eds.), *Handbook of Autism and Developmental Disorders* (pp. 880–893). New York: John Wiley & Sons.

Bauminger, N., & Kasari, C. (2000). Loneliness and friendship in high-functioning children with autism. *Child Development, 71,* 447–456.

Bauminger, N., & Shulman, C. (2001). *Friendship in High-Functioning Children with Autism: Child's and Parent's Perspectives.* Paper presented at the Promised Childhood Congress, April, Israel.

Belchic, J. K., & Harris, S. L. (1994). The use of multiple peer exemplars to enhance the generalization of play skills to the siblings of children with autism. *Child and Family Behavior Therapy, 16,* 1–25.

Bemporad, J. R. (1979). Adult recollections of a formerly autistic child. *Journal of Autism and Developmental Disorders, 9,* 179–197.

Berndt, T. J. (1982). The features and effects of friendship in early adolescence. *Child Development, 53,* 1447–1469.

Bormann-Kischkel, C., Vilsmeier, M., & Baude, B. (1995). The development of emotional concept in autism. *Journal of Psychology and Psychiatry and Allied Disciplines, 36,* 1243–1259.

Bowlby, J. (1973). *Attachment and Loss: Separation Anxiety and Anger.* New York: Basic Books.

Bronfenbrenner, U. (1979). *The Ecology of Human Development: Experiment in Nature and Design.* Cambridge, MA: Harvard University Press.

Bronfenbrenner, U. (1992). Ecological systems theory. In R. Vasta (Ed.), *Annals of Child Development. Six Theories of Child Development: Revised Formulations and Current Issues* (pp. 178–249). London: Jessica Kingsley.

Burgess, K. B., Ladd, G. W., Kochenderfer, B. J, Lambert, S. F., & Birch, S. H. (1999). Loneliness during early childhood: The role of interpersonal behaviors and relationships. In K. J. Rotenberg, & S. Hymel (Eds.), *Loneliness in Childhood and Adolescence* (pp. 109–134). Cambridge: Cambridge University Press.

Buysse, V. (1993). Friendships of preschoolers with disabilities in community-based child care settings. *Journal of Early Intervention, 17,* 380–390.

Cairns, R. B., McGuire, A., & Gariepy, J. L. (1993). Developmental behavior genetics: Fusion, correlated constraints, and timing. In D. Hay & A. Angold (Eds.), *Precursors in Developmental Psychopathology* (pp. 78–122). Chichester, UK: John Wiley & Sons.

Capps, L., Sigman, M., & Mundy, P. (1994). Attachment security in children with autism. *Developmental Psychopathology, 6,* 249–261.

Capps, L., Yirmiya, N., & Sigman, M. (1992). Understanding of simple and complex emotions in non-retarded children with autism. *Journal of Child Psychology and Psychiatry and Allied Disciplines, 33,* 1169–1182.

Cassidy, J., & Asher, S. R. (1992). Loneliness and peer relations in young children. *Child Development, 63,* 350–365.

Cassidy, J., & Berlin, L. J. (1999). Understanding the origins of childhood loneliness: Contributions of attachment theory. In K. J. Rotenberg & S. Hymel (Eds.), *Loneliness in Childhood and Adolescence* (pp. 56–79). Cambridge: Cambridge University Press.

Celani, G., Battacchi, M. W., & Arcidiacono, L. (1999). The understanding of the emotional meaning of facial expressions in people with autism. *Journal of Autism and Developmental Disorders, 29,* 57–66.

Dissanayake, C., & Crossley, S. A. (1996). Proximity and sociable behaviors in autism: Evidence for attachment. *Journal of Child Psychology and Psychiatry, 37,* 149–156.

Dunn, J. (1993). *Young Children's Close Relationships: Beyond Attachment.* London: Sage.

Evans, I. M., Salisbury, C. L., Palombaro, M. M., Berryman, J., & Hollowood, T. M. (1992). Peer interactions and social acceptance of elementary-age children with severe disabilities in an inclusive school. *Journal of the Association for Persons with Severe Handicaps, 17,* 205–212.

Farmer, T. W., Pearl, R., & Van Acker, R. M. (1996). Expanding the social skills deficit framework: A developmental synthesis perspective, classroom social networks, and implications for the social growth of students with disabilities. *The Journal of Special Education, 30*, 232–256.

Field, T. (1984). Play behaviors of handicapped children who have friends. In T. Field, J. L. Roopnarine, & M. Siegal (Eds.), *Friendship in Normal and Handicapped Children* (pp. 153–163). Nortwood, NJ: Ablex.

Fromm-Reichmann, F. (1980). Loneliness. In J. Hartog, J. R. Audy, & Y. A. Cohen (Eds.), *The Anatomy of Loneliness* (pp. 338-361). New York: International Universities Press.

Furman, W., & Bierman, K. L. (1983). Developmental changes in young children's conceptions of friendship. *Child Development, 54*, 549–556.

Furman, W., & Buhrmester, D. (1985). Children's perceptions of the personal relationships in their social networks. *Developmental Psychology, 21*, 1016–1024.

Gaylord-Ross, R. J., Haring, T. G., Breen, C., & Pitts-Conway, V. (1984). The training and generalization of social interaction skills with autistic youth. *Journal of Applied Behavior Analysis, 17*, 229–247.

Grenot-Scheyer, M., Staub, D., Peck, C.A., & Schwartz, I. S. (1998). Reciprocity and friendships: Listening to the voices of children and youth with and without disabilities. In L. H. Meyer, P. Hyun-Sook, M. Grenot-Scheyer, I. S. Schwartz, & B. Harry (Eds.), *Making Friends* (pp. 149–168). Baltimore: Paul H. Brooks.

Harris, S. L., & Handleman, J. S. (1997). Helping children with autism enter the mainstream. In D. J. Cohen & F. R. Volkmar (Eds.), *Handbook of Autism and Developmental Disorders* (pp. 901–919). New York: John Wiley & Sons.

Hart, K. J., & Morgan, J. R. (1993). Cognitive behavioral therapy with children: Historical context and current status. In A. J. Finch, W. M. Nelson, & E. S. Ott (Eds.), *Cognitive Behavior Procedures with Children and Adolescents: A Practical Guide*. Boston: Allyn Bacon.

Hartup, W. W., & Sancilio, M. F. (1986). Children's friendships. In E. Schopler & G. Mesibove (Eds.), *Social Behavior and Autism* (pp. 61–79). New York: Plenum.

Hauck, M., Fein, D., Waterhouse, L., & Feinstein, C. (1995). Social initiations by autistic children to adults and other children. *Journal of Autism and Developmental Disorders, 25*, 579–595.

Hermelin, B., & O'Connor, N. (1985). Logico-affective states and nonverbal language. In E. Schopler, & G. B. Mesibov (Eds.), *Communication Problems in Autism* (pp. 283–309). New York: Plenum.

Hinde, R. (1976). On describing relationships. *Journal of Child Psychology and Psychiatry, 17*, 1–19.

Hinde, R. (1979). *Towards Understanding Relationships*. New York: Academic Press.

Hobson, R. P. (1993). The emotional origins of social understanding. *Philosophical Psychology, 6*, 227–245.

Howes, C. (1992). *The Collaborative Construction of Pretend*. Albany, NY: SUNY Press.

Howes, C. (1996). The earliest friendships. In W. M. Bukowski, A. F. Newcomb, & W. W. Hartup (Eds.), *The Company They Keep: Friendships in Childhood and Adolescence* (pp. 66–86). Cambridge: Cambridge University Press.

Hurley-Geffner, C. M. (1995). Friendship between children with and without developmental disabilities. In R. L. Koegel, & L. K. Koegel (Eds.), *Teaching Children with Autism: Strategies for Initiating Positive Interactions and Improving Learning Opportunities* (pp. 105–127). Baltimore: Brooks.

Jaedicke, S., Storoschuk, S., & Lord, C. (1994). Subjective experience and causes of affect in high-functioning children and adolescents with autism. *Development and Psychopathology, 6*, 273–284.

Kanner, L. (1943). Autistic disturbances of affective contact. *Nervous Child, 2*, 217–250.

Kanner, L., Rodriguez, A., & Ashenden, B. (1972). How far can autistic children go in matters of social adaptation? *Journal of Autism and Childhood Schizophrenia, 2*, 9–33.

Kasari, C., Chamberlain, B., Paparella, T., & Bauminger, N. (1999). *Self-evaluative social emotions in children with autism*. Poster presented at the Society of Research of Child and Adolescent Psychiatry, Barcelona, Spain.

Kasari, C., Paparella, T., & Bauminger, N. (1999). *Pride in High-Functioning Children with Autism*. Manuscript submitted for publication.

Kendall, P. C., & Panichelli-Mindel, S. (1995). Cognitive–behavioral treatments. *Journal of Abnormal Child Psychology, 23*, 107–124.

Koegel, R. L., & Frea, W. D. (1993). Treatment of social behavior in autism through the modification of pivotal social skills. *Journal of Applied Behavior Analysis, 26*, 369–377.

Koegel, L. K., Koegel, R. L., Hurley, C., & Frea, W. D. (1992). Improving social skills and disruptive behavior in children with autism through self-management. *Journal of Applied Behavior Analysis, 25*, 341–353.

Lord, C. (1984). The development of peer relations in children with autism. In F. J. Morrison, C. Lord, & D. P. Keating (Eds.), *Advances in Applied Developmental Psychology* (pp. 165–229). New York: Academic Press.

Margalit, M. (1994). *Loneliness Among Children with Special Needs*. New York: Springer-Verlag.

McGee, G. B., Krantz, P. J., & McClannahan, L. E. (1984). Conversational skills for autistic adolescents: Teaching assertiveness in naturalistic game setting. *Journal of Autism and Developmental Disorders, 14,* 319–330.

Mesibov, G., & Handlan, S. (1997). Adolescents and adults with autism. In D. J. Cohen, & F. R. Volkmar (Eds.), *Handbook of Autism and Developmental Disorders* (pp. 309–324). New York: John Wiley & Sons.

Newcomb, A. F., & Bagwell, C. L. (1995). Children's friendship relations: A meta-analytic review. *Psychological Bulletin, 117,* 306–347.

Niemtimp, E. G., & Cole, C. L. (1992). Teaching socially valid social interaction responses to students with severe disabilities in an integrated school setting. *Journal of School Psychology, 30,* 343–354.

Odom, S. L., & Strain, P. S. (1986). A comparison of peer initiation and teacher antecedent interventions for promoting reciprocal social interactions of autistic preschoolers. *Journal of Applied Behavior Analysis, 19,* 59–71.

Odom, S. L., & Watts, P. S. (1991). Reducing teacher prompts in peer-mediated interventions for young children with autism. *Journal of Special Education, 25,* 26–43.

Oke, N., & Schreibman, L. (1990). Training social initiations to a high functioning autistic child: Assessment of collateral behavior change and generalization in a case study. *Journal of Autism and Developmental Disorders, 20,* 479–497.

Parker, J. G., & Gottman, J. M. (1989). Social and emotional development in a relational context: Friendship interaction from early childhood to adolescence. In T. Brendt, & G. Ladd (Eds.), *Peer Relationships in Child Development* (pp. 95–131). New York: John Wiley & Sons.

Parker, J. G., Rubin, K. H., Price, J. M., & DeRosier, M. E. (1995). Peer relationships, child development, and adjustment: A developmental psychopathology perspective. In D. Cicchetti, & D. J. Cohen (Eds.), *Developmental Psychopathology* (pp. 96–161). New York: John Wiley & Sons.

Parker, J. G., Saxon, J. L., Asher, S. R., & Kovacs, D. M. (1999). Dimensions of children's friendship adjustment: Implications for understanding loneliness. In K. J. Rotenberg & S. Hymel (Eds.), *Loneliness in Childhood and Adolescence* (pp. 201–224). Cambridge: Cambridge University Press.

Parker, J. G., & Seal, J. (1996). Forming, losing, renewing, and replacing friendships: Applying temporal parameters to the assessment of children's friendship experiences. *Child Development, 67,* 2248–2268.

Perlman, D., & Peplau, L. A. (1982). Theoretical approaches to loneliness. In L. A. Peplau & D. Perlman (Eds.), *Loneliness: A Source Book of Current Theory, Research and Therapy* (pp. 123–134). New York: John Wiley & Sons.

Roeyers, H. (1996). The influence of non-handicapped peers on the social interactions of children with pervasive developmental disorders. *Journal of Autism and Developmental Disorders, 26,* 303–320.

Rogers, S., Ozonoff, S., & Masline-Cole, C. (1991). A comparative study of attachment behavior in children with autism and children with other disorders of behavior and development. *Journal of American Academy of Child and Adolescence Psychiatry, 30,* 433–438.

Rogers, S., Ozonoff, S., & Masline-Cole, C. (1993). Developmental aspects of attachment behavior in young children with pervasive developmental disorder. *Journal of American Academy of Child and Adolescence Psychiatry, 32,* 1274–1282.

Rotenberg, K. J. (1999). Parental antecedents of children's loneliness. In K. J. Rotenberg & S. Hymel (Eds.), *Loneliness in Childhood and Adolescence* (pp. 176–200). Cambridge: Cambridge University Press.

Russo, D. C., & Koegel, R. L. (1977). A method of integrating an autistic child into a normal public school classroom. *Journal of Applied Behavior Analysis, 10,* 579–590.

Sameroff, A. J. (1983). Developmental systems: Contexts and evolution. In P. H. Mussen (Series Ed.) & W. Kessen (Vol. Ed.), *Handbook of Child Psychiatry,* Vol. 1. *History, Theories, and Methods* (pp. 237–294). New York: John Wiley & Sons.

Shapiro, T., Sherman, M., Calamari, G., & Koch, D. (1987). Attachment in autism and other developmental disorders. *Journal of American Academy of Child and Adolescence Psychiatry, 26,* 480–484.

Sigman, M., & Capps, L. (1997). *Children with Autism: A Developmental Perspective.* London: Harvard University Press.

Sigman, M., & Mundy, P. (1989). Social attachment in autistic children. *Journal of American Academy of Child and Adolescence Psychiatry, 28,* 74–81.

Sigman, M., & Ruskin, E. (1999). Continuity and change in the social competence of children with autism, Downs syndrome, and developmental delays. *Monographs of the Society for Research in Child Development, 64* (1, Serial No. 256).

Sigman, M., & Ungerer, J. (1984). Attachment behaviors in autistic children. *Journal of Autism and Developmental Disorders, 14,* 231–243.

Siperstein, G. N., & Bak, J. J. (1989). Social relationships of adolescents with moderate mental retardation. *Mental Retardation, 27,* 5–10.

Sontag, J. C. (1996). Toward a comprehensive theoretical framework for disability research: Bronfenbrenner revisited. *The Journal of Special Education, 30,* 319–344.

Strain, P. (1984). Social behavior patterns of nonhandicapped and developmentally disabled friend pairs in mainstream preschools. *Analysis and Intervention in Developmental Disabilities, 4,* 15–28.

Sullivan, H. S. (1953). *The Interpersonal Theory of Psychiatry.* New York: Horton.

Terrell-Deutsch, B. (1999). The conceptualization and measurement of childhood loneliness. In K. J. Rotenberg & S. Hymel (Eds.), *Loneliness in Childhood and Adolescence* (pp. 11–33). Cambridge: Cambridge University Press.

Ungerer, J. (1989). The early development of autistic children. In G. Dawson (Ed.), *Autism: Nature, Diagnosis and Treatment.* New York: Guilford.

Volkmar, F. R., & Cohen, D. J. (1985). The experience of infantile autism: A first-person account by Tony W. *Journal of Autism and Developmental Disorders, 15,* 47–54.

Waterhouse, L., & Fein, D. (1997). Perspectives on social impairment. In D. J. Cohen & F. R. Volkmar (Eds.), *Handbook of Autism and Developmental Disorders* (pp. 901–919). New York: John Wiley & Sons.

Weiss, R. S. (1973). Loneliness: *The Experience of Emotional and Social Isolation.* Cambridge, MA: The MIT Press.

Wing, L. (1992). Manifestation of social problems in high-functioning autistic people. In E. Schopler & G. Mesibov (Eds.), *High-Functioning Individuals with Autism* (pp. 129–142). New York: Plenum.

World Health Organization. (1990). International classification of diseases (10th ed., ICD-10). *Diagnostic Criteria for Research (DRAFT).* Geneva: Author.

Yirmiya, N., Sigman, M., Kasari, C., & Mundy, P. (1992). Empathy and cognition in high functioning children with autism. *Child Development, 63,* 150–165.

IV

Education and Interventions

12

Issues in Early Diagnosis and Intervention with Young Children with Autism

Lee M. Marcus, Ann Garfinkle, and Mark Wolery

In the past few years, the reported incidence of autism has increased at a remarkably high rate across the world. There are at least two reasons for this: broader boundaries of the definition, including high functioning persons with autism (and Asperger's syndrome) and the diagnosis of very young children (Filipek et al., 1999; Stone et al., 1999). These two trends have increased the numbers from the historical 4–5 per 10,000 to as high as 1 per 200 (depending on how loosely the criteria are applied). This dramatic explosion in the number of diagnoses may be attributable to more knowledge of the parameters, better trained clinicians, a broader definition of the condition, an actual increase in affected cases, and possibly false-positives diagnoses. Nonetheless, the practical reality is that this disorder and its variants have shifted from a low-incidence problem to a significant diagnostic and treatment challenge to the wide professional community. This rise is especially noted in the area of early intervention, which has become both a fertile ground for the development of innovative and effective techniques (Dawson & Osterling, 1997; Harris & Handleman, 1994; Hurth, Shaw, Izeman, Whaley, & Rogers, 1999) and a battleground for controversial claims and disputes (Gresham & MacMillan, 1998; see Schopler, Chapter 2, this volume).

Although it is not exactly clear what differentiates effective from ineffective early intervention, there is little doubt that providing education and treatment to very young children can have a very positive effect on their future development and prognosis (Rogers, 1996). There is consensus that early intervention should target those areas of weakness (social, communicative, cognitive) that form the constellation of characteristics of autism (Dawson & Osterling, 1997). It appears equally true that although there are many programs and approaches that report good outcomes, no comparative studies exist, so that at this stage in our knowledge it would be premature and unwise to consider any one method a treatment

LEE M. MARCUS • Division TEACCH, School of Medicine, University of North Carolina at Chapel Hill, Chapel Hill, North Carolina 27599-6305.   ANN GARFINKLE • Department of Special Education, Peabody College, Vanderbilt University, Nashville, Tennessee 37203.   MARK WOLERY • Frank Porter Graham Child Development Center, University of North Carolina at Chapel Hill, Chapel Hill, North Carolina 27599-8180.

The Research Basis for Autism Intervention, edited by Schopler, Yirmiya, Shulman, and Marcus. Kluwer Academic / Plenum Publishers, New York, 2001.

of choice. Unfortunately, in the long and checkered history of autism research and practice, many therapies have been touted as the best or key approach and, currently, in the excitement of the early identification movement, "most effective" has become an obsession for parents and many professionals. To avoid this trap, regardless of the age of the child, intervention should always be based on a combination of a thorough understanding of the nature of autism, in general; an awareness of the range of best practices; and individualizing the program for the child based on a careful, comprehensive assessment. Another consideration in early intervention is the real or imagined distinction between programs for children under 3 and those from 3 to 5 years of age. In the United States, funding for infants and toddlers is typically directed to the health and human service system, whereas funding for preschool age children is directed to the public schools. Does this imply that the needs and methods for these two age groups are different? Much of the published research has investigated children 3 years and older and then extrapolated to children under 3. It is not obvious if strategies developed for older children with autism can be generalized to very young children. While much has been learned about early intervention in the past decade, there remain more questions than answers. In this chapter we review critical factors in early diagnosis, summarize trends and recommended practices in early intervention, and describe a new program for very young children with autism.

FACTORS IN EARLY DIAGNOSIS

The trend toward very early diagnosis has been fueled by increased knowledge of typical and atypical social and communication developmental patterns (Mundy, Sigman, Ungerer, & Sherman, 1987; Stone, Ousley, Yoder, Hogan, & Hepburn, 1997; Trepagnier, 1996), legally mandated services for young children with special needs, and greater sophistication of parents, coupled with the Internet-based information explosion. In the past, a diagnosis by age 5 (more or less the age at which Kanner diagnosed and defined his cases) was considered reasonable, even though most parents had suspected that something (e.g., speech and language development) was wrong 2 or 3 years earlier (Short & Schopler, 1988). Currently, it is common to have diagnoses established at least by age 3 (Rogers, 2000; Stone et al., 1999). Given that some of the primary symptoms of autism may not manifest themselves unequivocally before age 3, it is interesting that a number of researchers are convinced that a meaningful diagnosis can be made in children as young as 12 months (Baranek, 1999a; Teitelbaum, Teitelbaim, Nye, Fryman, & Maurer, 1998). From the parental perspective, any delay in obtaining the correct diagnosis is costly. In a recent informal survey of parents involved with the TEACCH program in North Carolina, parents interviewed unanimously strongly regretted that they had not been given an early diagnosis, even though their children had been diagnosed by age 3 (Marcus & Reagan, 1998). With better understanding of significant developmental markers such as joint attention, eye contact and gaze, and other aspects of nonverbal communication and greater awareness in the professional community of what constitutes the boundaries of autism-spectrum disorders, we will continue to see more emphasis on early diagnosis. At the same time, caution is needed about overdiagnosis or premature diagnosis on the basis of too few signs or developmental irregularities or delays that may improve spontaneously (see Burack et al., Chapter 3, this volume, for further discussion of developmental issues).

Atypical Behaviors in Children under 36 Months

Stone (1997) reported a number of behaviors that distinguished infants and toddlers with autism from other children. With respect to social behaviors, early signs of autism included poor imitation, abnormal eye contact, ignoring or being unresponsive to others, little interest in social games, bland affective expression, and a preference for being alone. Osterling and Dawson (1994, 1999) and others who have done videotape studies of very young children (Baranek, 1999a; Mars, Mauk, & Dowrick, 1998) have also noted atypical social development in orienting to own name calling, aversion to social touch, failure to point, and showing. Filipek et al. (1999), in their comprehensive review of screening and diagnostic issues, emphasized the importance of parental concerns, such as the child being in his or her own world, being too "independent," tuning out, and lacking interest in other children.

Atypical communication behaviors include delays in speech, little use of gestures, and failure to attract attention of others to own activities (Lord & Paul, 1997; Mundy, Sigman, & Kasari, 1990). Nonverbal aspects of communication, including facial expression and body language, may be even more important as an index of autistic development for very young children than for older children. By contrast, children with other developmental problems, but not autism, will also show speech and language delays, but fewer problems with gestural communication. Concerns reported by parents include their child appearing deaf or inconsistently responsive to sounds at times, not following directions, loss of speech, and parental difficulty understanding what the child wants.

With regard to repetitive and restricted interests, the following behaviors have been noted to be significant for very young children: motor stereotypies, attachment to unusual objects, unusual play, unusual visual interests, and inconsistent response to sounds. Parents report concerns with toe walking, getting stuck on things over and over, lining things up, and odd movement patterns Filipek et al., 1999).

In considering how diagnostic features may differ between younger and older children with autism, Stone (1997) identifies three possible characteristics that are not seen in very young children: disordered peer relationships (the expectations for peer interactions at this age are much less), abnormal language features (harder to differentiate from other developmentally delayed children), and need for sameness and routines (perhaps too young for such patterns to be established or for the child to be that aware of his environment).

Atypical Behaviors in Preschool-Age Children

As the young child matures, certain developmental aspects of social, communication, and other behavioral characteristics emerge or sharpen and have been studied (Marcus & Stone, 1993; Mundy & Crowson, 1997; Sigman & Rhonda, 1993; Stone, Lemanek, Fishel, Fernandez, & Altemeier, 1990). Among these patterns are eye-to-eye gaze, joint attention, understanding and expression of affect, motor imitation, and functional and symbolic play. Although also relevant for children under 3 years of age, researchers have focused on and found that these behaviors seem to differentiate the preschooler with autism from his peers. These characteristics have not been studied as much in older persons with autism, although it is likely that developmental irregularities in these areas persist.

In addition to the social and communication deficits observed in young autistic children, there are a number of problematic learning characteristics that affect cognitive functioning and are important to recognize if proper intervention planning is to occur. These learning problems have been documented in theoretical constructs such as executive function, theory of mind, and central coherence (Bailey, Phillips, & Rutter, 1996; Baron-Cohen & Swettenham, 1997; Ozonoff, 1997) as well as based in clinical practice and experience (Mesibov & Shea, in press).

Among the cognitive (or thinking) problems are: difficulties in interpreting the meaning of events, difficulties in organization and sequencing, poor or weak ability to attend to relevant stimuli (or becoming overly focused on irrelevant or extraneous details), an uneven pattern of development such that visual skills tend to be stronger than auditory skills, and a poor sense of time. Children with autism tend to be literal or concrete in their thinking. Problem-solving skills are weak, and inflexibility in play and daily routines, in part, stems from these cognitive deficits. Often, what is seen as a behavioral problem (e.g., not following through with a parental request) is better understood as a cognitive shortcoming such as not understanding the sequence of events or being able to organize a set of responses.

Correctly diagnosing the young child with autism requires a thorough understanding of the dimensions of this disorder across the spectrum of levels of severity and mental and chronological ages. In addition to in-depth knowledge of the specific social, communication, and cognitive characteristics of autism, the clinician and researcher must have an appreciation for normal development of young children as well as delayed development. The purposes of early diagnosis are to clarify the nature of the child's developmental problems and obtain appropriate intervention services that can help reduce the long-term impact of the disorder. Perhaps most important of all, early diagnosis provides parents with helpful information and support to enable them to cope successfully with their child's disability (Marcus, Kunce, & Schopler, 1997). In the next sections, we review the relevance of these learning characteristics for intervention strategies, basic components of effective preschool programs, examples of program models, and specific techniques.

INTERVENTION STRATEGIES BASED ON LEARNING CHARACTERISTICS

The learning and cognitive/thinking problems outlined in the preceding (e.g., organization and sequencing, generalization, imitation, focusing on relevant information) have implications for intervention strategies for young autistic children across functioning levels that can be carried out at home, or in a school or community setting. The following list is intended to be illustrative, not necessarily exhaustive.

1. *Clarifying meaningful information.* Highlighting, color coding, and labeling can help the child focus on what is meaningful and overcome the tendency to focus on irrelevant details. Demonstrating the appropriate use of a toy, within the child's developmental level of understanding, can shift his or her attention away from tangential aspects of the material.

2. *Organization and scheduling.* Given the young autistic child's organizational and temporal processing problems, providing him or her with a way of understanding

what is coming next and how to go about sequencing an activity can reduce stress and teach independence. Most young children with autism who are nonverbal might need a transition object to know where to go next (e.g., a cup for a snack), while a verbal child might be able to associate a picture with the next activity.

3. *Teaching across settings and people.* The generalization problems of children with autism necessitates that skills and desired behaviors are taught in different settings and with different people. For example, if a child has learned to hand a cup for juice at school, that response should be encouraged at home and at different times.

4. *Active and directed instruction.* Given the autistic child's problems of attending to relevant stimuli, problem-solving, and initiation, teaching needs to more directed than with the typical child. If left to their own devices, most young children with autism will engage in repetitive, nonconstructive play and will need a guided, at times somewhat intrusive, approach to learn new skills.

5. *Individualization of teaching methods and curriculum.* An implication of the unevenness of the child's development and heterogeneity of their autism is the importance of tailoring a program, including both teaching techniques and curriculum content. Two children of the same age with the same diagnosis may have a very different program, if individualization is considered. One child may need to start with learning cause-and-effect sequences, while another may benefit from categorization tasks. One child might need a long processing time to understand a demonstration or direction, while another will process quickly.

6. *Providing visual supports.* Given the characteristically weak auditory processing and relatively strong visual skills, it makes sense and has been demonstrated to be effective (Schopler, Mesibov, & Hearsey, 1995) for autistic children to be provided with visual cues or supports. Particularly in the early years when language understanding is very tenuous and communication abilities quite limited, adding a visual cue in the form of an object or picture or other meaningful item can greatly assist their understanding of what is expected. On the expressive side, giving the child something tangible to communicate with can facilitate their connection to people and make the communication process effective (Watson, Lord, Schaffer, & Schopler, 1989).

7. *Teaching imitation at a developmentally appropriate level.* Since imitation is a core skill related to social development, language, and imagination and a deficit in young children with autism (Stone et al., 1990), it should be a basic part of a curriculum. However, the decision about how to teach imitation should be based on an assessment of the child's level and understanding of the process. For example, a child at a very early stage should not be expected to imitate unfamiliar or novel actions, but rather to have his or her own behaviors copied by the adult. Meaningless and repetitive copying by the child is not a means of teaching the concept of imitation.

8. *Using strengths and interests to help with weak areas of development.* One implication of having an uneven pattern of development is that a child will have strengths and weaknesses, and the strengths (e.g., visual memory) can be used to work on the weaker area (e.g., sequencing). What this means is that direct teaching in the deficit area without recognizing and utilizing the child's better skills and high interests is likely to cause frustration and resistance. For example, requiring the child to follow

a verbal direction when he or she does not have adequate language comprehension, without a concrete or visual cue, will end not only in a failure to respond, but, perhaps, in an angry outburst. Combining the verbal direction with an understandable cue in an area of interest will result in more success and a calmer reaction.

BASIC COMPONENTS OF A PRESCHOOL PROGRAM

The strategies described in the preceding have been incorporated into many preschool and early intervention programs, although their philosophies and approaches may differ. Dawson and Osterling (1997) comprehensively reviewed early intervention programs and identified a list of general components that these model programs shared in common regardless of the philosophy (also see Handleman & Harris, 2000, for detailed descriptions of model programs). These components have been utilized by school systems and other service providers in helping to develop new programs for preschoolers with autism. Dawson and Osterling divided these components into two categories: basic components and other recommended components, with the former being considered a part of each of the models they reviewed. Since their review provides an objective, unbiased, and thorough account, it is worth listing these components as an overall framework for what are the current practices in the field. As noted earlier, no meaningful distinctions have been made, with regard to intervention, between young children under 3 years and those older than 3 years; although the reviewed programs are almost exclusively designed for children older than 3 years, the strategies and components are likely to be relevant for the very young as well. Basic components include:

1. *Curriculum emphasizes attention/compliance, imitation, language, and social skills.* Although different programs might vary with respect to how they teach these areas, this curriculum is consistent with the areas identified as unique needs in autism and of greatest importance for development.
2. *Works to establish "core processes" (e.g., imitation and attention) in a highly structured teaching environment.* Again, although the definition of how to provide structure might differ from model to model, there is general acceptance of the principle that intervention must be directly guided by the adult and not by the child. There is room for flexibility and incorporating the child's interests and perspective, but the lead is externally promoted and directed.
3. *Addresses the child's need for predictability and routine.* This component involves consistent daily schedules and activities, systematic ways of presenting information and communicating with the child, and teaching daily chores and self-help routines that are familiar and repetitive.
4. *Programs for generalization of skills.* As noted earlier, generalization is a fundamental weakness in autistic children and strategies for both response and stimulus generalization are built into model programs.
5. *Decrease behavior problems by increasing communication skills.* This component reflects the crucial principle that most behavior problems in autistic children, particularly young children, are the result of some aspect of their disorder and

communication is a primary factor. By improving the child's ability to communicate, behaviors such as temper tantrums can be reduced.

6. *Programs for transition to kindergarten.* If the preschool child is going to make a smooth transition to the next level program, steps need to be taken by the current preschool to maximize his chances for success. Such steps may include visiting various program options with the parents; identifying what the structure, curriculum, and behavioral expectations might be; finding out what resources are available; and establishing a follow-up plan of support. Typically the Individualized Education Plan for the kindergarten year is written in the spring of the final preschool year and should incorporate how the transition will be facilitated as well as the basic goals and objectives. Although most parents and preschool staffs hope that the next step will be regular education, with or without support, other special education alternatives need to be considered as well.

7. *Encourage family involvement.* The crucial role of parents in the education of their autistic child cannot be overestimated, especially during the preschool years. Schopler, Mesibov, Shigley, and Bashford (1984) have noted that parents can be trainers as well as trainees, provide as well as receive emotional support from staff, and learn to be effective advocates. The early years, during which services to the child and family can be the most intense and personalized, should lay the foundation for a lifetime of positive experiences for parents as they navigate the multiple service systems.

Other Recommended Components of a Preschool Program

Dawson and Osterling also noted important strategies or methods not utilized by all the models reviewed, but worth considering.

1. *Provides augmentative communication methods.* Because many, if not most, young autistic children lack meaningful speech as they begin their program, providing an alternative or augmentative approach, such as pictures, objects, or manual signs (Prizant & Wetherby, 1989), should be considered.

2. *At least 15 hours per week.* An unfortunate aspect of the early intervention movement is the emphasis on the number of hours per week that is necessary for positive changes to be seen. The concept of "intensity," although superficially equated with hours of direct teaching, is complex. Meaningful engagement (McWilliam & Bailey, 1992) is a term that may better reflect what is important, since it does not depend on a child interacting with others or being taught by an adult, but applies to useful time spent with materials and activities such as climbing on playground equipment. A lower limit of 15 hours per week makes sense and avoids the rhetoric of the hour numbers game that distracts from focusing on the more relevant factors of curriculum and content of instruction.

3. *Provides Occupational Therapy (OT) services.* Not all children with autism have fine or gross motor or sensori-integration difficulties, but those who do can benefit from the services of an occupational therapist who provides service either directly or through consultation to the teacher and/or parents. Most children enjoy the

activities designed by OTs and parents are usually enthusiastic about their child's participation.

4. *Includes normally developing peers*. It seems axiomatic that, with their serious communication and social difficulties, young autistic children need to be actively involved with typical peers, yet the nature of their imitation and learning characteristics significantly hampers their ability to benefit from peer experiences. Still, most programs make efforts to find ways and develop innovative strategies to capitalize on the natural teaching and modeling skills of nondisabled peers or peers with mild disabilities other than autism. Parents desperately desire their autistic child to "make it" in the regular world, although most understand that this adjustment does not come easily. The critical point, not always acknowledged by professionals, is that successful integration requires as much, if not more, structured teaching and systematic planning as other curriculum areas.

5. *Emphasizes child independence, initiative, and choice-making*. Given the tendency of the autistic child's to become cue dependent, passive, and struggle with making informed choices, building in systems and strategies for overcoming these problems makes sense as part of the child's program. Examples of how to develop these skills include following an individualized daily schedule, a work or study system (Schopler, Mesibov, & Hearsey, 1995), and having a choice board in a play area.

BRIEF REVIEW OF PROGRAM MODELS

Although, as Dawson and Osterling (1997) effectively documented, diverse programs across the United States share a number of common ideas and methods, the philosophical frameworks may differ and these need to be recognized. In this review, we provide one way of classifying the majority of early intervention programs that are well documented and that articulate their model. Our review is intended as illustrative of an organizational scheme. Handleman and Harris (2000) provide more in-depth details and descriptions about these programs.

1. *Primarily behavioral (ABA)*. Examples of program models that are based on applied behavioral analysis are Douglass Development Center (Handleman & Harris, 1994), Princeton Child Developmental Center (McClannahan & Krantz, 1994), and the Young Child Project at UCLA (Lovaas, 1987). Although built around the principles of ABA, these programs are not carbon copies or monolithic forms of one another. The UCLA program, for example, strongly emphasizes discrete trial training (DTT), home-based therapy, and 40 hours per week minimum with the expectation that the child will move next to a regular preschool or kindergarten setting. The other programs use DTT as a key method of delivering direct instruction, but also include other methods, do not necessarily prescribe a certain number of hours, and utilize a classroom setting. However, all the programs derive from the behavioral framework and tradition whose roots lie in the work of B. F. Skinner and the learning theorists and researchers who followed.

2. *Primarily developmental (social–emotional theory)*. Examples of programs whose techniques are grounded in developmental theory are Greenspan's "floortime" (Greenspan & Weider, 1998) [recently described in workshops and trainings as the

Developmental, Individual-Difference, Relationship-Based (DIR) model] and the project at the University of Colorado Health Sciences Center (Rogers & Lewis, 1989). Although the specific theoretical framework of these two programs may slightly differ, both proceed from the assumption that understanding and dealing with the social–emotional variables in the child is the key to improving development. There is less emphasis on directed intervention and more on following the child's lead. Relationship-building with the therapist and parent is central, as is the notion that affective development precedes and promotes cognitive and language development. This therapeutically oriented approach to child development does not preclude other intervention strategies such as speech and language, OT, or a preschool classroom, but it is viewed as, perhaps, a prerequisite to the successful mastery of abstract concept and skill learning.

3. *Inclusive/behavioral.* Examples of programs that combine principles of ABA and inclusive education are the LEAP (Strain & Cordisco, 1994) and Walden School (McGee, Daly, & Jacobs, 1994) projects. Although other behaviorally based classroom programs such as Douglass are committed to peer involvement at some point, LEAP and Walden design their curriculum and instructional methodologies to be carried out in a carefully organized inclusive classroom setting. Each program has a fixed number of typical and autistic students and a systematic process for teaching a full range of skills, although the primary goal is social and communication development. The expectation is that, by providing an ABA-type program in an inclusive setting, the young autistic child will benefit from the "best of both worlds" and be well prepared for the transition to a regular kindergarten or preschool.

4. *Integrative.* Examples of a holistic or integrative approach are the TEACCH program at the University of North Carolina (Marcus, Schopler & Lord, 2000; Schopler, 1987) and the TRIAD project at Vanderbilt University (Stone & Ruble, 1999). By integrative we mean a blending of empirically based methodologies and conceptual frameworks that include developmental, social cognition, behavioral, and neuropsychological perspectives. Rather than drawing from one theoretical model or set of principles, these programs take what is known from current research and practice in a variety of areas and apply these ideas in an individualized way. Not only are strategies of intervention meant to reflect a broad spectrum of sound concepts, but the contexts in which the instruction is given are varied and flexibly organized. For example, in the TEACCH program, some preschoolers are judged to learn best in a highly specialized setting with five children, a teacher, and an assistant; another child may do better in a regular preschool appropriately adapted; and a third may do best in a preschool with language-handicapped or developmentally delayed but not autistic students. Regardless of the setting, instruction is based on an individualized developmental and functional assessment (Schopler, Reichler, Bashford, Lansing, & Marcus, 1990) and the use of structured teaching (Schopler et al., 1995).

EXAMPLES OF SPECIFIC INTERVENTION STRATEGIES

Within the context of the models listed in the preceding section, a number of specific techniques can be utilized, although most programs are likely to choose strategies considered compatible with their approach. Some examples of such techniques that have been shown to be of value in programs for young children with autism are briefly described.

1. *Structured teaching.* As noted earlier, most programs emphasize structure, but the term may differ across models. TEACCH has developed the concept of structured teaching as both a curriculum domain and a set of instructional strategies. Structured teaching is organized around four components: physical structure, the individualized daily schedule, the work system, and visual structure (Schopler et al., 1995). By incorporating all four dimensions of structure into the classroom, home, and community, the child's chances of learning, becoming independent, and behaviorally adjusted are enhanced.

2. *Discrete trial training (DTT).* DTT is a central component in ABA programs because of its emphasis on teaching of basic skills in a step-by-step fashion. The technique involves breaking down a skill such as learning colors by having the child select a card among a series and touching or giving it to the teacher. It is based on a stimulus, response and consequence sequence with importance on reinforcing a correct response. By successively shaping correct responses, users of DTT hope to teach fundamental learning skills across a wide range of functions (e.g., imitation, expressive language) so that eventually the child will be an independent learner.

3. *Picture Exchange Communication System (PECS).* PECS is a systematic, behaviorally based approach that is intended to enable the student to overcome the basic communication understanding and intent problems common in autism (Frost & Bondy, 1994). As a nonverbal technique, it initially bypasses the verbal challenges faced by the autistic student. A key component of PECS is the emphasis on two-way communication as the child is prompted and guided to hand a picture of a desired object or activity to the teacher. Unlike DTT, it does not direct the child to give an answer, but starts with the child's observed interests and builds on them.

4. *Floortime.* Floortime is a play-based technique that emphasizes engaging the child at the level where he or she is socially and emotionally functioning and builds on that with the expectation that the child will develop improved play, communication, and cognitive skills (Greenspan & Weider, 1998). In contrast to the other techniques, floortime is not considered a structured approach, but one in which the child's lead is followed. In practice, the child, therapist, and parent work together with the therapist, guiding and coaching the parent to make the experience as positive and successful as possible. Although floortime can be used in a classroom, its main focus has been in the home to promote the child–parent relationship and development of the child's affective experience.

5. *Incidental learning or teaching.* Incidental learning is the process whereby the child is indirectly taught concepts and skills in a natural context as the teacher or parent capitalizes on a situation that occurs (McGee et al., 1994). It is a systematic approach because the teacher is looking for opportunities to expose the child to a learning activity that is not formally set up. For example, in the play area, the child might pick up some blocks in a random fashion and the teacher might redirect the child to stack them or construct a pattern. Like DIR, it can start with the child's initiation, but it is more directed with specific and defined goals.

Having reviewed a number of programs and strategies, the next section of the chapter will describe a new project for children under 3 years. Most of the programs previously reviewed have been implemented with young children over age 3.

THE CENTER-BASED EARLY INTERVENTION DEMONSTRATION PROJECT FOR CHILDREN WITH AUTISM

This project is a partnership between the Frank Porter Graham Child Development Center and Division TEACCH, both at the University of North Carolina—Chapel Hill. The project is supported by North Carolina's Department of Health and Human Services, Division of Early Intervention and Education and has three broad goals: (1) to design, implement, and evaluate a program for children under the age of 3 who have been diagnosed with autism; (2) to describe the model, in particular, its principles and practices as they pertain to the classroom and support for families; and (3) to provide outreach and technical assistance to Early Interventionists in North Carolina.

For each funded year of the model program, a total of six children are targeted for intervention. Each of the six children has a diagnosis of autism and is younger than 30 months of age. Children who meet these criteria are offered enrollment in the program on a first-come, first-served basis. Even when enrollment is offered, the decision to participate is made by the family.

The six target children attend one of four project classrooms, located at the Frank Porter Graham Child Development Center's Childcare. All of the project classroom are inclusive—that is, there are more typically developing children than children with disabilities enrolled in each class. Three of the classrooms have seven children total (five typically developing children; one child with autism; one child with a disability other then autism) and are staffed by a head teacher and a teaching assistant. The fourth classroom has nine children enrolled (six typically developing children; three children with autism) and are staffed with a head teacher and two teaching assistants. The target children spend between 20 and 40 hours a week in these classrooms.

The Frank Porter Graham Child Care Program (including the project classrooms) is accredited by the National Association for the Education of Young Children (NEAYC). As a result, the classes are structured and operated following the guidelines of developmentally appropriate practices that are sanctioned and recommended by NEAYC; guidelines are described in detail in many sources (Bredekamp & Copple, 1997). Further, the quality of the classroom environment is rated using the Infant/Toddler Environmental Rating Scale (I/TERS) (Harms, Clifford, & Cryer, 1990). It is these guidelines and standards that describe the basis of each project classroom. It is recognized, however, that even though these standards and guidelines help create classrooms that support the development and learning of typically developing children, it is not sufficient to support the development and learning of children who develop atypically, particularly children with autism. The target children therefore received specialized instruction or therapy. This therapy is delivered using an integrated therapy approach wherein the therapists (e.g., speech–language pathologist, occupational therapist, special educator, and so forth) come into the child's classroom and provide services in the child's context. The goal of the therapist is not only to interact with the target child, but also to guide the teacher and help the teacher integrate the therapeutic programs throughout the child's day. In this way the classroom can also be described as using a transdisciplinary model of service delivery (McWilliam, 1996).

The project's curriculum is unique to each classroom in that teachers, in consultation with the special service providers, develop the themes and plan learning activities to meet the needs of the children in their classroom. For the target children, their learning experiences are guided by the goals and objectives developed by the school staff and the parents. These goals and objectives are formalized in the Individualized Family Service Plan (IFSP) and reviewed with the parents at least every 6 months. By definition, the IFSP is individualized; thus, every target child has a program designed to meet his individualized needs. However, all of the target children have individual goals in each of the following five areas: language, toy play, attention, social interactions, and imitation. These five areas are targeted because they have been identified as being deficit areas for young children with autism (Dawson & Osterling, 1997).

In addition to the classroom (or center-based) component, the program provides family support. At a minimum families receive one home visit each month. Families may receive more support based on the needs of the child and the family. Just as the child's classroom program is individualized, so is the family support. Family support is given in many ways: parents are taught ways to interact with their children; parents are shown ways to help their children learn; parents are supplied with respite; and parents are given information about other community resources that may be helpful to their family. All families are encouraged to participate in peer support.

Given that there is a paucity of information about effective programs for very young children with autism and that this is a new program, many scales and assessments are being used to help evaluate the effectiveness of the program. The scales being used are as follows: Mullen Scales of Early Learning (Mullen, 1995), Vineland ABS and SEEC (Sparrow, Balla, & Cicchetti, 1984, 1998), Child Behavior Checklist (Achenbach, 1992), Temperament and Atypical Behavior Scale (TABS) (Neisworth, Bagnato, Salvia, & Hunt, 1999), Parent Stress Index (Abidin, 1995), Preschool Language Scale-3 (Zimmerman, Steiner, & Pond, 1992), MacArthur Language Sample (Fenson et al., 1993), Structured Play Assessment (Reinhartsen, Baranek, Pretzel, & Teplin, 1998), Knox Preschool Play Scale (Knox, 1997), and the Sensory Supplement Questionnaire (Baranek, 1999b). Each of these assessments is administered as children enter the program, after they have been enrolled in the program for 6 months, and as they exit the program (children exit the program when they turn 3). The project is in its early stage and it is too soon to evaluate its effectiveness, aside from the very positive responses of the families who have participated so far; in the future, we expect to document critical factors in this type of early intervention program.

IMPLICATIONS FOR FUTURE INTERVENTION RESEARCH AND PRACTICE

There appear to be at least four trends affecting issues in early diagnosis and intervention, mostly positive: (1) Diagnoses and are being made at earlier and earlier ages with increasing degrees of confidence and clarity. (2) Researchers are identifying important underlying mechanisms that affect learning and behavioral characteristics and these mechanisms, such as social referencing and joint attention, can be a focus for intervention. (3) Parents have greater exposure than ever to current practices, both positive and negative;

are more sophisticated in their knowledge than in the past; and, perhaps, as a result, have become very critical consumers. (4) There is a dangerous fractionalization in the field where promotion of an approach or program seems to take precedence over what is in the best interests of the child and family.

In addition to being aware of these and other trends, professionals and parents need to continue to work collaboratively, researchers and practitioners must meaningfully translate and share their findings for one another, and good faith efforts need to be taken to avoid the negativism and harsh rhetoric that sometimes mark the arguments among professionals. Constructs from neuropsychological, developmental, and behavioral research have the potential to infuse instructional techniques, especially if the conceptual knowledge is transformed into practical strategies and different models incorporate overlapping ideas. Parents, who are the consumers and a primary beneficiary of helpful information, should not be caught in the crossfire of conflicting methodologies. They do not really care about professional turfism, other than how it interferes with obtaining good services. They are not invested in any one framework. The professional community is obligated not only to investigate, develop, and provide the best practices available, but to do so in a spirit of cooperation and mutual respect. To that end, overstated claims of success or most effectiveness need to be tempered by a realistic cautiousness and open-mindedness to the work of others in the field. The new decade promises more exciting developments in early diagnosis and intervention which, hopefully, will be accomplished as a partnership between researchers, practitioners, and parents.

REFERENCES

Abidin, R. R. (1995). *Parenting Stress Index*. Odessa, FL: Psychological Assessment Resources.

Achenbach, T. M. (1992). *Manual for the Child Behavior Checklist and 1992 Profile*. Burlington: University of Vermont Department of Psychiatry.

Bailey, A., Phillips, W., & Rutter, M. (1996). Autism: Towards an integration of clinical, genetic, neuropsychological, and neurobiological perspectives. *Journal of Child Psychology and Psychiatry, 37*, 89–126.

Baranek, G. T. (1999a). Autism during infancy: A retrospective video analysis of sensory-motor and social behaviors at 9–12 months of age. *Journal of Autism and Developmental Disorders, 29*, 213–224.

Baranek, G. T. (1999b). *Sensory Supplemental Questionnaire*. Chapel Hill: University of North Carolina.

Baron-Cohen, S., & Swettenham, J. (1997). Theory of mind: Its relationship to executive function and central coherence. In D. J. Cohen and F. R. Volkmar (Eds.), *Handbook of Autism and Pervasive Developmental Disorders*, 2nd ed. (pp. 880–893) New York: John Wiley & Sons.

Bredekamp, S., & Copple, C. (Eds.) (1997). *Developmentally Appropriate Practice in Early Childhood Program*, 2nd ed. Washington, DC: National Association for the Education of Young Children.

Dawson, G., & Osterling, J. (1997). Early intervention in autism: Effectiveness and common elements of current approaches. In M. J. Guralnick (Ed.), *The Effectiveness of Early Intervention: Second Generation Research* (pp. 307–326). Baltimore, MD: Paul H. Brookes.

Fenson, L., Dale, P., Reznick, S., Thal, D., Bates, E., Hartung, J., Pethick, S., & Reilly, J. (1993). *MacArthur Communication Development Inventories*. San Diego, CA: Singular.

Filipek, P. A., & (in alphabetical order) Accardo, P. J., Baranek, G. T., Cook, E. H., Dawson, G., Gordon, B., Gravel, J. S., Johnson, C. P., Kallen, R. J., Levy, S. E., Minshew, N. J., Prizant, B. M., Rapin, I., Rogers, S. J., Stone, W. L., Teplin, S., Tuchman, R. F., & Volkmar, F. R. (1999). The screening and diagnosis of autism spectrum disorders. *Journal of Autism and Developmental Disorders, 29*, 439–484.

Frost, C., & Bondy, A. (1994). PECS: *The Picture Exchange Communication Manual*. Cherry Hill, NJ: Pyramid Educational Consultants.

Greenspan, S. I., & Weider, S. (1998). *The Child with Special Needs: Intellectual and Emotional Growth*. Reading, MA: Addison Wesley Longman.

Gresham, F. M., & MacMillan (1998). Early intervention project: Can its claims be substantiated and its effects replicated? *Journal of Autism and Developmental Disorders, 28,* 5–12.

Handleman, J. S., & Harris, S. (1994). The Douglass Developmental Disabilities Center. In S. Harris & J. S. Handleman (Eds.), *Preschool Education Programs for Children with Autism* (pp. 71–86). Austin, TX: PRO-ED.

Harms, T., Clifford, R. M., & Cryer, D. (1990). *Infant/Toddler Environmental Rating Scale*. New York: Teachers College Press.

Harris, S., & Handleman, J. S. (Eds.) (1994). *Preschool Education Programs for Children with Autism*. Austin, TX: PRO-ED.

Handleman, J. S., & Harris, S. (Eds.) (2000). *Preschool Education Programs for Children with Autism*, 2nd ed. Austin, TX: PRO-ED.

Hurth, J., Shaw, E., Izeman, S., Whaley, K. & Rogers, S. (1999). Areas of agreement about effective practices among programs serving young children with autism spectrum disorders. *Infants and Young Children, 12,* 17–26.

Knox, S. (1997). Development and current use of the Knox Preschool Play Scale. In D. Parham & L. Fazio (Eds.), *Play in Occupational Therapy for Children*. (pp. 35–51). St. Louis, MO: Mosby.

Lord, C., & Paul, R. (1997). Language and communication in autism. In D. J. Cohen and F. R. Volkmar (Eds.), *Handbook of Autism and Pervasive Developmental Disorders*, 2nd edit (pp. 195–225). New York: John Wiley & Sons.

Lovaas, O. I. (1987). Behavioral treatment and normal educational and intellectual functioning in young autistic children. *Journal of Consulting and Clinical Psychology, 55,* 3–9.

Marcus, L. M., Kunce, L. J., & Schopler, E. (1997). Working with families. In D. J. Cohen and F. R. Volkmar (Eds.), *Handbook of Autism and Pervasive Developmental Disorders*, 2nd ed. (pp. 631–649). New York: John Wiley & Sons.

Marcus, L., & Reagan, C. (1998). *Interpreting diagnostic information to parents of young children with autism*. Paper presented at the 10th Annual Leo M. Croghan Conference, Raleigh, NC.

Marcus, L. M., Schopler, E., & Lord, C. (2000). TEACCH Services for Preschool Children. In J. S. Handleman & S. L. Harris (Eds.), *Preschool Education Programs for Children with Autism*, 2nd ed. (pp. 215–232). Austin, TX: PRO-ED.

Marcus, L. M., & Stone, W. L. (1993). Assessment of the young autistic child. In E. Schopler, M. E. Van Bourgondien, & M. Bristol (Eds.), *Preschool Issues in Autism and Related Developmental Handicaps* (pp. 149–173). New York: Plenum.

Mars, A. E., Mauk, J. E., & Dowrick, P. (1998). Symptoms of pervasive developmental disorders as observed in prediagnostic home videos of infants and toddlers. *Journal of Pediatrics, 132,* 500–504.

McClannahan, L., & Krantz, P. (1994). The Princeton Child Development Institute. In S. Harris & J. S. Handleman (Eds.), *Preschool Education Programs for Children with Autism* (pp. 107–126). Austin, TX: PRO-ED.

McGee, G., Daly, T., & Jacobs, H. A. (1994). The Walden Preschool. In S. Harris & J. S. Handleman (Eds.), *Preschool Education Programs for Children with Autism* (pp. 127–162). Austin, TX: PRO-ED.

McWilliam, R. A. (1996). *Rethinking Pull-Out Services in Early Intervention: A Professional Resource*. Baltimore, MD: Paul H. Brookes.

McWilliam, R. A., & Bailey, D. B. (1992). Promoting engagement and mastery. In D. B. Bailey & M. Wolery (Eds.), *Teaching Infants and Preschoolers with Disabilities*, 2nd ed. (pp. 229–255). Columbus, OH: Macmillan.

Mesibov, G. B., & Shea, V. (in press). The culture of autism. In G. B. Mesibov & E. Schopler (Eds.), *The TEACCH Approach to Working with Students with Autism*. New York: Kluwer.

Mullen, E. M. (1995). *Mullen Scales of Early Learning*. Circle Pines, MN: American Guidance Service.

Mundy, P., & Crowson, M. (1997). Joint attention and early social communication: Implications for research on intervention with autism. *Journal of Autism and Developmental Disorders, 27,* 653–676.

Mundy, P., Sigman, M., & Kasari, C. (1990). A longitudinal study of joint attention and language development in autistic children. *Journal of Autism and Developmental Disorders, 20,* 115–128.

Mundy, P., Sigman, M., Ungerer, J., & Sherman, T. (1987). Defining the social deficits of autism: The contribution of non-verbal communication measures. *Journal of Child Psychology and Psychiatry, 27,* 657–669.

Neisworth, J. T., Bagnato, S. J., Salvia, J., & Hunt, F. M. (1999). *Temperament and Atypical Behavior Scale: Early Childhood Indicators of Developmental Dysfunction*. Baltimore, MD: Paul H. Brookes.

Osterling, J., & Dawson, G. (1994). Early recognition of children with autism: A study of first birthday home videotapes. *Journal of Autism and Developmental Disorders, 24,* 247–257.

Osterling, J., & Dawson, G. (1999). *Early identification of 1-year-olds with autism versus mental retardation based on home videotapes of first birthday parties*. Paper presented at the Proceedings of the Society for Research in Child Development, Albuquerque, NM.

Ozonoff, S. (1997). Causal mechanisms of autism: unifying perspectives from an information-processing frame- work. In D. J. Cohen and F. R. Volkmar (Eds.), *Handbook of Autism and Pervasive Developmental Disorders*, 2nd ed. (pp. 868–879). New York: John Wiley & Sons.

Prizant, B., & Wetherby, A. (1989). Enhancing language and communication in autism: From theory to practice. In G. Dawson (Ed.), *Autism: Nature, Diagnosis, and Treatment* (pp. 282–309). New York: Guilford.

Reinhartsen, D., Baranek, G. T., Pretzel, R., & Teplin, S. (1998). *Structured Play Assessment*. Unpublished manuscript. Chapel Hill, NC: University of North Carolina.

Rogers, S. J. (1996). Brief report: Early intervention in autism. *Journal of Autism and Developmental Disorders*, *26*, 243–247.

Rogers, S. J. (2000). Differential diagnosis of autism before age 3. *International Review of Research in Mental Retardation*, *23*, 1–31.

Rogers, S. J., & Lewis, H. (1989). An effective day treatment model for young children with pervasive develop- mental disorders. *Journal of the American Academy of Child and Adolescent Psychiatry*, *28*, 207–214.

Schopler, E. (1987). Specific and non-specific factors in the effectiveness of a treatment system. *American Psychologist*, *42*, 376–383.

Schopler, E., Mesibov, G. B., & Hearsey, K. (1995).Structured teaching in the TEACCH system. In E. Schopler & G. B. Mesibov (Eds.). *Learning and Cognition in Autism* (pp. 243–268). New York: Plenum

Schopler, E., Mesibov, G. B., Shigley, R. H., & Bashford, A. (1984). Helping autistic children through their parents: The TEACCH model. In E. Schopler & G. B. Mesibov (Eds.), *The Effects of Autism on the Family* (pp. 65–81). New York: Plenum.

Schopler, E., Reichler, R. J., Bashford, A., Lansing, M., & Marcus, L. M. (1990). *Individualized Assessment and Treatment for Autistic and Developmentally Disabled Children*, Vol. I. *Psychoeducational Profile Revised (PEP-R)*. Austin, TX: PRO-ED.

Short, A. B., & Schopler, E. (1988). Factors relating to age of onset in autism. *Journal of Autism and Developmen- tal Disorders*, *18*, 207–216.

Sigman, M., & Rhonda, S. (1993). Pretend play in high-risk and developmentally delayed children. *New Directions for Child Development*, *59*, 29–42.

Sparrow, S. S., Balla, D. A., & Cicchetti, D. V. (1984). *Vineland Adaptive Behaviors Scales—Interview Edition*. Circle Pines, MN: American Guidance Service.

Sparrow, S. S., Balla, D. A., & Cicchetti, D. V. (1998). *Vineland Social-Emotional Early Childhood Scales*. Circle Pines, MN: American Guidance Service.

Stone, W. L. (1997). Autism in infancy and early childhood. In D. J. Cohen and F. R. Volkmar (Eds.), *Handbook of Autism and Pervasive Developmental Disorders*, 2nd ed. (pp. 266–282). New York: John Wiley & Sons.

Stone, W. L., Lee, E. B., Ashford, L., Brissie, J., Hepburn, S. L., Coonrod, E. E., & Weiss, B. H. (1999). Can autism be diagnosed accurately in children under three years? *Journal of Child Psychiatry and Psychiatry*, *40*, 219–226.

Stone, W. L., Lemanek, K. L., Fishel, P. T., Fernandez, M. C., & Altemeier, W. A. (1990). Play and imitation skills in the diagnosis of autism in young children. *Pediatrics*, *86*, 267–272.

Stone, W. L., Ousley, O. Y., Yoder, P. J., Hogan, K. L., & Hepburn, S. L. (1997). Nonverbal communication in two- and three-year old children with autism. *Journal of Autism and Developmental Disorders*, *27*, 677–696.

Stone, W. L., & Ruble, L. (1999). *Early identification for children with autism*. Workshop sponsored by the Pennsylvania Departments of Health Education and Public Welfare through Early Intervention Technical Assistance, Gibsonia, PA.

Strain, P. S., & Cordisco, L. K. (1994). LEAP Preschool. In S. Harris & J. S. Handleman (Eds.), *Preschool Education Programs for Children with Autism* (pp. 225–252). Austin, TX: PRO-ED.

Teitelbaum, P., Teitelbaum, O., Nye, J., Fryman, J., & Maurer, R. G. (1998). Movement analysis in infancy may be useful for early diagnosis of autism. *Proceedings of the National Academy of Science USA*, *95*, 13982–12987.

Trepagnier, C. (1996). A possible origin for the social and communicative deficits of autism. *Focus on Autism and Other Developmental Disabilities*, *11*, 170–182.

Watson, L., Lord, C., Schaffer, B., & Schopler, E. (1989). *Teaching Spontaneous Communication to Autistic and Developmentally Handicapped Children*. New York: Irvington.

Zimmerman, I., Steiner, V., & Pond, R. (1992). *Preschool Language Scale-3*. San Antonio, TX: The Psychological Corporation.

13

Evaluating Treatment Effects for Adolescents and Adults with Autism in Residential Settings

Mary E. Van Bourgondien and Nancy C. Reichle

Learning is a lifelong activity for individuals with autism. Adults with autism continue to need treatment to maximize the quality of their lives and their ability to function in the community as independently as possible. Historically, the primary treatment approach for adults has been through residential programs. The goal of this chapter is to describe the existing research on the effectiveness of residential programs for adults with autism. By examining the treatment goals of adult services and the research to date, directions and approaches for future research are outlined.

A current emphasis in outcome research within the field of autism is on the effects of early intervention with children with autism (Dawson & Osterling, 1997). Researchers have attempted to determine how different types of educational and behavioral interventions affect the development of young children with autism. Outcome measures have included measures of cognitive and adaptive development, behavioral functioning, social and communication skills, and educational placements as well as parent satisfaction. This focus on early development follows naturally from the belief that during the preschool years the child has the greatest capacity to learn and grow.

In contrast, there has been very little research on the effectiveness of treatment interventions with adolescents and adults with autism. Historically, the major treatment milieu for adults with autism and other developmental disabilities was residential programs or institutions (Hilton, 1987). There is limited research that documents the effectiveness of residential treatment models for individuals with autism.

This chapter reviews the goals of residential programs, and then summarizes the available literature on the effects of treatment approaches for adults with autism. The results

MARY E. VAN BOURGONDIEN and NANCY C. REICHLE • Division TEACCH, School of Medicine, University of North Carolina at Chapel Hill, Chapel Hill, North Carolina 27599-7180.

The Research Basis for Autism Intervention, edited by Schopler, Yirmiya, Shulman, and Marcus. Kluwer Academic/Plenum Publishers, New York, 2001.

of this review are synthesized to give direction for both content issues and methodological considerations for future studies.

DETERMINANTS OF OUTCOME MEASURES

To evaluate the effectiveness of a residential treatment program, it is important to first recognize the purpose of the placements. The goals of residential treatment programs for individuals with autism may vary depending on the interests and needs of an individual, his or her family, and the philosophy of the program (Van Bourgondien & Reichle, 1997).

INDIVIDUAL/FAMILY/PROGRAM GOALS

Individual Goals

Each adult with autism is an individual with her or his own personality, preferences, and needs. Like any adults who leave home, one would expect that adults with autism will value living and work opportunities that enable them to pursue their interests and areas of strength. While others may have expectations of growth and positive changes in behaviors, these may not be the primary objective for persons with autism. The degree of control or autonomy the individuals have in using their skills is more apt to be an important goal for them. To reflect the individual perspective, outcome measures need to determine the degree to which the individual can communicate preferences and engage in high interest activities that utilize his or her strengths.

Family Goals

For many families of children with autism, the highest priority in a group home is a family atmosphere with caring, concerned staff members who will keep their children safe and interact with them as if they were the parents (Sloan & Schopler, 1977). Another major goal for parents is to have a permanent placement for their sons and daughters where they can stay long after the parents are deceased (Wall, 1990). In discussions with parents seeking services, many families express the desire for a program where the staff members understand autism and utilize the successful treatment techniques for these individuals. The families would also like for their adult children to be as involved in their communities as possible.

Program Goals

From a program perspective, programs specifically designed for individuals with autism also emphasize the importance of understanding autism and providing an individualized program based on a careful assessment of the adults' skills, needs, and interests (Holmes, 1990; Kay, 1990; LaVigna, 1983; Lettick, 1983; Wall, 1990). The goals of these programs are typically to increase an individual's skills while decreasing problem behavior, with the ultimate objective being to enhance the individual's involvement and acceptance in the community (Van Bourgondien & Reichle, 1997). Specific skill areas addressed in residential programs for adults include self-help and domestic skills, communication skills, leisure, recreation, and social skills. In addition, these programs are often either directly or indirectly involved in developing vocational skills and behaviors.

Based on both the objectives of the individuals and the families and the stated goals of the residential treatment programs, program evaluation research needs to examine the effectiveness of residential treatment options from several perspectives. From the perspective of the treatment programs, outcome measures should address whether specific skills are increased and whether inappropriate behaviors are decreased. While family members may share these objectives, they are also looking for other benefits. The family's general satisfaction with this alternative living situation is an equally important consideration. From the family's perspective, outcome measures need to examine the degree of supervision, stimulation, and autism-specific structure that are provided to the residents. Socialization and community involvement are also important areas to assess. To maintain the individual's perspective, all measures need to take into account individually defined skills, behaviors, needs, and preferences.

PROGRAM EVALUATION RESEARCH

Skill Acquisition in Adults

Several studies have investigated the acquisition of specific skills by adults with autism living in residential treatment settings (LaVigna, 1983; Smith & Belcher, 1985). LaVigna (1983) reported successful skill acquisition by the first six adult residents of the Jay Nolan Center in California. All six men had spent a significant portion of their lives in an institutional setting. Utilizing a training program based on Marc Gold's task analysis procedures (Gold, 1976), tasks were reduced to sequential steps and trainers provided the minimal assistance required for the resident to complete each step successfully. Staff members encouraged the residents to "try another way" prior to providing assistance.

The results indicated that as a group, the six residents mastered 105 skills in 2½ years in the areas of self-help, home care, and cooking. Two residents achieved the skills needed to move into a home with fewer staff members. Utilizing the same training approach the residents also mastered a variety of ground maintenance skills in the vocational program.

In a similar study, Smith and Belcher (1985) examined the impact of a life skills training program on five adults with autism in community-based group home settings in the Community Services for Autistic Adults and Children (CSAAC) program in Maryland. Each of the residents was assigned an individualized treatment objective based on the assessment of the interdisciplinary team. The target behaviors included cleaning the sink, cooking spaghetti, hair combing, face washing, and tooth brushing. Utilizing task analyses and systematic training procedures, the direct care staff members provided ongoing training to the residents. Over time, all residents gradually increased the number of steps they could perform without assistance.

Both the LaVigna (1983) and the Smith and Belcher (1985) studies suggest that task analysis and systematic prompt hierarchies are helpful for increasing the skills of adults with autism. The lack of comparison groups or multiple baseline designs makes it difficult to establish with certainty the exact reason for the residents' improvements.

Reduction in Inappropriate Behaviors in Adults

Brown (1991); Elliot, Dobbin, Rose, and Soper (1994); and Reese, Sherman, and Sheldon (1998) have examined how specific treatment approaches have reduced the behavior problems of individual residents. Brown (1991) utilized case studies to demonstrate the importance of lifestyle preferences when designing daily activities for individuals in residential settings. Many of the case examples included individuals with autism and demonstrated that utilizing the concepts of communication, choice, and refusal within their daily routine proved to be effective strategies for reducing challenging behaviors. She recommended examining the individual's preferences regarding time, content, and sequences when setting up a daily schedule. For example, some individuals perform best when the schedule has no fixed times for when an activity needs to be performed. Recognizing a person's need to go at his or her own pace may reduce behavior problems. Some individuals need to know exactly what activities they will do that day, while others prefer more choices about the content of their daily schedule. The sequence dimension looks at whether an individual prefers to do a single activity followed by a break versus a series of activities that are linked together in a predictable sequence. To be able to detect individuals' preferences regarding their schedules, measurement of outcome needs to include progress in following the schedule in addition to assessing the acquisition of skills and the reduction in challenging behavior.

Elliot et al. (1994) examined the impact of antecedent exercise conditions on the maladaptive and stereotypic behaviors of six adults with both autism and moderate to profound mental retardation. The behaviors were observed before and after three levels of exercise—aerobic, general motor exercise, and no exercise. Each participant experienced each of these conditions five times in a randomly assigned order with at least 48 hours between each session. Only the aerobic exercise significantly reduced maladaptative and stereotypic behaviors in the controlled setting. Although there were significant group findings, three of the six participants accounted for most of the effect, suggesting that there are individual differences in response to exercise. Studies with adolescents with autism (Rosenthal-Malek & Mitchell, 1997) and with adults with other types of developmental disabilities (McGimsey & Favell, 1988) have also supported the effectiveness of exercise in reducing inappropriate behaviors.

Reese et al. (1998) utilized single-subject methodology to study the impact of differentially reinforcing other behaviors (DROs) to reduce the frequency of aggressive and disruptive behavior (hitting, kicking, cursing, verbal threats, and throwing things) in an adult with autism. The treatment package included DROs, token fines, and prompted relaxation. The study design included an initial baseline session followed by treatment sessions, reversal to baseline, treatment sessions, return to baseline, treatment session, reversal to baseline, treatment, and then maintenance. The aggressive and disruptive behaviors were measured during three different activities in the group home—household jobs, leisure time, and individual instruction time. The baseline rates of the negative behavior varied between activities. During each activity an initial reduction of the problem behaviors was dependent on choosing an appropriate DRO interval, with shorter DRO intervals required during activities in which the baseline rates of the agitated–disruptive behavior were higher. Teaching counselors delivered tokens during the household chores and individual instruction activities. A peer with Down syndrome and mental retardation gave the reinforcement during the leisure time. Once shorter DRO intervals had been used to reduce the agitated–disruptive behavior, longer intervals between reinforcers were effective in maintaining those reductions. Reductions in problem behaviors were maintained for up to 6 months.

EFFECTS OF RESIDENTIAL TREATMENT ON CHILDREN WITH AUTISM

Sherman, Barker, Lorimer, Swinson, and Factor (1988) investigated the relative effectiveness of three different treatment approaches—Home-Based, Outpatient, and Residential for children with autism. Fifteen children were divided into three treatment groups—Home-Based, Outpatient, and Residential. The goal of each setting was to improve the child's self-help, social, and leisure skills and to reduce inappropriate behaviors. The Home-Based model involved intensive work directly with the child as well as parent training and school consultation. The outpatient model was a less intensive version of the home-based intervention. The trainers primarily trained the parent and did not work directly with the children. In the residential program, the five participants received direct training in the residential setting, but parents were not involved in the treatment. Behavior observations and psychometric evaluations of basic functional skills were collected during initial baseline period, after a 6-month treatment period and after a return to the baseline condition. The results indicated that all three types of treatments had comparable effectiveness, with slightly more significant changes in the Home-Based group. Based on both clinical and economic factors, the authors recommended outpatient and home-based treatment for children with autism.

Daily Life Therapy is the primary treatment approach at the Higashi School in Massachusetts, where a majority of students participate in the residential program (Larkin & Gurry, 1998). Daily Life Therapy emphasizes group-oriented instruction, highly structured routine activities, imitation, rigorous physical exercise, and a curriculum that focuses on movement, music, and art (Quill, Gurry, & Larkin, 1989). An observational study over 2 years of three students ages 15, 11, and 6 found that the students increased their attending behavior and decreased their inappropriate behaviors. Appropriate skills were either unchanged or in one case declined over the course of the study. Therefore, while the Daily Life Therapy helped the children to watch the teacher, be quiet, well behaved, and to sit at their desks in a group context, they did not increase their ability to follow directions or to comprehend what the teacher was asking them to do. No comparison group or multiple baseline design was used in this study.

A MULTIDIMENSIONAL APPROACH TO EVALUATING A RESIDENTIAL TREATMENT PROGRAM FOR ADULTS

Van Bourgondien, Reichle, Schopler, and Mesibov (1996) evaluated the effectiveness of a residential program, based on the TEACCH psychoeducational model, in improving the stimulation, care, and adaptation of adults with autism who had severe handicaps and behavioral problems. This study is reviewed in depth as an example of how to examine treatment effectiveness from individual, family, and program perspectives.

The Carolina Living and Learning Center (CLLC) is a combination residential and vocational treatment program developed by Division TEACCH. The program utilizes the individually defined interests and visual strengths of individuals with autism to improve their self-care and domestic skills, communication skills, and social experiences. The vocational program is integrated with the residential program and emphasizes farming, landscaping, and baking activities (Van Bourgondien & Reichle, 1996, 1997).

The treatment study involved 32 adults with autism who had applied for admission to the CLLC. Six participants were admitted to the special treatment program (CLLC) based on a part random, part clinical assignment process. The comparison participants lived in three different types of settings: group homes—10 participants, institutions—6 participants, family homes—nd 10 participants. Baseline analyses indicated that all groups were generally comparable and that subjects on average had moderate to severe autism and their adaptive skills were in the severe to profound range of disability. Most participants had a history of challenging behaviors.

The outcome measures in this study attempted to address the variety of objectives of residential treatment. Changes in participant's skills and behaviors were measured through direct assessment and observational measures as well as through interviews and questionnaires that were completed by the primary caregivers. The Adolescent and Adult Psychoeducational Profile (AAPEP) (Mesibov, Schopler, Schaffer, & Landrus, 1988) was used to assess the participants skills in six domains: vocational skills, independent functioning, leisure skills, vocational behavior, functional communication, and interpersonal behavior. A single index of adaptive skills was empirically created. The behaviors of the adults were assessed through two questionnaire measures—the Autism Behavior Inventory (Van Bourgondien & Mesibov, 1989) and the Vineland Maladaptive Scale (Sparrow, Balla, & Cicchetti, 1984). A single index of Negative Behavior was created empirically based on these two measures. A modified version of Landesman's Behavior Observation Scale (Landesman, 1987) that included individually defined problem behaviors was used to record observed behaviors during work, meal, and transition times.

To assess the nature of the living and treatment settings, the Environmental Rating Scale (ERS) (Van Bourgondien, Reichle, Campbell, & Mesibov, 1998) was utilized as a measure of environmental adaptation and individualized programming based on the TEACCH philosophy. The ERS consists of five subscales: Communication, Structure, Social and Leisure Skill Development, Developmental Assessment and Planning, and Behavior Management. The scoring of the ERS is based on a semistructured interview of the caregiver and a tour of the living environment.

In addition, at the conclusion of the study all families completed a Family Satisfaction Questionnaire. The families were asked to rate their overall satisfaction with the placement and their offsprings' general well being as well as their satisfaction with the physical environment, direct care staff, and administrative staff members.

Each study participant was assessed at four time periods of 6-month intervals. The two baseline assessments occurred 6 months and 1 month prior to the participants in the treatment group moving into the CLLC. The final two assessments occurred 6 to 12 months following the move the to CLLC.

Environmental Treatment Activities

Participants who entered the specialized treatment setting received significantly more individualized environmental adaptation and treatment programming at the study's conclusion from the CLLC than they had in their baseline settings in all areas—communication, use of visual structure, socialization, developmental assessment and planning, positive, preventive behavior, and management. No significant changes occurred in any of the other comparison groups' environments over time. When the final environments of all four groups were compared, the participants at the CLLC were receiving significantly more communicative adaptations, structure, socialization experiences, and positive, preventative approaches to managing behaviors than were the participants in group homes, family homes, or institutions. The CLLC was also significantly more likely to engage in developmental assessments and individualized planning activities than were either the institutions or the family homes.

Family Satisfaction

Families whose adult offspring were placed at the CLLC were significantly more satisfied than parents whose children were in other group homes in terms of their general satisfaction, as well as satisfaction with direct care staff members and administration and with the impact the placement had on the family. The ratings of the parents of the adults in institutional settings were generally between the other two groups (CLLC and group homes) and did not differ significantly from either group. There was no difference between groups in their satisfaction with the physical settings.

Skills

The results of the study indicated that there were no significant changes in skills as measured by the AAPEP regardless of setting. When all the subjects were grouped together and the Environmental Rating Scale (ERS) was treated as a continuous variable, there was no relationship between treatment approach and change in skills over time. Given the severity of the sample, the short duration of the study, and the fact that most of the subjects had received treatment for many years, it is not surprising that there were no detectable changes in skills over time by any group given the use of this general measure of adaptive behavior (AAPEP).

Behaviors

The results of the behavior questionnaires indicated that there were generally no changes over time in any group. Regardless of setting, however, the best predictor of negative behavior at the study's conclusion was aggression at baseline.

When all the subjects were grouped together and the ERS was used as a continuous variable, there were significant relationships between the outcome of the negative behavior index and the current environment and the changes in the environment over time. The use over time of visual structure, positive preventative behavioral approaches, and adaptive communication strategies was related to a decrease in negative behaviors over time. The reduction in use of these techniques was related to an increase in negative behaviors over time.

The results of this study clearly demonstrated that the participants in the specialized treatment setting received significantly more stimulation, individualized instruction, and socialization experiences in the community than participants in other settings. The families were significantly more satisfied with this setting than with the group homes. Changes in skills were not documented on a general measure of adaptive behavior, while interactions between treatment approaches and changes in behaviors over time were suggestive of areas for further study. The authors caution that given the small sample size the results of the interactions should be considered exploratory in nature.

CONCLUSIONS BASED ON AVAILABLE RESEARCH

Behavior Problems

The effectiveness of treatment programs designed to reduce the behavior problems of adults with autism has the strongest research support to date. Taken together, the studies cited in this chapter suggest the effectiveness of a multidimensional positive/preventative behavioral approach in reducing the behavior problems of adults with autism. Differential reinforcement of other behaviors (Reese et al., 1998), use of exercise (Elliot et al., 1994), adapting communication techniques, providing choices, and using visual structure to make the environment more predictable (Brown, 1991; Van Bourgondien et al., 1996) can all play a role in reducing negative behaviors. Both Reese et al. (1998) and Van Bourgondien et al. (1996) suggest that the intervention for negative behaviors needs to be maintained on an ongoing basis to sustain the reduction in behavior problems.

Skill Acquisition

Demonstrating the effectiveness of a residential program in the acquisition of skills by adults with autism is a more challenging area. Both LaVigna (1983) and Smith and Belcher (1985) gave clinical examples of how the residents' skills increased over time with systematic training. Given the lack of control groups or single-subject multiple baseline designs, it is hard to determine what element of the treatment environment is responsible for change, and whether the change generalized to other skills or was maintained over time. Van Bourgondien et al.'s (1996) lack of change in skills as measured by the AAPEP was not surprising given the general nature of the instrument and the severity of the cognitive challenges of participants. Interviews with staff members of the various programs indicated that many of the participants were gaining specific skills; however, the AAPEP was too general to pick up on these highly individualized treatment effects. It appears that the best approach to evaluating the effects of treatment programs on the acquisition of skills will build on the work of LaVigna (1983) and Smith and Belcher (1985) while employing more experimental controls. Concrete and individually defined teaching goals seem to be the most appropriate targets given the diversity of skills and previous learning experiences of adults with autism. Utilizing more single-subject multiple baseline designs will help to determine the specificity of the success of treatment techniques and the generalizability of the treatment outcomes.

Quality of Living Environment

Based on observations of the individual preferences of adults with autism and discussions with family members, there are other important dimensions to consider in a residen-

tial setting in addition to whether the program increases skills or decreases problem behaviors. They are also looking for a "home" for their adults with autism—a place where they
can be happy, have fun, pursue their special interests, be safe, have privacy, make choices,
have friends, and be as independent and as involved in the community as possible. They
would like their children to be responsible adults who are involved in meaningful activities
both at home and at work.

Given these goals, outcome measures need to be expanded as mentioned by Brown
(1991) and in the Van Bourgondien et al. (1996) study to include measures of the daily
schedule and the living environment. These authors suggest that factors that may be
important are the degree of individualization in the daily schedule, socialization experiences both at home and in the community, communication programming and choice
making, the degree to which the staff members understand autism and know how to adapt
activities to the strengths and interests of each individual, and the frequency and types of
family involvement. From the results of the studies that examined how to reduce problem
behaviors (Elliot et al., 1994; Reese et al., 1998; Van Bourgondien et al., 1996), it is apparent
that an effective treatment environment will employ ongoing individualized, positive
intervention strategies that will emphasize preventing the occurrence of negative behaviors.

Given the heterogeneity of adults with autism, it is unlikely that one setting or type
of setting will be appropriate for all individuals. Therefore, measures of the individual and
family's satisfaction with the treatment/living setting will be very important to include in
any outcome study.

METHODOLOGICAL CONSIDERATIONS

A major challenge in this research area is how to conduct methodologically sound
research that allows us to first have confidence in the results in terms of the reliability and
validity of the findings. Second, it is important to be able to determine what factor(s)
contributed to the outcome.

As mentioned previously, it appears that studies that employ subjects as their own
controls utilizing single-subject methods such as a multiple baseline design (Kazdin, 1982)
are very appropriate for examining approaches to increasing the skills or reducing the
behavior problems of individuals with autism. More single-subject studies would help to
delineate for whom and for what skills or behaviors a particular treatment approach
provides benefits. The difficulty will continue to be the issue of the generalizability of these
findings across the variety of individuals with autism.

Are large group comparison studies an appropriate approach to evaluating the
effectiveness/success of a program? The answer to the question is a cautious yes. The three
major issues to consider are the nature of the comparison group, the measures or outcome
variables, and the time frame of the study.

While Sherman et al. (1988) in their study of a group of children compared a residential program to home-based and outpatient treatment programs, this comparison seems
less meaningful for an adult population. The reality for most families is that at some point
their adult children need to leave the family home and live in some type of community
setting. As parents get older, they often begin to seek an alternative living arrangement that
will attend to all their adult children's needs for a happy, healthy, safe environment where
they can grow and learn and participate in meaningful activities at home and in the com-

munity. Therefore, comparison studies will need to include different types of residential settings.

A comparison study of different residential options would need to actually measure the environments to determine how they are different. One cannot assume that just because a program differs in the number of inhabitants, location of the home, or funding source there are actually day-to-day differences in the experiences of those who live there. Brown (1991) strongly recommends measuring the individual's ability/willingness to follow his or her daily schedule. Variation from the schedule gives important information about the individual's preferences. The ERS (Van Bourgondien et al., 1998) is another approach to documenting the differences between living environments for adults with autism. The amount of individualization based on interests and strengths, stimulation, teaching of new skills, exposure to new experiences, and the degree to which the individuals are involved in socialization activities in the community are some of the factors that need to be compared. Individualized programming that takes into account the interests and preferences of each resident is an essential area to assess.

More difficult will be choosing or developing measures of skill acquisition that can allow for comparisons across the variety of individuals with autism in different settings. Some combination of individually defined objectives together with some uniform measures of performance needs to be explored. Skill acquisition studies need to distinguish whether individuals have learned skills that they can independently initiate and perform versus skills that require another person to be present in order to prompt the person with autism to initiate and complete the activity. For changes in behavior, it appears that global measures of behavior problems such as the Aberrant Behavior Scale or Vineland Maladaptive Behavior Scale are of help in detecting changes in a diverse sample. Still, individually defined goals that are observable would be a helpful addition. Defining and comparing the techniques used to reduce the negative behaviors is as important as the actual reduction in problem behaviors.

Finally, the length of the study period is an important consideration. In Van Bourgondien et al.'s (1996) group comparison study, we found that adults within this study were mobile and did not necessarily stay in the same treatment setting for the entire length of the study (18 months). In addition, in another study (Van Bourgondien & Reichle, 1993), we found that moving an adult with autism into a new treatment environment (regardless of the setting) frequently led to a decline in skills and an increase in behavior problems for up to 18 months following the move. For future studies, it will be important to follow the participants long enough to take into account transient responses to changes in the living situation.

SUMMARY

The effects of residential treatment approaches on adults with autism needs to be evaluated from a variety of perspectives. The living environments should be examined in terms of the qualities related to being both a home and a learning environment. One aim is to determine the degree to which adults are able to express preferences and to engage in preferred activities. Changes in the individuals with autism need to examine the acquisition and independent use of adaptive skills as well as the reduction of inappropriate behaviors.

The limited research to date has shown that there are some techniques that successfully increase skills and decrease behavior problems of specific individuals with autism. The specificity and generalizability of these techniques has yet to be documented empirically. More information is needed about which techniques are helpful for which individuals with autism.

Preliminary research has also shown that it is possible to create a positive, proactive environment that takes into account the unique interests and needs of an adult with autism, and that families value settings that have these attributes.

REFERENCES

Brown, F. (1991). Creative daily scheduling: A nonintrusive approach to challenging behaviors in community residences. *Journal of the Association for Persons with Severe Handicaps, 16,* 75–84.

Dawson, G., & Osterling, J. (1997). Early intervention in autism. In J. J. Guralnick (Ed.), *The Effectiveness of Early Intervention.* Baltimore, MD: Brooks.

Elliot, R. O., Dobbin, A. R., Rose, G. D., & Soper H. V. (1994). Vigorous, aerobic exercise versus general motor training activities: Effects on maladaptive and stereotypic behaviors of adults with both autism and mental retardation. *Journal of Autism and Developmental Disorders, 24*(5), 565–576.

Gold, M. W. (1976). Task analysis of a complex assembly task by the retarded blind. *Exceptional Children, 43,* 78–84.

Hilton, A. (1987). Residential facilities. In C. R. Reynolds & C. Mann (Eds.), *Encyclopedia of Special Education* (pp. 1350–1351). New York: John Wiley & Sons.

Holmes, D. L. (1990). Community-based services for children and adults with autism: The Eden family of programs. *Journal of Autism and Developmental Disorders, 20,* 339–351.

Kay, B. R. (1990). Bittersweet farms. *Journal of Autism and Developmental Disorders, 20,* 309–322.

Kazdin, A. E. (1982). *Single-Case Research Designs.* New York: Oxford University Press.

Landesman, S. (1987). The Changing structure and function of institutions: A search for optimal group care environments. In S. Landesman & P. Vietze (Eds.), *Living Environments and Mental Retardation* (pp. 79–126). Washington, DC: American Association on Mental Retardation.

Larkin, A. S., & Gurry, S. (1998). Brief report: Progress reported in three children with autism using daily life therapy. *Journal of Autism and Developmental Disorders, 28*(4), 339–342.

LaVigna, G. W. (1983). The Jay Nolan Center: A community-based program. In E. Schopler & G. B. Mesibov (Eds.), *Autism in Adolescents and Adults* (pp. 381–410). New York: Plenum.

Lettick, A. L. (1983). Benhaven. In E. Schopler & G. B. Mesibov (Eds.). *Autism in Adolescents and Adults* (pp. 355–379). New York: Plenum.

McGimsey, J. F. & Favell, J. E. (1988). The effects of increased physical exercise on disruptive behavior in retarded persons. *Journal of Autism and Developmental Disorders, 18,* 167–180.

Mesibov, G., Schopler, E., Schaffer, B., & Landrus, R. (1988). *Individualized Assessment and Treatment for Autistic and Developmentally Disabled Children,* Vol. IV: *Adolescent and Adult Psychoeducational Profile (AAPEP).* Austin, TX: PRO-ED.

Quill, K., Gurry, S., & Larkin, A. (1989). Daily life therapy: A Japanese model for educating children with autism. *Journal of Autism and Developmental Disabilities, 19,* 625–635.

Reese, R. M., Sherman, J. A., & Sheldon, J. B. (1998). Reducing disruptive behavior of a group home resident with autism and mental retardation. *Journal of Autism and Developmental Disorders, 28,* 159–165.

Rosenthal-Malek, A., & Mitchell, S. (1997). Brief report: The effects of exercise on the self-stimulatory behaviors and positive responding of adolescents with autism. *Journal of Autism and Developmental Disorders, 27*(2), 193–202.

Sherman, J., Barker, P., Lorimer, P., Swinson, R., & Factor, D. C. (1988). Treatment of autistic children: Relative effectiveness of residential out-patient, and home-based interventions. *Child Psychiatry and Human Development, 19,* 109–125.

Sloan, J. L., & Schopler, E. (1977). Some thoughts about developing programs for autistic adolescent. *Journal of Pediatric Psychology, 2,* 187–190.

Smith, M. D., & Belcher, R. (1985). Teaching life skills to adults disabled by autism. *Journal of Autism and Developmental Disorders, 15*, 163–175.

Sparrow, S. S., Balla, D. A., & Cicchetti, D. V. (1984). *Vineland Adaptive Behavior Scales*. Circle Pines, MN: American Guidance Service.

Van Bourgondien, M. E., & Mesibov, G. B. (1989). Diagnosis and treatment of adolescents and adults with autism. In G. Dawson (Ed.), *Autism: Nature, Diagnosis and Treatment* (pp. 367–385). New York: Guilford.

Van Bourgondien, M. E., & Reichle, N. C. (1993, June). *Making changes: Adolescents and adults with autism in transition*. A presentation at the annual conference of the American Association on Mental Retardation (AAMR), Washington, DC.

Van Bourgondien, M. E., & Reichle, N. C. (1996). The Carolina Living and Learning Center: An example of the TEACCH approach to residential and vocational training for adults with autism. In G. Kristoffersen & E. Kristoffersen (Eds.), *Status Pa Garden* (pp. 155–169). Copenhagen: Parentes.

Van Bourgondien, M. E., & Reichle, N. C. (1997). Residential treatment for individuals with autism. In D. J. Cohen & F. R. Volkmar (Eds.), *Handbook of Autism and Pervasive Developmental Disorders* (pp. 691–706). New York: John Wiley & Sons.

Van Bourgondien, M. E., Reichle, N. C., Campbell, D., & Mesibov, G. (1998). The environment rating scale (ERS): A measure of the quality of the residential environment for adults with autism. *Research in Developmental Disabilities, 19*, 381–394.

Van Bourgondien, M. E., Reichle, N. C., Schopler, E., & Mesibov, G. B. (1996). *The Effectiveness of a Model Treatment Program on Adults with Autism*. Manuscript in preparation, University of North Carolina at Chapel Hill.

Wall, A. J. (1990). Group homes in North Carolina for children and adults with autism. *Journal of Autism and Developmental Disorders, 20*, 353–366.

14

Psychopharmacologic Treatment Studies in Autism

Linmarie Sikich

Autism is a developmental disorder that results in lifelong disability. It is frequently associated with problematic behaviors such as self-injurious behaviors (SIB) and aggression that harm both the affected individuals and those around them. There is widespread consensus that autism is a physical disorder in which the functioning of the brain is subtly disrupted, leading to very significant changes in behavior. In many other brain disorders, such as epilepsy and depression, specific medications have been of tremendous benefit and frequently lead to complete resolution of symptoms. The combination of these two factors (the severe, persistent manifestations of autism and its biological basis) has led many individuals to hope that pharmacologic treatments can greatly reduce the symptoms of autism and perhaps even "cure" the illness. There have been frequent announcements of treatments with dramatic benefits, which are almost inevitably followed by families rushing to secure the touted treatment. Unfortunately, the efficacy and safety of these treatments are seldom scientifically examined prior to such announcements. Thus far none of these treatments has proved to be as beneficial as initially hoped when examined more rigorously.

In this chapter existing criteria for evaluating the evidence supporting psychological and medical treatments are reviewed and specific criteria for assessing the empirical support of pharmacologic treatments in autism are proposed. Then, the evidence regarding the use of several medications in autism is reviewed using these criteria. The limitations of these studies are discussed. Finally, approaches for strengthening and refining future pharmacologic studies in autism are explored.

LINMARIE SIKICH • Division TEACCH, School of Medicine, University of North Carolina at Chapel Hill, Chapel Hill, North Carolina 27599-7160.

The Research Basis for Autism Intervention, edited by Schopler, Yirmiya, Shulman, and Marcus. Kluwer Academic/Plenum Publishers, New York, 2001.

CRITERIA FOR EMPIRICALLY SUPPORTED TREATMENTS

Research examining the effects of new medications and treatments can be done in many different ways. Often community physicians will make an observation about the effects of a treatment in one or more of their patients. These anecdotal observations are usually referred to as *case reports*. Such case reports are generally *retrospective* and describe the results of the medication using observations made fortuitously during the course of treatment. Often the observations have limited salience and differ between patients, thus limiting meaningful comparisons. Typically, a particularly dramatic response is described without regard for its generalizability or prevalence. Case reports do identify potentially useful drugs or treatments that should be investigated in more detail.

In a *case series*, investigators retrospectively examine the effects of a given treatment in all patients who received the treatment during a given time frame. Case series are somewhat more compelling than case reports because the researcher does not omit cases in which the patients responded to the treatment in a different way than expected. However, because they are retrospective, important information is often missing.

In a *prospective* study, the researcher decides ahead of time how to assess the effects of the medication and does so in the same way at the same points for all individuals in the study. This allows for much more meaningful comparisons between people.

In an *open* trial, both the participants and researchers are aware of the treatment each person receives. Most often, all participants receive the study treatment. The effects of the treatment are assessed by determining the amount of change in specific symptom areas immediately before starting treatment and at the end of treatment. Naturally occurring variations in symptom severity may confound the interpretation of open trials. In addition, in open studies, there is great potential for improvement in symptoms simply as a result of increased contact with health care professionals and the hopes of all involved that the study treatment will be beneficial. The likelihood of falsely attributing such improvements to the experimental treatment may be diminished somewhat using *discontinuation* or *crossover* designs. In a discontinuation study, assessments are made prior to the experimental treatment, during the treatment, and after the treatment. If the observed benefits are a result of the experimental treatment, they should diminish when the treatment is discontinued. In a crossover study, two treatments, such as the experimental treatment and a placebo, are compared within the same individual. The order of the treatments is varied among different participants in the study to account for duration of treatment effects. Benefits attributable to the experimental treatment should be evident only when an individual is receiving it and should be absent or greatly reduced when the individual receives the comparison treatment. In both discontinuation and crossover studies, it is very important to know how long the drug is likely to remain in the body and the duration of the drug's expected effect. For instance, fluoxetine (Prozac™) usually takes 6 weeks to be cleared from the body. Therefore, the efficacy of fluoxetine in a discontinuation trial would likely be underestimated in a discontinuation trial if the final assessment was made 2–4 weeks following the last fluoxetine dose. Often the results of open studies are viewed skeptically because of the potential biases of both researchers and participants.

A modification of the open trial design is a *cohort study* in which two groups, one that receives the research treatment and one that does not, are followed prospectively. In this case, everyone is aware of the specific treatment a particular individual receives. Advantages of cohort studies include the possibility of recruiting large numbers of individuals and the ability to assess long-term treatment effects.

In *double-blind* studies, participants are randomly assigned to different treatments and neither the researcher nor the participants know what treatment a particular individual is receiving so as to increase the objectivity of assessments. In especially rigorous studies, an *independent evaluator* who is uninvolved in treatment and unaware of side effects assesses the efficacy of treatment.

Double-blind studies are also referred to as randomized controlled trials (RCTs). In all double-blind studies, the study treatment is compared to at least one other intervention. There are three main types of interventions used for such comparisons. A *placebo* medication is an inert substance (such as gelatin or sugar) that is packaged to look like the experimental treatment and believed to have no direct pharmacologic effects. Placebos provide the most rigorous comparison. Although counterintuitive, placebo treatments frequently lead to greater improvements between the initial and final assessments than are seen in individuals who have received no intervention at all (Benkert & Maier, 1990; Laporte & Figueras, 1994; Quitkin, 1999). An *active medication comparator* is another drug thought to be effective in the condition. A *behavioral comparator* is a specific non-pharmacological treatment that is thought to be effective. Ideally when an active medication or behavioral comparator is used, its efficacy in treating the condition should already be well established. Because few, if any, treatments have been rigorously demonstrated to be effective in autism, many investigators feel a placebo should be included to eliminate the possibility that improvements observed are not simply the result of participating in a study or the passage of time. When an active comparator is used, the goal of the study can be to determine either the experimental treatment's *equivalence* to the already established treatment or its *superiority* to the already established treatment. Studies that show equivalence are often viewed skeptically because small to moderate differences that may be clinically important are unlikely to be statistically detected unless very large numbers of individuals are examined.

Double-blind studies may use crossover or discontinuation designs as in open studies or a *parallel* design involving at least two distinct treatment groups (e.g., experimental treatment and placebo). Parallel design studies and open-cohort design studies are both also referred to as group design studies. Crossover and discontinuation designs compare changes within specific individuals and are likely to have decreased variability. Parallel designs compare the mean values between each treatment group and often have considerable variability. Statistically it is easier to detect a difference between groups when the variability within each group is small. Thus, parallel studies are often considered to be more robust than crossover studies.

The Food and Drug Administration (FDA) has ultimate responsibility in the United States for determining whether a drug is efficacious and safe for treating a given disorder. Typically, the FDA is more confident in trials that show superiority of the experimental treatment than in equivalence trials that find no difference between the experimental treatment and the comparator. Therefore, the FDA finds "it highly desirable for a claim to be convincingly demonstrated in at least one trial showing superiority of the test agent over placebo or active control. If a claim of superiority over a specific comparator is sought, rather than just straightforward efficacy, the claim should be substantiated by two adequate and well-controlled trials showing superiority" (FDA, 1999). These criteria are so stringent that pharmaceutical companies frequently choose not to get specific approval for use in autistic individuals and physicians prescribe the medication in an "off-label" fashion.

Over the past decade, physicians, psychologists, health economists, and the general public have increasingly emphasized the use of rigorous evidence to guide treatment interventions. Criteria to evaluate the evidence supporting psychotherapy interventions were recently defined by The American Psychological Association's Task Force on Promotion and Dissemination of Psychological Procedures (1995) and elaborated by Chambless et al. (1996). These were modified for use in pediatric populations by another task forces of child psychologists (Lonigan, Elbert, & Johnson, 1998). They considered "well established" psychosocial interventions to be based upon either (1) at least two well designed, parallel group studies done by different investigators showing superiority of the intervention or equivalence to a well established treatment in a sufficiently large sample; or (2) more than nine consistent crossover or cohort studies in which the effects of the intervention in single persons was compared to other treatments. They felt a treatment should be regarded as "probably efficacious" if there were (1) at least two studies demonstrating superiority to a no-treatment control group, (2) two well conducted group design studies in different samples done by the same investigator, or (3) three to eight consistent crossover or cohort studies. They also discussed the difficulties involved in determining an adequate sample size despite the Chambless et al. (1996) guidelines that "about" 30 children per group is sufficient.

A number of groups within the general medical community have also established criteria for evaluating the strength of treatment research (Ball, Phillips, & Shenker, 2000; Cho & Bero, 1994; Edwards, Russell, & Stott, 1998; Guyatt, Sackett, & Cook, 1994, 1995; Hayward, Wilson, Runis, Bass, & Guyatt, 1995; Michaud, McGowan, Van der Jagt, Wells, & Tugwell, 1998; Sackett, Strauss, Richardson, Rosenberg, & Haynes, 2000). Highest confidence is placed upon systematic reviews or meta-analyses that demonstrate consistent results across multiple randomized controlled trials. However, one should be aware that, since it is more difficult to publish negative randomized controlled trials than positive ones, early meta-analyses may place undue emphasis on positive results. The next highest level of confidence is assigned to randomized controlled trials with clear findings and narrow confidence limits. Midlevel confidence is given to systematic reviews of cohort studies that demonstrate consistent results, an individual cohort study with compelling results or a low quality randomized controlled trial. Some also view a case series with all or none results as moderately compelling. However, typically case series and single case reports are viewed skeptically.

Synthesis of the hierarchy suggested for assessing general medical treatments and the criteria developed for assessing pediatric psychotherapeutic interventions suggests the following guidelines for evaluating pharmacological treatments in autism. The cornerstones of compelling studies are (1) clear specification of the sample being studied, (2) clear specification of the study treatments, and (3) random assignment to treatment. Meta-analyses are unlikely to be helpful given the small number of controlled studies and the relative lack of standardized outcome measures.

Criteria for unsupported but potentially useful treatments:

- A limited number of case reports of efficacy
- An open study reporting improvement using retrospective measures

Criteria for possibly efficacious treatment:

- A large number of case reports
- Two or more case series reporting efficacy
- Two or more open studies reporting significant improvement on prospective measures
- Double-blind studies with limited sample sizes that show equivalence to an active agent

Criteria for probably efficacious treatment:

- Two or more well designed, crossover studies showing a distinct effect of the treatment on prospective measures
- One double-blind study with a large sample size showing equivalence to an active agent
- One double-blind study showing superiority to placebo

Criteria for well established treatment:

- Two or more double-blind studies showing superiority to placebo or another active treatment, ideally from different research groups
- Two or more large double-blind studies showing equivalence to an active treatment

This approach emphasizes the importance of consistent findings across different studies so that isolated positive results are not given undue emphasis. However, it also seeks to recognize clinically important observations that may initially be made during a poorly designed study and not to overvalue statistical significance. Ideally effective treatments will have both clinical and statistical significance. Unfortunately, there are a number of challenges in conducting well controlled clinical trials that may prevent accumulation of sufficient data to consider some highly effective treatments "well established." This is especially true in autism.

Autistic individuals are frequently unable to consent to the studies themselves because of their age or intellectual disabilities. Consequently, the amount of potential risk to which they are exposed in research is often limited, thus weakening a study's experimental design. The rigor of the experimental design may be further compromised because the behavioral problems associated with autism are often so disabling that many feel uncomfortable participating in placebo-controlled research. In addition, autistic individuals are often unable to provide feedback about their internal state, despite the fact that this is frequently the target of psychopharmacologic interventions. In addition, autism is a highly heterogeneous disorder. It is likely that specific treatments will be most effective in specific subgroups. Hence, a central challenge will be to define the subset of autistic individuals who are most likely to respond to a given treatment.

REVIEW OF PSYCHOPHARMACOLOGIC TREATMENTS IN AUTISM

Typical Antipsychotics

Typical antipsychotics or neuroleptics have been the mainstay of treatment for psychotic disorders such as schizophrenia. They often have significant side effects including sedation and effects on the extrapyramidal motor system that may lead to stiffness (dystonia), restlessness (akathisia), or involuntary movements (dyskinesias). Transient dyskinesias are common when typical neuroleptics are withdrawn. Tardive dyskinesias (TD) persist for long periods and may never disappear even if neuroleptic use is discontinued. Agents in this class include haloperidol (Haldol™), fluphenazine (Prolixin™), thiothixene (Navane™), and thioridazine (Mellaril™).

The evidence supporting the use of typical antipsychotics in autism is fairly strong and meets the criteria for a "probably efficacious" treatment. Joshi and colleagues (1988) conducted an open label study of haloperidol or fluphenazine in 12 autistic children (7 to 11 years) and observed clinically meaningful improvements in hyperactivity, aggression, and peer relatedness. There have also been two well designed, double-blind studies of haloperidol in autistic children using crossover designs done by the same research group (Anderson, Campbell, Adams, Small, Perry, & Shell, 1989; Anderson, Campbell, Greya, Perry, Small, & Green, 1984). In the first, 40 young autistic children between the ages of 2 and 7 years received between 0.5 and 3.0 mg/day of haloperidol. Significant improvements were seen in overall functioning, discrimination learning, withdrawal, stereotypies, irritability, and hyperactivity as compared to placebo treatment. In the 1989 study, 45 autistic children between 2 and 8 years of age were studied. A significant effect of haloperidol was noted in the Clinician's Global Impressions scale (CGI—Guy, 1976). However, improvements on specific symptom scales did not reach statistical significance and the previous effects on learning were not replicated. It is quite possible that the absence of effects on particular symptoms reflects an inadequate sample size.

The research group at New York University Medical Center has also examined the long-term safety of haloperidol in autistic children (Campbell, Armenteros, Malone, Adams, Eisenberg, & Overall, 1997). They found that 31% of participants developed withdrawal dyskinesias when haloperidol was abruptly stopped and nearly 10% developed tardive dyskinesia. Most who developed tardive dyskinesia had previously had withdrawal dyskinesias. Dyskinesias were more likely with prolonged treatment and in girls.

These studies suggest that haloperidol and other typical antipsychotics may frequently be useful in modestly improving the overall functioning of autistic children. However, these medications should be gradually discontinued to avoid withdrawal dyskinesias. Further, longterm use, particularly in individuals who have experienced withdrawal dyskinesias, should be undertaken cautiously given the potential for the development of tardive dyskinesia. Individuals on these agents should be monitored regularly (every 3 to 6 months) for the development of tardive dyskinesia.

Atypical Antipsychotics

Atypical antipsychotics were developed over the last 20 years, primarily in an effort to minimize the extrapyramidal side effects observed with typical agents. They are rapidly becoming the standard of care for treating psychoses. Currently available atypical antipsychotics include clozapine (Clozaril™), risperidone (Risperdal™), olanzapine (Zyprexa™), ziprasidone (Geodon™), and quetiapine (Seroquel™). In addition to having fewer extrapyramidal side effects, atypical antipsychotics appear to reduce negative symptoms such as social withdrawal and cognitive problems in schizophrenia to a greater extent than typical antipsychotics. The similarity between the negative symptoms of schizophrenia and the core social deficits in autistic individuals, as well as the benefits observed with typical antipsychotic treatment, have led to great optimism that the atypical antipsychotics may be particularly useful in treating autism.

The evidence supporting the efficacy of atypical antipsychotics in autism is fairly strong and meets the criteria for a "probably efficacious treatment." Risperidone has been most widely studied with a case series in very young children, three open studies, and one randomized controlled trial. In two toddlers, open risperidone treatment significantly improved social relatedness and reduced aggression (Posey, Walsh, Wilson, & McDougle. (1999b). There have been four open studies of risperidone treatment in autistic children. All found that risperidone treatment was associated with substantial clinical improvements over baseline whether assessed qualitatively or with standardized rating scales (Findling, Maxwell, & Wiznitzer, 1997; Horrigan & Barnhill, 1997; McDougle et al., 1997; Nicolson, Award, & Sloman, 1998). McDougle and colleagues (1998b) have conducted the only double-blind, placebo-controlled trial in a heterogeneous group of 31 autistic adults. Risperidone treatment over 12 weeks was associated with clinically significant improvement in half of the individuals treated. In contrast, none of those treated with placebo responded. Improvements were seen in repetitive behaviors, aggression, irritability, and anxiety. However, no changes in language or social behaviors were observed. An NIMH-sponsored multisite study of risperidone in autistic children is currently underway (McDougle et al., 2000).

There has also been one consistent open study of olanzapine in eight autistic individuals (5 to 42 years old), which observed significant improvements in overall functioning, language use, and social relatedness but not repetitive behaviors (Potenza, Holmes, Kanes, & McDougle, 1999). In contrast to these positive findings, an open study of quetiapine in six boys with mental retardation and autism failed to show a positive treatment effect (Martin et al., 1999). This raises the possibility of differences in the efficacy among atypical antipsychotics.

The side effects most frequently observed with the atypical antipsychotics were sedation and weight gain, which was quite significant in some individuals. In addition, risperidone use was associated with cardiac changes in one of the toddlers and quetiapine use was associated with a seizure in one individual.

These studies suggest that atypical antipsychotics, particularly risperidone, are often quite helpful in moderately improving overall behavior, especially aggression, in autistic individuals. It remains unclear to what extent these agents may be useful in improving social relatedness. It also remains unclear to whether quetiapine has similar effects to risperidone and olanzapine. Finally, the usefulness of these agents in children is not yet clear. When these agents are used, it is important to adjust the dose to minimize sedation and to monitor weight gain.

Serotonin Reuptake Inhibitors

The serotonin reuptake inhibitors were initially developed as antidepressants and have also had great efficacy in reducing the symptoms of obsessive–compulsive disorder (OCD). Potent serotonin reuptake inhibitors include the tricyclic antidepressant clomipramine

(Anafranil™) and the mixed antidepressant venlaflaxine (Effexor™) and all selective serotonin reuptake inhibitors (SSRIs) including fluoxetine (Prozac™), sertraline (Zoloft™), paroxetine (Paxil™), fluvoxamine (Luvox™), and citalopram (Celexa™). The hypothesis that se otonin reuptake inhibitors will reduce autistic symptomatology is based upon the parallels between repetitive behaviors in autism and OCD, serotonergic abnormalities in many autistic individuals, and altered patterns of brain serotonin synthesis.

The evidence supporting the use of serotonin reuptake inhibitors in older individuals with autism is quite strong and approaches being well established. There have been numerous case reports of improvements with these agents in autistic individuals of all ages (Harvey & Cooray, 1995; Koshes, 1997; Ozbayrak, 1997; Posey, Litwiller, Koburn, & McDougle, 1999a; Snead, Boon, & Presberg, 1994; Todd, 1991). In adults and adolescents, there have also been several positive case series and open label studies with various agents (Brodkin, McDougle, Naylor, Cohen, & Price, 1997; Cook, Rowlett, Taselskis, 1992; Fatemi, Realmuto, Khan, & Thuras, 1998; Hellings, Kelly, Gabrielli, Kilgore, & Shah, 1996; Holander, Kaplan, Cartwright, & Reichman, 2000; McDougle, Brodkin, Naylor, Carlson, 1998a). Finally there have been two positive double-blind, placebo-controlled trials with clomipramine and fluvoxamine, respectively. The initial double-blind crossover trial compared clomipramine to placebo in 12 individuals and to desipramine in 12 others. In both cases, clomipramine reduced autistic symptoms to a significantly greater degree than the comparators did (Gordon, State, Nelson, Hamburger, & Rapoport, 1993). In the second double-blind study, fluvoxamine led to significant improvements in the overall functioning of 53% of the 16 people treated, while none of those in the placebo group responded. Specific improvements were noted in repetitive thoughts and behaviors, maladaptive behavior, aggression, and language usage (McDougle, Naylor, Cohen, Volkmar, Heninger, & Price, 1996). Thus far the therapeutic efficacy of serotonin reuptake inhibitors in autistic adults appears to generalize to all such agents.

Evidence supporting the efficacy of serotonin reuptake inhibitors in children is more equivocal. This may relate to differential effects of the different medications, differences in the age of people studied or to the very small number of participants in reported studies. No randomized controlled trials with serotonin reuptake inhibitors have been undertaken in children. The available studies of clomipramine have reported conflicting findings. One open study of eight younger children (3 to 9 years old) observed improvement in only one child and worsening in six others (Sanchez, Campbell, Small, Cueva, Armenteros, & Adams, 1996). This contrasts with the improvements observed in Brasic and colleagues' (1994) open study of five prepubertal boys and the NIMH double-blind study which included seven older children (Gordon, Rapoport, Hamburger, State, & Mannheim, 1992). Clinically significant improvements have been more uniformly observed in open studies of the selective serotonin reuptake inhibitors (SSRIs) (DeLong, Teague, & McSwain Kamran, 1998; Fatemi et al., 1998; Steingard, Zimjnitzky, DeMaso, Bauman, Bucci, 1997). DeLong and colleagues' (1998) case series of 37 autistic children between 2 and 7 years old is particularly provocative. Twenty-two (59%) showed significant overall improvement with striking gains in language skills. In 11 children, the improvements are reported to be so large that only "vestiges of [autism] remained." Several of these patients showed behavioral deterioration when fluoxetine was stopped. Similar striking improvements in social functioning and increased interest in the environment were reported in an open prospective study of six autistic children between 4 and 8 years (Peral, Alxami, & Gilaberte, 1999).

These two studies suggest that treatment of autistic preschoolers may have greater effects on the core symptoms of autism than the treatment of adults. However, there are also anecdotal reports that SSRIs may be more activating in younger children.

The different serotonin reuptake inhibitors have different side effect profiles. Clomipramine is notable for significant anticholinergic effects such as urinary retention. The SSRIs are better tolerated in general, but may be more likely to result in behavioral agitation or insomnia, especially in young children (Friedman, 1991).

The serotonin reuptake inhibitors appear quite useful in improving the functioning of autistic adults. Improvements are seen in language use and aggression as well as repetitive behaviors. These agents, with the possible exception of clomipramine, are quite well tolerated and safe in adults. However, the use of these agents in children is more controversial with both beneficial and adverse effects frequently reported. Again the newer selective serotonin reuptake inhibitors are likely to be better tolerated than clomipramine.

Secretin

Secretin is a peptide hormone secreted by the small intestine which increases pancreatic secretions. As of yet, secretin has not been reported to have activity in the brain. However, several other peptides initially identified in the gastrointestinal system have subsequently been found in the brain where they act as neurotransmitters to [e.g., vasoactive intestinal peptide (VIP)]. Interest in secretin as a treatment for autism was evoked by a report of three individuals who had received secretin in the context of a medical workup for chronic diarrhea. All three had a dramatic improvement in both their gastrointestinal symptoms and their behavior particularly with regard to eye contact and expressive language (Horvath, Stefanatos, Sokolski, Wachtel, Nabors, & Tildon, 1998). Since that report, there have been further anecdotal reports of autistic individuals who have both responded and not responded (Sidney Baker, MD website (http://www.sbakermd.com); (Horvath, 2000; Perry & Bangaru, 1998; Rimland, 2000).

However, three double-blind, placebo controlled studies have failed to demonstrate the efficacy of secretin (Owley et al., 1999; Sandler, Sutton, DeWeese, Girardi, Sheppard, & Bodfish, 1999; Chez et al., 2000). The first involved 20 autistic children 3 to 12 years old who were treated in a crossover fashion with porcine secretin for 4 weeks and placebo for 4 weeks. No significant differences were observed between secretin and placebo treatment on the CGI, Autism Diagnostic Observation Schedule-Generic (ADOS-G), Aberrant Behavior Checklist (ABC), Gilliam Autism Rating Scale (GARS) or Vineland Adaptive Behavior Scales (Owley et al., 1999). Similarly a larger study involving 60 individuals in a parallel group design failed to find any difference in the effects of treatment with a single injection of synthetic human secretin (Sandler et al., 1999). Significantly both secretin and placebo treatment were associated with 15% to 25% reductions in the total aberrant behavior checklist scores in this study. The third study was a double-blind, placebo-controlled crossover study in which each subject received both secretin and placebo for 4 weeks. The majority (17) of the 25 subjects were selected based on robust response to open treatment with secretin and were young (mean age 6.4 years). Overall, there were few children showed meaningful improvements and there was no significant difference between secretin and placebo treatment on gastrointestinal symptoms, language, awareness, or social interactions (Chez et al., 2000). None of the studies observed significant side effects although their design did not permit assessment of allergic sensitization with repeated injections.

Controversy about the efficacy of secretin in autism persists, fueled by individuals who feel the signal present in the initial case reports is too strong to be ignored. These people argue that difficulties with patient selection and assessment time points resulted in the randomized clinical trials missing a real and important difference. While this is possible, it does not seem likely since other treatments for autism have been able to demonstrate efficacy using similar measures with smaller equally heterogeneous samples. At the present time, secretin appears unlikely to provide significant benefit to the majority of autistic individuals. The potential adverse effects of its use appear fairly insignificant although there are concerns that repeated use of the porcine form may lead allergic responses.

Vitamin B$_6$ and Magnesium

Linus Pauling (1968) proposed that some psychiatric disorders might be the result of relative deficiencies in certain vitamins and minerals and that these disorders might be ameliorated by supplementation with the missing vitamins. There has been particular interest in vitamin B$_6$ because it is involved in the biosynthesis of several neurotransmitters. This has prompted two major research groups, led by Rimland and LeLord respectively, to investigate the use of megadoses of vitamin B$_6$ and magnesium in autism. In a double-blind, placebo-controlled withdrawal study of 15 autistic children selected because they had responded in open trials, investigators were able to correctly predict whether participants were receiving vitamin B$_6$ or placebo in 11 of 15 cases (Rimland, Callaway, & Dreyfus, 1978). However, the absence of random selection and of standardized rating scales in this study limit its significance. LeLord and colleagues have also published several reports using crossover designs or control cohorts which have recently been reviewed (Pfeiffer, Norton, Nelson, & Shott, 1995). Although, there are concerns that the same individuals may have participated in multiple studies and standard rating scales were not used, significant improvement across multiple symptom areas were found in about one third to one half of participants (Barthelemy et al., 1981, 1983; LeLord, Muh, Barthelemy, Martineau, & Garreau, 1981; Matineau, Barthelemy, Garreau, & LeLord, 1985). Recently, a small study of 10 autistic individuals using a double-blind placebo-controlled crossover design failed to detect a difference with vitamin B$_6$ and magnesium treatment (Findling, Maxwell, Scotese-Wojtila, Huang, Yamashita, & Wiznitzer, 1997). However, this is not surprising given the extremely small sample size of the study (Rimland, 1998). No side effects are reported, but compliance is difficult due to the bitter taste. Taken together these studies suggest that vitamin B$_6$ and magnesium are possibly to probably efficacious in some autistic individuals. The potential difficulties administering the agents and their relatively small effect even in individuals who do respond limit the use of this agent.

Naltrexone

Naltrexone (ReVia™) is an opiate antagonist that has been hypothesized to be helpful in autism by blocking endogenous opiods that may be released during self-injurious repetitive behaviors. There is fairly consistent evidence that naltrexone is possibly to probably efficacious in reducing hyperactivity and impulsivity to a limited degree in children with autism. However, the long-term clinical importance of these changes has been questioned (Willemsen-Swinkels, Buitelaar, van Berckelaer-Onnes, & van Engeland, 1999). Specifically two open studies (Cazzullo, Musetti, Musetti, Bajo, Sacerdote, & Panerai, 1999; Willemsen-Swinkels et al., 1999) and three double-blind, placebo-controlled crossover studies involving 10 to 23 individuals each have demonstrated small but statistically significant improvements with naltrexone treatment (Bouvard et al., 1995; Kolmen, Feldman, Handen, & Tanosky, 1995; Willemsen-Swinkels, Buitelaar, Weijnen, & van Engeland, 1995). However, Kolmen and colleagues (1998) were unable to replicate their initial findings in a second sample of eleven people and instead found that both naltrexone and placebo showed improvements from baseline, and that the magnitude of these improvements was not statistically different between the two groups. The one controlled study in autistic adults also failed to show a significant benefit and instead showed consistent worsening with naltrexone treatment (Willemsen-Swinkels et al., 1995). This suggests that response to naltrexone may be a function of the patient's age. Significant side effects are not reported, but the medicine is extremely bitter. These results suggest that naltrexone may be useful in some autistic children with significant hyperactivity who are able to tolerate the taste of the medication.

Biopterin

Tetrahydrobiopterin is a cofactor for tyrosine hydroxylase in the biosynthetic pathway of catecholamines and serotonin. Some have speculated that inadequate amounts of biopterin may reduce levels of serotonin and dopamine in autistic individuals. Thus, biopterin supplementation might reduce autistic symptoms. Three open-label studies involving a total of 156 autistic children have described significant benefits of biopterin treatment with improvements in social function and language in about half of the children treated (Fernell et al., 1997; Komori, Matsuishi, Yamada, Yamashita, Ohtaki, & Kato, 1995; Nagahata et al., 1992). A double-blind, placebo-controlled study in 41 individuals also found improvements were significantly more frequent in the biopterin group than in the placebo group (Nakane, Naruse, Takesada, & Yamazaki, 1992). This suggests that biopterin is possibly to probably an efficacious treatment in autism.

Biopterin treatment appears to elicit small improvements particularly in language and social functioning in some autistic individuals. Few side effects have been reported. However, in this country biopterin is seldom used. This suggests that the effects of biopterin may be clinically insignificant or may not be sustained with prolonged use. A trial of biopterin appears appropriate in most autistic individuals.

Methylphenidate

Methylphenidate (Ritalin™) is the mainstay of treatment of attention deficit hyperactivity disorder. Because many autistic children have significant problems with attention, hyperactivity and impulsivity, stimulants may be helpful in the autistic population. There is one double-blind, placebo-controlled crossover study with two doses of methylphenidate, which demonstrated modest but statistically significant improvements in hyperactivity with no adverse events associated with methylphenidate treatment (Quintana et al., 1995). This result is promising and should be explored further. A trial of methylphenidate in autistic individuals with significant attentional problems seems warranted.

Immunoglobulin

A significant number of autistic individuals have immunologic abnormalities. Therefore some have speculated that treatment with immunoglobulin might ameliorate some of the symptoms of autism. This hypothesis has been examined in two open-label studies. Gupta, Aggarwal, and Heads (1996) administered immunoglobulin to 10 young autistic children every 4 weeks over 6 months or more and observed dramatic improvements in unstructured behavioral ratings in half the children with one child appearing "almost normal." The remaining children were reported to have milder improvements. The second study examined the effect of injections given every 6 weeks over a 6-month period in 10 children, many of whom were older. One child experienced a dramatic improvement which dissipated when treatment was stopped. Four others had mild, clinically insignificant improvements, while five demonstrated no changes (Plioplys, 1998). Gupta and colleagues plan to examine the effects of immunoglobulin in a randomized controlled trial (Gupta, 1999).

At the present time, use of immunoglobulin is unlikely to be beneficial in most autistic individuals. However, there do appear to be rare individuals who experience dramatic improvements with immunoglobulin treatment. Research is needed to develop ways to identify these individuals. The potential traumatic effects of repeated intravenous infusions must be considered before initiating or continuing immunoglobulin treatments. At this time, immunoglobulin use should probably be reserved for individuals with significant immune abnormalities and severe behavioral problems who have not responded to other treatments.

Summary of Published Psychopharmacologic Research

Psychopharmacologic research in autism is punctuated by initial case reports and open studies that demonstrate dramatic treatment benefits. However, when these treatments have been examined more rigorously, the benefits appear much more modest and often can not be substantiated in randomized controlled trials. This might reflect the very limited sample sizes of most trials or the limited magnitude of the potential benefits. Clinical significance is also hard to establish because most of the agents studied thus far have elicited a positive response in a minority of individuals. The best treatments seem to work in only 50% to 60% of participants. Unfortunately the small size and heterogeneity of most study samples precludes meaningful analyses of clinical subgroups which may preferentially respond to a specific treatment. In addition, placebo responses are prominent in many of the studies. Further there are not widely agreed-upon standards or rating scales to assess potential improvements. Time-sensitive measures of the core features of autism are not available and many of the problem behaviors assessed with rating scales such as the Aberrant Behavior Checklist (Aman, Singh, Stewart, & Field, 1985) are not specific to autism. Finally, almost all studies are relatively short term even though autism is a chronic disorder resulting in lifelong symptomatology which often requires lifelong treatment.

Despite these limitations, there are a surprising number of pharmacologic treatments whose use in subsets of autistic individuals is supported by clinical trials. These results are summarized in Table 14-1. The most well supported treatments include typical antipsychotics, atypical antipsychotics, and serotonin reuptake inhibitors. Vitamin B_6/magnesium and methylphenidate are supported by weaker evidence. However, most of these treatments appear to provide only modest symptomatic relief. No treatment has yet been rigorously shown to change the core features of autism to a sufficient extent that the affected individual is able to achieve normative levels of functioning.

Implications for Treatment

There is no evidence at this time that any particular pharmacologic treatment will dramatically change the core symptoms or course of autism. However, suggestions that very early treatment with agents such as the selective serotonin reuptake inhibitors may have more profound effects are promising and must be investigated further.

In the meantime, there is good evidence that many different pharmacologic treatments can be beneficial in improving the overall functioning of a significant number of autistic individuals. Improvement of the overall functioning of an individual is likely to have additional benefits by enhancing other behavioral and educational interventions. With the exception of naltrexone, it has been difficult to determine particular symptoms which respond to particular medications. In some cases the efficacy of a particular agent seems to be dependent upon the individual's age. In general, the order in which various treatments are utilized is determined by the distinctive side effect profiles of the various agents.

It seems quite reasonable to conduct a trial of one of the selective serotonin reuptake inhibitors (e.g., fluoxetine, fluvoxamine, sertraline, paroxetine, citolpram) in most autistic adults because of the significant chance of improvement with relatively few side effects. If this is not effective, a trial of an atypical antipsychotic such as risperidone or olanzapine is warranted. However, close monitoring for sedation, which may impair overall functioning, and for large amounts of weight gain, which might jeopardize the individual's general health, is needed. If these treatments are ineffective and symptoms sufficiently severe, trials of other treatments with more significant side effects should be considered. The typical antipsychotics appear most likely to be useful in generally improving functioning, but one must be vigilant for extrapyramidal side effects including restlessness and dystonias. Naltrexone may be useful in children but not adults for reducing hyperactivity and impulsiveness. The utility of ritalin is less well established for these symptoms, but it is likely to be easier to administer and might be efficacious in adults as well as children. Vitamin B_6, magnesium, and biopterin all seem to have some benefit with a very benign side effect profile. However, the clinical significance of these effects is unclear. The benefits of secretin and immunoglobulin treatment, both of which are administered intravenously, are not well supported. Further research is needed to identify the rare autistic individuals who may respond to these invasive treatments. Ultimately the use of medication in a particular person must be evaluated in sequential trials that consider both the magnitude and clinical significance of observed improvements, the difficulty administering the treatment on a consistent basis and the particular side effects experienced. Each autistic person and/or their family will need to individually decide whether a very small chance of great improve-

TABLE 14-1. Summary of Psychopharmacologic Treatment Studies in Autism Spectrum Disorders

Treatment	Case series (n)	Open studies (n)	Double-blind studies (n)	Negative studies
TYPICAL ANTIPSYCHOTICS: Effective for multiple symptoms, studies limited to children, significant side effects				
	Joshi et al., 1988 (12)		Anderson et al., 1984 (40)	No
			Anderson et al., 1989 (45)	
ATYPICAL ANTIPSYCHOTICS: Effective for multiple symptoms across all ages, Risperidone best studied				
Risperidone	Posey et al., 1999b (2)	Findling et al., 1997 (6)	McDougle et al., 1998b (31)	No
		Horrigan and Barnhill, 1997 (11)		
		Nicolson et al., 1998 (10)		
		McDougle et al., 1998b (18)		
		Potenza et al., 1999 (8)		
Olanzapine				
SEROTONIN REUPTAKE INHIBITORS: Consistent evidence in adults, but not children esp. with clomipramine				
Clomipramine	Brasic et al., 1994 (5)	Brodkin et al., 1997 (35)	Gordon et al., 1993 (24)	Sanchez et al., 1997 (8)
Fluvoxamine			McDougle et al., 1996 (16)	
Fluoxetine	Fatemi et al., 1998 (7)	Peral et al., 1999 (5)		
	DeLong et al., 1998 (37)	Cook et al., 1992 (23)		
Sertraline		McDougle et al., 1998a (42)		
		Steingard et al., 1997 (9)		
		Hellings et al., 1996 (9)		
Venlafaxine	Hollander et al., 2000 (10)			

SECRETIN: Dramatic results in initial case series

Horvath et al., 1998 (3)

Sandler et al., 1999 (60)
Owley et al., 1999 (40)
Chez et al., 2000 (25)

VITAMIN B_6/Mg: Most studies support general improvement but use nonstandard measures, bitter taste

Many

Rimland et al., 1978 (15)
LeLord multiple

Findling et al., 1997 (10)

NALTREXONE: Effects appear limited to children and ADHD symptoms, ? clinical significance

Cazzullo et al., 1999 (11)

Bouvard et al., 1995
Kolmen et al., 1995 (13)
Willemson et al., 1995 (23)

Willemson. et al., 1995 (33) adults
Willemson et al., 1996 (23) chronic
Kolmen et al., 1997 (11)

BIOPTERIN: Modest improvements, few side effects

Nagahata et al., 1992 (136)
Fernell et al., 1997 (6)
Komori et al., 1995 (14)

Nakane et al., 1992 (41)

No

METHYLPHENIDATE: Modest effect on ADHD symptoms

Quintana et al., 1995 (10)

No

IMMUNOGLOBULINS: Dramatic responses in ~10%, invasive administration

Gupta et al., 1996 (10)

Plioplys et al., 1998 (10) mixed

ment justifies a trial of relatively poorly supported treatments such as secretin and immuno-globulin.

Directions for Future Research

It is essential that the treatment of autistic individuals become as evidence-based as possible. Such evidence will ensure that all autistic individuals have broad access to potentially efficacious treatments, and will reduce exposure to unsubstantiated treatments that may have adverse effects or limit access to more efficacious treatments. Further, evidence supporting specific treatments will support families trying to obtain these treatments in their negotiations with insurance companies and school systems. Investigations into the efficacy of pharmacologic treatments can be relatively easily implemented and should lead the way.

Particular effort should be given to defining subgroups of responsive individuals. Such subgroups might be defined by cognitive abilities, age, symptom profiles, and biological markers such as immune abnormalities or genetic factors. Age is likely to be a particularly important factor for agents that modify brain structure during specific development periods. Although the role of genetic factors in increasing vulnerability is frequently discussed, genetic factors may also play an important role in determining the efficacy of specific drugs in particular individuals because naturally occurring variations, known as polymorphisms, in the genes for different neurotransmitters and receptors are associated with different levels of functional activity. For instance, depressed individuals with two copies of the polymorphism for the low activity form of the serotonin transporter are much less likely to respond to SSRI treatment than those with at least one copy of the polymorphism associated with high activity form of the transporter (Smeraldi, Zanardi, Benedetti, DiBella, Perz, & Catalano, 1998; Zanardi, Benedetti, DiBella, Catalano, & Smeraldi, 2000).

It is also important to move beyond the current studies, which are seriously compromised by the small number of participants, the failure to use comparable outcome measures across studies, and their limited duration. Multisite collaborations using standardized assessment protocols with objective and reliable rating scales will very effectively address these concerns. In addition, it will be important to conduct long-term studies of agents found to be effective in brief trials to fully assess the medication's safety and tolerability when used chronically.

REFERENCES

Aman, M. G., Singh, N. N., Stewart, A. W., & Field, C. J. (1985). The aberrant behavior checklist: a behavior rating scale for assessment of treatment effects. *American Journal of Mental Deficiency, 89*, 485–491.

American Psychological Association, Task Force on Psychological Intervention Guidelines. (1995). *Template for Developing Guidelines: Interventions for Mental Disorders and Psychosocial Aspects of Physical Disorders.* Washington, DC: American Psychological Association.

Anderson, L. T., Campbell, M., Adams, P., Small, A. M., Perry, R., & Shell, J. (1989). The effects of haloperidol on discrimination learning and behavioral symptoms in autistic children. *Journal of Autism and Developmental Disorders, 19*, 227–239.

Anderson, L. T., Campbell, M., Grega, D. M., Perry, R., Small, A. M., & Green, W. H. (1984). Haloperidol in the treatment of infantile autism: Effects on learning and behavioral symptoms. *American Journal of Psychiatry, 141*, 1195–1202.

Ball, C., Phillips, R., & Shenker, N. (2000). *Evidence-Based On-Call.* Churchill Livingston, London.

Barthelemy, C., Garrequ, B., Leddet, I., Ernouf, D., Muh, J. P., & Lelord, G. (1981). Behavioral and biological effects of oral magnesium, vitamin B$_6$ administration in autistic children. *Magnesium Bulletin, 2,* 150–153.

Barthelemy, C., Garrequ, B., Leddet, I., Ernouf, D., Muh, J. P., Lelord, G., & Callaway, E. (1983). Interest of behavioral scales and determination levels of urinary homovanillic acid for the control of the effects of a treatment associating vitamin B$_6$ and magnesium in children presenting an autistic behavior. *Neuropsychiatrie de L'Enfance, 31,* 289–301.

Benkert, O., & Maier, W. (1990). The necessity of placebo application in psychotropic drug trials. *Pharmacopsychiatry, 23,* 203–205.

Bouvard, M. P., Leboyer, M., Launay, J. M., Recasens, C., Plumet, M. H., Waller-Perotte, D., Tauteau, F., Bondoux, D., Dugas, M., & Lensing, P., et al. (1995). Low-dose naltrexone effects on plasma chemistries and clinical symptoms in autism: A double-blind placebo-controlled study. *Psychiatry Research, 58,* 191–201.

Brasic, J. R., Barnett, J. Y., Kaplan, D., Sheitman, B. B., Aisemberg, P., Larargue, R. T., Kowalik, S., Clark, A., Tsaltas, M. O., & Young, J. G. (1994). Clomipramine ameliorates adventitious movements and compulsions in prepubertal boys with autistic disorder and severe mental retardation. *Neurology, 44,* 1309–1312.

Brodkin, E. S., McDougle, C. J., Naylor, S. T., Cohen, D. J., & Price, L. H. (1997). Clomipramine in adults with pervasive developmental disorders: A prospective open-label investigation. *Journal of Child and Adolescent Psychopharmacology, 7,* 109–121.

Campbell, M., Armenteros, J. L., Malone, R. P., Adams, P. B., Eisenberg, Z. W., & Overall, J. E. (1997). Neuroleptic-related dyskinesias in autistic children: A prospective, longitudinal study. *Journal of the American Academy of Child and Adolescent Psychiatry, 36,* 835–843.

Cazzullo, A. G., Musetti, M. C., Musetti, L., Bajo, S., Sacerdote, P., & Panerai, A. (1999). Beta-endorphin levels in peripheral blood mononuclear cells and long-term naltrexone treatment in autistic children. *European Neuropsychopharmacology, 9,* 361–366.

Chambless, D. L., Sanderson, W. C., Shoham, V., Johnson, S. B., Pope, K. S., Crits-Cristoph, P., Baker, M., Johnson, B., Woods, S. R., Sue, S., Beutler, L., Williams, D. A., & McCurry, S. (1996). An update on empirically validated therapies. *The Clinical Psychologist, 49,* 5–18.

Cho, M. K., & Bero, L. A. (1994). Instruments for assessing the quality of drug studies published in the medical literature. *Journal of the American Medical Association, 272,* 101–104.

Cook, E. H., Jr., Rowlett, R., Jaselskis, C., & Leventhal, B. L. (1992). Fluoxetine treatment of children and adults with autistic disorder and mental retardation. *Journal of the American Academy of Child and Adolescent Psychiatry, 31,* 739–745.

DeLong, G. R., Teague, L. A., & McSwain Kamran, M. (1998). Effects of fluoxetine treatment in young children with idiopathic autism. *Developmental Medicine and Child Neurology, 40,* 551–562.

Edwards, A. G. K., Russell, I. T., & Stott, N. C. H. (1998). Signal versus noise in the evidence base for medicine: An alternative to hierarchies of evidence? *Family Practice 15,* 319–322.

Fatemi, S. H., Realmuto, G. M., Khan, L., & Thuras, P. (1998). Fluoxetine in treatment of adolescent patients with autism: A longitudinal open study. *Journal of Autism and Development, 28,* 303–307.

Fernell, E., Watanabe, Y., Adolfsson, I., Tani, Y., Bergstrom, M., Hartvig P., Lilja A., vonKnorring A. L., Gillberg C., & Langstrom B. (1997). Possible effects of tetrahydrobiopterin treatment in six children with autism— clinical and positron emission tomography data: A pilot study. *Developmental Medicine and Child Neurology, 39,* 313–318.

Findling, R. L., Maxwell, K., Scotese-Wojtila, L., Huang, J., Yamashita, T., & Wiznitzer, M. (1997). High-dose pyridoxine and magnesium administration in children with autistic disorder: An absence of salutary effects in a double-blind, placebo-controlled study. *Journal of Autism and Developmental Disorders, 27,* 467–478.

Findling, R. L., Maxwell, K., & Wiznitzer, M. (1997). An open clinical trail of risperidone monotherapy in young children with autistic disorder. *Psychopharmacology Bulletin, 33,* 155–159.

Food and Drug Administration. (1999). *Guidance for Industry. Clinical development programs for drugs, devices, and biological products intended for the treatment of rheumatoid arthritis (RA).* www.fda.gov/cder/guidance/1208fnl.htm.

Friedman, E. H. (1991. Adverse effects of fluoxetine. *Journal of the American Academy of Child and Adolescent Psychiatry, 30,* 508.

Gordon, C. T., Rapoport, J. L., Hamburger, S. D., State, R. C., & Mannheim G. B. (1992). Differential response of seven subjects with autistic disorder to clomipramine and desipramine. *American Journal of Psychiatry, 149,* 363–366.

Gordon, C. T., State, R. C., Nelson, J. E., Hamburger, S. D., & Rapoport, J. L. (1993). A double-blind comparison of clomipramine, desipramine, and placebo in the treatment of autistic disorder. *Archives of General Psychiatry, 50,* 441–447.

Gupta, S. (1999). Treatment of children with autism with intravenous immunoglobulin [letter]. *Journal of Child Neurology, 14,* 203–205.

Gupta, S., Aggarwal, S., & Heads, C. (1996). Brief report: Dysregulated immune system in children with autism: Beneficial effects of intravenous immune globulin on autistic characteristics. *Journal of Autism and Developmental Disorders, 26,* 439–452.

Guy, W. (1976). *ECDEU Assessment Manual for Psychopharmacology, revised, DHEW Pub. No. (ADM) 76–338.* Rockville, MD: National Institute of Mental Health.

Guyatt, G. H., Sackett, D. L., Cook, D. J., for the Evidence-Based Medicine Working Group. (1994). Users' guide to the medical literature, II. How to use an article about therapy or prevention, B—what were the results and will they help me in caring for my patients? *Journal of the American Medical Association, 271,* 59–63.

Guyatt, G. H., Sackett, D. L., Sinclair, J. C., Hayward, R., Cook, D. J., Coo, R. J., for the Evidence-Based Medicine Working Group. (1995). Users' guide to the medical literature, IX. A method for grading healthcare recommendations. *Journal of the American Medical Association, 274,* 1800–1804.

Harvey, R. J., & Cooray, S. E. (1995). The effective treatment of severe repetitive behaviors with fluvoxamine in a 20 year old autistic female. *International Clinical Psychopharmacology, 10,* 201–203.

Hayward, R. S. A., Wilson, M. C., Runis, S. R., Bass, E. B., & Guyatt, G. H. (1995). Users' guide to the medical literature. VII. How to use clinical guidelines. A. Are the recommendations valid? *Journal of the American Medical Association, 274,* 570–574.

Hellings, J. A., Kelley, L. A., Gabrielli, W. F., Kilgore, E., & Shah, P. (1996). Sertraline response in adults with mental retardation and autistic disorder. *Journal of Clinical Psychiatry, 57,* 333–336.

Hollander, E., Kaplan, A., Cartwright, C., & Reichman, D. (2000). Venlafaxine in children, adolescents and young adults with autism spectrum disorders: An open retrospective clinical report. *Journal of Child Neurology, 15,* 132–135.

Horrigan, J. P., & Barnhill, L. J. (1997). Risperidone and explosive aggressive autism. *Journal of Autism and Developmental Disorders, 27,* 313–323.

Horvath, K. (2000). Secretin treatment for autism. *New England Journal of Medicine, 342,* 1216.

Horvath, K., Stefanatos, G., Sokolski, K. N., Wachtel, R., Nabors, L., & Tildon, J. T. (1998). Improved social and language skills after secretin administration in patients with autistic spectrum disorders. *Journal of the Association for Academic Minority Physicians, 9,* 9–15.

Joshi, P. T., Capozzoli, J. A., & Coyle, J. T. (1988). Low-dose neuroleptic therapy for children with childhood-onset pervasive developmental disorder. *American Journal of Psychiatry, 145,* 335–338.

Kolmen, B. K., Feldman, H. M., Handen, B. L., & Janosky, J. E. (1995). Naltrexone in young autistic children: A double-blind, placebo-controlled crossover study. *Journal of the American Academy of Child and Adolescent Psychiatry, 34,* 223–231.

Kolmen, B. K., Feldman, H. M., Handen, B. L., & Janosky, J. E. (1998). Naltrexone in young autistic children: Replication study and learning measures. *Journal of the American Academy of Child and Adolescent Psychiatry, 36,* 1570–1578.

Komori, H., Matsuishi, T., Yamada, S., Yamashita, Y., Ohtaki E., & Kato, H. (1995). Cerebrospinal fluid biopterin and biogenic amine metabolites during oral R-THBP therapy for infantile autism. *Journal of Autism and Developmental Disorders, 25,* 183–193.

Koshes, R. J. (1997). Use of fluoxetine for obsessive–compulsive behavior in adults with autism. *American Journal of Psychiatry, 154,* 578.

Laporte, J. R., & Figueras, A. (1994). Placebo effects in psychiatry. *Lancet, 344,* 1206–1209.

Lelord, G., Muh, J. P., Barthelemy, C., Martineau, J., & Garreau, B. (1981). Effects of pyridoxine and magnesium on autistic symptoms—initial observations. *Journal of Autism and Developmental Disorders, 11,* 219–230.

Lonigan, C. J., Elbert, J. C., & Johnson, S. B. (1998). Empirically supported psychosocial interventions for children: An overview. *Journal of Clinical Child Psychology, 27,* 138–145.

Martin, A., Koenig, K., Seahill, L., & Bergman, J. (1999). Open-label quetiapine in the treatment of children and adolescents with autistic disorders. *Journal of Child and Adolescent Pharmacology, 9,* 99–107.

Martineau, J., Barthelemy, C., Garreau, B., & Lelord, G. (1985). Vitamin B6, magnesium and combined B6-magnesium: Therapeutic effects in childhood autism. *Biological Psychiatry, 20,* 467–478.

McDougle, C. J., Brodkin, E. S., Naylor, S. T., Carlson, D. C., Cohen, D. J., & Price, L. H. (1998a). Sertraline in adults with pervasive developmental disorders: A prospective open-label investigation. *Journal of Clinical Psychopharmacology, 18,* 62–66.

McDougle, C. J., Holmes, J. P., Bronson, M. R., Anderson, G. M., Volkmar, F. R., Price, L. H., & Cohen D. J. (1997). Risperidone treatment of children and adolescents with pervasive developmental disorders: A prospective open-label study. *Journal of the American Academy of Child and Adolescent Psychiatry*, *36*, 685–693.

McDougle, C. J., Holmes, J. P., Carlson, D. C., Pelton, G. H., Cohen, D. J., & Price, L. H. (1998b). A double-blind, placebo-controlled study of risperidone in adults with autistic disorder and other pervasive developmental disorders. *Archives of General Psychiatry*, *55*, 633–641.

McDougle, C. J., Naylor, S. T., Cohen, D. J., Volkmar, F. R., Heninger, G. R., & Price, L. H. (1996). A double-blind, placebo-controlled study of fluvoxamine in adults with autistic disorder. *Archives of General Psychiatry*, *53*, 1001–1008.

McDougle, C. J., Scahill, L., McCracken, J. T., Aman, M. G., Tierney, E., Arnold, L. E., Freeman, B. J., Martin, A., McGough, J. J., Cronin, P., Posey, D. J., Riddle, M. A., Ritz, L., Swiezy, N. B., Vitiello, B., Volkmar, F. R., Votolato, N. A., & Walson, P. (2000). Research units on pediatric psychopharmacology (RUPP) autism network. background and rationale for an initial controlled study of risperidone. *Child and Adolescent Psychiatric Clinics of North America*, *9*, 201–224.

Mehlinger, R., Scheftner, W. A., & Poznanski, E. (1991). Fluoxetine and autism. *Journal of the American Academy of Child and Adolescent Psychiatry*, *29*, 985.

Michaud, G., McGowan, J. L., van der Jagt, R., Wells, G., & Tugwell, P. (1998). Are therapeutic decisions supported by evidence from health care research? *Archives of Internal Medicine*, *158*, 1665–1668.

Nagahata, M., Kazamaturi, H., Nuruse, H., Yamazaki, K., Takesada, M., Nakane, Y., Kaihara S., & Ohashi, Y. (1992). Clinical evaluation of apropterin hydrochloride (R-THBP) on infantile autism: A multicenter cooperative study. In H. Naruse and E. M. Ornitz (Eds.), *Neurobiology of Infantile Autism* (pp. 351–354). Amsterdam: Elsevier.

Nakane, Y., Naruse, H., Takesada, M., & Yamazaki, K. (1992). Clinical effect of R-THBP on infantile autism. In H. Naruse and EM Ornitz (Eds.), *Neurobiology of Infantile Autism* (pp. 337–350). Amsterdam: Elsevier.

Nicolson, R., Awad, G., & Sloman, L. (1998). An open trial of risperidone in young autistic children. *Journal of the American Academy of Child and Adolescent Psychiatry*, *37*, 372–376.

Owley, T., Steele, E., Corsello, C., Risi, S., McKaig, K., Lord, C., Leventhal, B. L., & Cook, E. H., Jr. (1999). A double-blind, placebo-controlled trial of secretin for the treatment of autistic disorder. *Medscape-General Medicine*. www.medscape.com/Medscape/GeneralMedicine/journal/1999/v01.m10/mgm1006.owle/pn-mgm1006.owle.html.

Ozbayrak, K. R. (1997). Sertraline in PDD. *Journal of the American Academy of Child and Adolescent Psychiatry*, *36*, 7–8.

Pauling, L. (1968). Orthomolecular psychiatry. *Science*, *160*, 265–271.

Peral, M., Alxami, M., & Gilaberte, I. (1999). Fluoxetine in children with autism. *Journal of the American Academy of Child and Adolescent Psychiatry*, *38*, 1471–1472.

Perry, R., & Bangaru, B. S. (1998). Secretin in autism. *Journal of Child and Adolescent Psychopharmacology*, *8*, 247–248.

Pfeiffer, S. I., Norton, J., Nelson, L., & Shott, S. (1995). Efficacy of vitamin B6 and magnesium in the treatment of autism: A methodology review and summary of outcomes. *Journal of Autism and Developmental Disorders*, *25*, 481–493.

Plioplys, A. V. (1998). Intravenous immunoglobulin treatment of children with autism. *Journal of Child Neurology*, *13*, 79–82.

Posey, D. J., Litwiller, M., Koburn, A., & McDougle, C. J. (1999a). Paroxetine in autism. *Journal of the American Academy of Child and Adolescent Psychiatry*, *38*, 111–112.

Posey, D. J., Walsh, K. H., Wilson, G. A., & McDougle, C. J. (1999b). Risperidone in the treatment of two very young children with autism. *Journal of Child and Adolescent Psychopharmacology*, *9*, 273–276.

Potenza, M. N., Holmes, J. P., Kanes, S. J., & McDougle, C. J. (1999). Olanzapine treatment of children, adolescents, and adults with pervasive developmental disorders: An open label pilot study. *Journal of Clinical Psychopharmacology*, *19*, 37–44.

Quintana, H., Birmaher, B., Stedge, D., Lennon, S., Freed, J., Bridge, J., & Greenhill, L. (1995). Use of methylphenidate in the treatment of children with autistic disorder. *Journal of Autism and Developmental Disorders*, *25*, 283–294.

Quitkin, F. M. (1999). Placebos, drug effects, and study design: A clinician's guide. *American Journal of Psychiatry*, *156*, 829–836.

Rimland, B. (1998). High dose vitamin B6 and magnesium in treating autism: Response to study by Findling et al. *Journal of Autism and Developmental Disorders*, *28*, 581–582.

Rimland, B. (2000). Secretin treatment for autism. *New England Journal of Medicine, 342,* 1216–1217.

Rimland, B., Callaway, E., & Dreyfus, P. (1978). The effect of high doses of vitamin B6 on autistic children: A double-blind crossover study. *American Journal of Psychiatry, 135,* 472–475.

Sackett, D. L., Strauss, S. E., Richardson, W. S., Rosenberg, W., & Haynes, R. B. (2000). *Evidence-Based Medicine: How to Practice and Teach EBM,* 2nd edit., Churchill Livingston, London.

Sanchez, L. E., Campbell, M., Small, A. M., Cueva, J. E., Armenteros, J. L., & Adams, P. B. (1996). A pilot study of clomipramine in young autistic children. *Journal of the American Academy of Child and Adolescent Psychiatry, 35,* 537–544.

Sandler, A. D., Sutton, K. A., DeWeese, J., Girardi, M. A., Sheppard, V., & Bodfish, J. W. (1999). Lack of benefit of a single dose of synthetic human secretin in the treatment of autism and pervasive developmental disorder. *New England Journal of Medicine, 341,* 1801–1806.

Smeraldi, E., Zanardi, R., Benedetti, F., DiBella, D., Perz, J., & Catalano, M. (1998). Polymorphism within the promoter of the serotonin transporter gene and antidepressant efficacy of fluvoxamine. *Molecular Psychiatry, 3,* 508–511.

Snead, R. W., Boon, F., & Presberg, J. (1994). Paroxetine for self-injurious behavior. *Journal of the American Academy of Child and Adolescent Psychiatry, 33,* 909–910.

Steingard, R. J., Zimjnitzky, B., DeMaso, D. R., Bauman, M. L., & Bucci, J. P. (1997). Sertraline treatment of transition-associated anxiety and agitation in children with autistic disorder. *Journal of Child and Adolescent Psychopharmacology, 7,* 9–15.

Todd, R. (1991). Fluoxetine in autism. *American Journal of Psychiatry, 148,* 8.

Willemsen-Swinkels, S. H., Buitelaar, J. K., Nijhof, G. J., & van Engeland, H. (1995). Failure of naltrexone hydrochloride to reduce self-injurious and autistic behavior in mentally retarded adults. Double-blind placebo-controlled study. *Archives of General Psychiatry, 52,* 766–773.

Willemsen-Swinkels, S. H., Buitelaar, J. K., van Berckelaer-Onnes, I. A., & van Engeland, H. (1999). Brief report: Six months continuation treatment in naltrexone-responsive children with autism: An open-label case-control design. *Journal of Autism and Developmental Disorders, 29,* 167–169.

Willemsen-Swinkels, S. H., Buitelaar, J. K., Weijnen, F. G., & van Engeland, H. (1995). Placebo-controlled acute dosage naltrexone study in young autistic children. *Psychiatry Research, 58,* 203–215.

Zanardi, R., Benedetti, F., DiBella, D., Catalano, M., & Smeraldi, E. (2000). Efficacy of paroxetine in depression is influenced by a functional polymorphism within the promoter of the serotonin transporter gene. *Journal of Clinical Psychopharmacology, 20,* 105–107.

15

Sleep Problems in Autism

Shoshana Arbelle and Itezhak Z. Ben-Zion

Children spend almost half of a 24-hour day sleeping. Although much research and effort have been directed at investigating the physiologic basis and the need for sleep, it is still not well understood. Our knowledge of sleep problems in children in general and in autism in particular is still lacking. In this chapter we summarize the present knowledge on sleep problems in autism and on the known interventions.

NORMAL SLEEP

Sleep is a state marked by a characteristic immobile posture and reversible diminished sensitivity to stimuli, during which volition and consciousness are in partial or complete abeyance and bodily functions are partly suspended. When measured by electroencephalography (EEG), brain electrical activity shows specific changes during sleep (Figure 15-1) (Anders, 1994; Armstrong, Quinn, & Dadds, 1994).

There are two major types of sleep: NREM, which is quiet, synchronized sleep with no rapid eye movements, and REM, which is desynchronized, paradoxical sleep with rapid eye movements. Generally, during the night there are four to six cycles of quiet sleep alternating with REM sleep. During the later part of the night the REM sleep becomes more prominent (Figure 15-2).

Sleep onset latency (SOL) refers to the interval between the time the child is put to bed and the time she or he falls asleep. During the transition from wakefulness to sleep there are typical physiological changes: (1) On the EEG the signal changes from an alpha rhythm to a mix of frequencies and (2) muscle relaxation is shown with a slight decrease in the amplitude of the muscle tone. Before the onset of sleep, slower eye movements are observed and soothing movements are noticed.

The establishment of a mature sleep–wake rhythm is a developmental phenomenon. In babies the sleep–wake cycle is not well adapted, but during the first 2 years of life,

SHOSHANA ARBELLE and ITEZHAK Z. BEN-ZION • Ben-Gurion University Soroka Medical Center, Beer-Sheva, 84777 Israel.

The Research Basis for Autism Intervention, edited by Schopler, Yirmiya, Shulman, and Marcus. Kluwer Academic/Plenum Publishers, New York, 2001.

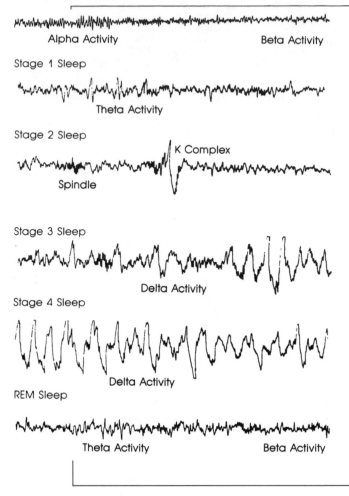

FIGURE 15-1. Electroencephalogram (EEG) of human of human sleep stages. The first trace illustrates alpha activity seen in quiet wakefulness (eyes closed) and the beta activity of an alert person. Stage 1 theta activity is seen in the second trace. Stage 2 sleep (with associated K complex and sleep spindle) is in the third trace. The fourth and fifth traces show slow-wave sleep (stages 3 and 4), with prominent delta activity. Thus synchronous activity is absent in REM sleep (sixth trace), which resembles stage 1 EEG. The REM sleep is accompanied by rapid eye movements and muscle paralysis.

infants adapt a 24-hour schedule. The infant begins to sleep for the longest time during the night, and takes some shorter naps during the day. As a toddler, the child usually gives up daytime naps and night sleep becomes the sole sleep time. This period is longer for younger children as the total time required decreases during infancy to reach adult levels during teenage years (Ferber, 1996). Factors that entrain the sleep–wake rhythm include environmental and social signs such as feeding times, sounds, voices, dark–light cycle, and so forth. Studies of normal children suggest a link between sleep problems and the results

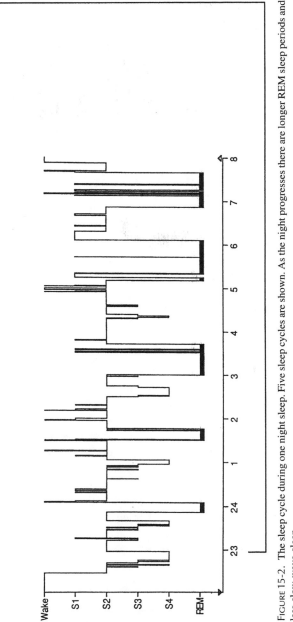

FIGURE 15-2. The sleep cycle during one night sleep. Five sleep cycles are shown. As the night progresses there are longer REM sleep periods and less slow wave sleep.

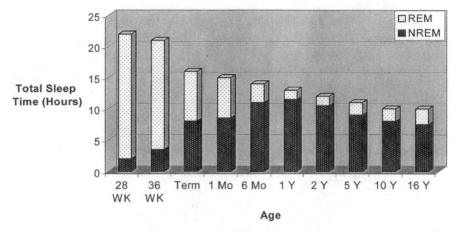

FIGURE 15-3. The development of REM, and of non-REM sleep. Total time spent in REM sleep decreases throughout infancy and early childhood. By 3 to 5 years of age the adult level of 25% of the total sleep time is reached though the total number of hours continues to decrease, reaching the adult level at about age 16.

of neuropsychological tests addressing attention, concentration, cognitive function, and precision.

The duration of SOL and its daily regulation were found to be good predictors of sleep problems of children in both early and late infancy (Van-Tassel, 1985). Infants who fall asleep on their own are more likely to sleep through the night than those who are actively soothed, nursed, rocked, or comforted by their parents (Anders 1994; Johnson, 1991; Richman 1981; Richman, Douglas, Heather, Landsdown, & Levere, 1985). The ability of the child to relax his or her body and then tune out external and internal stimulation is one of the factors influencing the length and nature of the SOL (Borkovec, Kaloupek, & Slama, 1975; Lacks, Bertelson, Gans, & Kunkel 1983; Shealy, 1979). If the child fails to fall asleep or to maintain it repetitively, a sleep problem is usually diagnosed.

Sleep disorders are divided into three major groups: dyssomnias, parasomnias, and sleep disorders that accompany medical or psychiatric disorders. Dyssomnias are sleep problems during the sleep period and are classified as either intrinsic, extrinsic, or circadian sleep disorders. Parasomnias are behavioral disorders that occur in conjunction with sleep and that are associated with brief or partial arousal, without marked sleep disruption or impaired daytime alertness. Almost every medical or psychiatric disease has an impact on the normal sleep pattern. The sleep abnormalities associated with these diseases are diverse (Barthlen & Stacy, 1994).

SLEEP PROBLEMS IN CHILDREN

Sleep problems are sleep behaviors that are disturbing in some way to the child him- or herself, his or her family, or others in his environment. Sleep problems are different than "sleep disorders," which imply an underlying physiological dysfunction. Sleep problems in children are common. They can be divided into problems in initiating and problems in maintaining a good and restful sleep. Overall one third of preschool children have a considerable degree of such problems. In young healthy children it is common to find arousals associated with confusion, nightmares, and sleep terrors. During adolescence sleep usually improves and the occurrence of sleep problems diminishes.

SLEEP PROBLEMS IN AUTISM

Sleep problems are among a number of secondary behavioral difficulties that occur in children with autism. There are little data concerning sleep problems in children with developmental disabilities in general and with autism specifically. We do know that sleep problems are common in children with mental retardation; 34% to 80% of these children are reported to have sleep difficulties (Hering et al., 1999; Jonson, 1996; Quine, 1991).

As with typically developing children, younger children have a greater occurrence of sleep problems than older children. In some of the different groups of mentally retarded individuals there is a correlation between the intellectual deficit and sleep problems. It is well documented that sleep disorders are associated with problematic behaviors, but it is hard to differentiate if the sleep disorder is the cause of the behavioral problem or one of its manifestations.

Studying sleep requires cooperation on the part of the child and his or her ability to tolerate the attachment of electrodes to his or her head. In addition, the child often has to sleep in a laboratory setting. These factors make the study of sleep in children with autism very difficult. As a result most of the available data on sleep patterns and sleep problems are based on parental reports on relatively older children with autism rather than on physiologic parameters (Keener, Zeanah, & Anders 1988; Minde, Popiel, Leos, Falkner, Parker, & Handley-Derry, 1993; Sadeh, Lavie, & Scher, 1994).

The exact causes of sleep problems in children with mental retardation are poorly understood, but are likely to be related to some factors that interfere with sleep control and maintenance. Likewise, they may be due to a lack of comprehension of environmental and social signs. Sleep problems are more prevalent in children with autism than in children with other developmental problems of scholastic skills or in children with mental retardation. It has been estimated that up to 90% of children with autism currently experience, or experienced in the past, from significant sleep problems (Taira, Takase, & Sasaki, 1998).

The more commonly reported severe sleep problems in the autism-spectrum disorders are those associated with sleep onset and maintenance: Irregular sleep–wake patterns, long sleep latencies, problems with sleep onset, poor sleep, early waking, and poor sleep routines. In addition, shortened night sleep, alteration in sleep onset and wake times, night walking, and irregular sleep patterns have been reported. In general sleep problems are more frequent in younger children (under 8 years of age). These high rates do not correlate significantly with either the degree of the disability or with the child's intelligence. The high rate of sleep problems in children with autism appears to occur at all IQ levels, with possible differences in the profile of disturbance. In some of the parental reports, children in the high functioning autistic group sleep less than those in the low functioning group, have longer sleep latencies, and if they wake up, spend longer time awake at night. The low functioning children take more frequent naps during the day and fall asleep earlier in the evening. Though, in other studies parents report that the likelihood of sleep problems such as increased sleep latency, multiple waking, and short night sleep is high for the lower functioning children, particularly those younger than 8 years of age. The same amount and quality of sleep disorders have been found in children with Asperger's disorder as in those with autism. There is some evidence of abnormalities of the sleep–wake cycle in children with Rett syndrome when compared to typically developing children (Richdale, 1999; Richdale & Priot, 1995).

Controversy exists regarding the incidence of parasomnia sleep disorders among children with autism. Some studies have found the same incidence as in children with mental retardation, but higher than in normal children, while other studies have found a higher likelihood of this disorder in children with autism, especially sleepwalking and nightmares. Unusual sleep routines may also be disruptive in that sleep problems are likely to occur when the conditions for the routine are not met. Unusual and problematic routines for settling to sleep have been reported in children with autism.

As for children with developmental disabilities, children with autism and sleep problems have a greater tendency to problematic daytime behaviors. More problematic, energetic, and exited behaviors during the day were associated with shorter night sleep length (Gozal, 1998). There is evidence that for older people with autism the EEG patterns of sleep were different from normal adults and showed higher REM density. In some studies the REM sleep in children and adults with autism (in comparison with typically developing children) showed some immaturity in the organization of the eye movements: the periods did not became longer during the night, and instead some irregular bursts were demonstrated (Diomedi, Curatolo, Scalise, Placidi, Caretto, & Gigli, 1999; Tanguay, Ornitz, Forsythe, & Rituo, 1976).

THE ETIOLOGY OF SLEEP PROBLEMS IN AUTISM

The reasons for the high incidence of sleep problems among children with autism is not well understood. A relationship between social and communication difficulties and sleep disorders is possible. The sleep–wake cycle is a circadian rhythm. There is evidence to suggest that as well as the light–dark cycle, humans use social cues to entrain circadian rhythms. Routine and social cues are thought to help the infant develop stable sleep–wake patterns, with the longest sleep occurring at night. Children with primary social–communication deficit may therefore have difficulty with their sleep–wake schedules. For a subgroup of children with autism the dysregulation of melatonin—the brain hormone released during the dark—may be the reason for sleep problems. The major physiologic role of melatonin relates to the synchronization of bodily rhythms to photoperiodic information. Melatonin is also important in the regulation of sleep initiation and maintenance. Low levels of melatonin have been found in only a small subgroup of children with autism, however. The neurotransmitter serotonin, which is further along the synthetic pathway of melatonin, is found to be elevated in a quarter to a third of the children with autism. However, the relationship between these two compounds is not yet clearly established. In addition, the higher incidence of abnormality of the hypothalamic–pituitary–adrenal axis in children with autism may also contribute to the circadian rhythm disturbance. High levels of anxiety are reported in children with autism. As in typically developing children and adults, anxiety may cause insomnia and can contribute to the sleep problems in autism.

It is still unclear whether children with autism have some specific brain abnormality. Recent studies have found abnormalities in the cerebellum and limbic system. If confirmed, these findings might provide a putative etiology for some of the sleep problems in these children.

Another area that is still not well explored is subthreshold epileptic activity in autism. Some investigators claim that in a subgroup of children with autism, careful and sensitive electroencephalograms show epileptic activity in areas of the brain that are responsible for alertness. Once again this might explain some of the sleep problems in these children.

TREATMENT OF SLEEP PROBLEMS IN AUTISM

Even though we do not understand the exact reasons, children with autism suffer from severe sleep problems. These problems are stressful to child, the family, and the caretakers. There are some interventions that might help and that are worthwhile trying. Sleep problems are one of the problems in autism that are amenable to therapy, and should not be seen as an inevitable consequence of autistic disorders (Takase, Taira, & Sasaki, 1998).

Interventions might be behavioral, environmental, or medical. In any event the therapeutic intervention should be based on a careful history and a sleep diary that documents actual problems rather than assumptions. Parents tend to remember only the bad sleepless nights, and keeping a diary might be therapeutic in itself, as the actual problem rather than the imagined one is defined.

Behavioral treatment of sleep disorders might also ameliorate other behavioral problems in these children. Behavioral techniques employ reinforcement of appropriate sleep behaviors and decreasing inappropriate behaviors, establishing strict wake and sleep schedules, appropriate bedtime routines, and strict constant approach to waking and sleeping problems. Parents are encouraged to deal with cries and pleas for attention in the same systematic and predetermined way, for example, coming to the room but not taking the child out of bed or giving a kiss and a hug and demanding return to sleep, leaving the room after a short while. The intervention needs constant readjustments to maximize the effect. Each intervention should be tailored to the individual child and family. The treatment has to take into account the needs and abilities of each family member.

Medical therapy is possible with drugs that are used to treat adult sleep disorders. Treatment with sedatives is possible, although not recommended owing to the problem of addiction and adaptation (Gilman & Tuchman, 1995). Melatonin supplementation may also be helpful, even though the studies on this intervention are still being debated. A single dose of 0.05–0.1 mg/kg is recommended before bedtime (Lord, 1998; Jan & O'Donnell, 1996). Antiepileptic drugs should be considered if an epileptiform disorder is suspected. Antipsychotic drugs are not a good choice for the treatment of sleep disorders per se, but might be helpful if used for other reasons (McDaniel, 1986).

Environmental interventions involve readjustment of the circadian sleep–wake cycle. This includes light therapy—employing bright light that may readjust the sleep cycle, presumably by altering the melatonin secretion. Chronotherapy is another environmental intervention that does not let the child sleep, delaying sleep little by little until the desired bedtime is reached (Keener et al., 1988; Richdale, 1999).

CONCLUSIONS

Sleep problems in autism specifically are common and need attention and treatment. Although very common, sleep problems are not part of the diagnostic criteria for autism. The exact reasons and mechanisms of this disorder are not well understood. It seems that children with autism have a specific profile of sleep problems, particularly in relation to onset and maintenance. Problems occur at a higher frequency and are more severe than those found in typically developing children and many children with other developmental disabilities. There are also associations between problematic behaviors and sleep problems, and more energetic daytime behavior and sleep problems. Sleep problems occur at all levels of intellectual functioning. These findings suggest that that sleep difficulties are probably related to some specific deficits found in autism, rather than to primary impairment in intellectual functioning.

It is difficult to accurately assess sleep in children with autism because of technical problems and the need for cooperation. More studies are needed both to define the etiology of the sleep problems in autism and to carefully assess different therapeutic interventions.

REFERENCES

Anders, T. F. (1994). Infant sleep, nighttime relationships, and attachment. *Psychiatry*, *57*, 11–21.

Armstrong, K. L, Quinn, R. A., & Dadds, M. R. (1994). The sleep patterns of normal children. *Medical Journal of Australia*, *161*, 202–205.

Barthlen, G. M., & Stacy, C. (1994). Dyssomnias, parasomnias, and sleep disorders associated with medical and psychiatric diseases. *The Mount Sinai Journal of Medicine*, *61*(2), 139.

Borkovec, T. D., Kaloupek, D. G., & Slama, K. M. (1975). The facilitative of muscle tension-release in the relaxation treatment of sleep disturbance. *Behavioral Therapy*, *6*, 301–309.

Diomedi, M., Curatolo, P., Scalise, A., Placidi, F., Caretto, F., & Gigli, G. L. (1999). Sleep abnormalities in mentally retarded autistic subjects: Down's syndrome with mental retardation and normal subjects. *Brain Development*, *21*(8), 548–553.

Ferber, R. (1996). Childhood sleep disorders. *Neurologic Clinics*, *14*, 493–511.

Gilman, J. T., Tuchman, R. F. (1995). Autism and associated behavioral disorders: Pharmacotherapeutic interventions. *Annals of Pharmacotherapy*, *29*, 47–56.

Gozal, D. (1998). Sleep disordered breathing and school performance in children. *Pediatrics*, *102*(3), 616–620.

Hering, E., Epstein, R., Elroy, S., Iancu, D. R., & Zelnik, N. (1999). Sleep patterns in autistic children. *Journal of Autism and Developmental Disorders*, *29*(2), 143–147.

Jan, J. E., & O'Donnell, M. E. (1996). Use of melatonin in the treatment of paediatric sleep disorders. *Journal of Pineal Research*, *21*(4), 193–199. Review.

Johnson, M. (1991). Infant and toddlers sleep: A telephone survey of parents in one community. *Journal of Developmental and Behavioral Pediatrics*, *12*, 108–114.

Jonson, C. R. (1996). Sleep problems of children with mental retardation and autism. *Child and Adolescent Psychiatric Clinic of North America*, *5*, 673–683.

Keener, M., Zeanah, C., & Anders, T. (1988). Infant temperament, sleep organization and nighttime parental intervention. *Pediatrics*, *81*, 762–771.

Lacks, P., Bertelson, A. D., Gans, L., & Kunkel, J. (1983). The effectiveness of three behavioral treatment for different degrees of sleep onset insomnia. *Behavior Therapy*, *14*(5), 593–605.

Lord, C. (1998). What is melatonin? Is it useful treatment for sleep problems in autism? *Journal of Autism and Developmental Disorders, 28*(4), 345–346.

McDaniel, K. D. (1986). Pharmacologic treatment of psychiatric and neurodevelopmental disorders in children and adolescents (Part 1). *Clinical Pediatrics, 25*(2), 65–71.

Minde, K., Popiel, K., Leos, N., Falkner, S., Parker, K. & Handley-Derry, M. (1993). The evaluation and treatment of sleep disturbances in young children. *Journal of Child Psychology and Psychiatry, 34*(4), 521–523.

Quine, L. (1991). Sleep problems in children with mental handicap. *Journal of Mental Deficiency Research. 35,* 269–290.

Richdale, A. L. (1999). Sleep problems in autism: Prevalence, cause, and intervention. *Developmental Medicine and Child Neurology, 41,* 60–66.

Richdale, A. L., & Priot, M. R. (1995). The sleep/wake rhythm in children with autism. *European Child and Adolescent Psychiatry, 4*(3) 175–186.

Richman, N. (1981). A community survey of characteristics of one- to two-year-olds with sleep disruptions. *Journal of the American Academy of Child Psychiatry, 20,* 281–291.

Richman, N., Douglas, J., Heather, H., Lansdown, R., & Levere, R. (1985). Behavioral methods in the treatment of sleep disorders-a pilot study. *Child Psychology and Psychiatry, 26,* 581–590.

Sadeh, A., Lavie, P., & Scher, A. (1994). Sleep and temperament maternal perceptions of temperament of sleep-disturbed toddlers. *Early Education and Development, 5*(4), 311–322.

Shealy, R. (1979). The effectiveness of various treatment techniques on different degrees and duration of sleep onset insomnia. *Behavior Research and Therapy, 17*(6), 541–546.

Taira, M., Takase, M., & Sasaki, H. (1998). Sleep disorder in children with autism. *Psychiatry Clinics in Neuroscience, 52*(2), 182–183.

Takase, M., Taira, M., & Sasaki, H. (1998). Sleep–wake rhythm of autistic children. *Psychiatry Clinics in Neuroscience, 52*(2), 181–182.

Tanguay, P. E., Ornitz, E. M., Forsythe, A. B. & Ritvo, E. R. (1976). Rapid eye movement (REM) activity in normal and autistic children during REM sleep. *Journal of Autism and Child Schizophrenia, 6*(3), 275–278.

Van Tassel, B. (1985). The relative influence of child and environmental characteristics on sleep disturbances in the first and second year of life. *Developmental and Behavioral Pediatrics, 6,* 81–86.

16

Concluding Comments

Cory Shulman, Robert Zimin, and Edna Mishori

Different philosophical and scientific approaches to the understanding of autism were presented in this book. In this conclusion, we discuss issues and recurring themes raised in the different chapters so as to enhance our understanding of this complex syndrome, and to be able to treat individuals with autism and their families more successfully as a result of this improved understanding. First, by focusing on typical and atypical developmental patterns, one of the proposed methodologies, we address some of the unique impairments manifested in autism. Next, we deal with some of the implications of the biological approach to the study of autism. Then, because we feel that better understanding of autism as a pervasive developmental disorder serves as the basis for establishing appropriate intervention strategies, we address various issues pertaining to intervention as presented in this volume, including the need for a multidisciplinary approach both in scientific research and clinical applications. In addition, we address the impact that cultural perceptions of autism can have on the manner in which members of a given society relate to the disorder. Finally, we conclude with some general thoughts regarding individuals with autism and their families in the study of autism.

THE DEVELOPMENTAL APPROACH IN AUTISM

The importance of investigating both universal developmental patterns and psychopathology to examine the specific impairments associated with autism is a recurring theme throughout this book. Communicative intent, language comprehension, and friendship—all reflective of primary deficits in autism—were discussed in this volume. For each topic, typical developmental patterns were compared with developmental patterns found in autism to establish a basis for understanding autism. Communicative intent was suggested as a significant construct for understanding the uniqueness of autism because intentional

---

CORY SHULMAN • School of Social Work and School of Education, The Hebrew University of Jerusalem, Mount Scopus, Jerusalem, 91905 Israel.   ROBERT ZIMIN • Child and Adolescent Psychiatry Unit, Sheba Medical Center, Tel Hashomer, Israel.   EDNA MISHORI • Yachdav School, Tel Aviv, Israel.

The Research Basis for Autism Intervention, edited by Schopler, Yirmiya, Shulman, and Marcus. Kluwer Academic/Plenum Publishers, New York, 2001.

behavior lies at the interface of linguistic, social, and cognitive development, which are the identified areas of impairments in autism. Likewise, communicative comprehension was discussed, because comprehension precedes expression, and while specific expressive deficits have been identified in autism, comprehension skills are less well studied. A survey of normal development of communicative comprehension was provided to arrive at a better understanding of autism. Since autism is also defined by marked qualitative impairments in social interactions, friendship, a salient social measure, was surveyed developmentally in children with typical development and in those with autism. The interplay of the development of language and social skills has not always been a major area of research in autism, as researchers seemed to investigate singular deficits as possible core deficits from which the other impairments stemmed. By placing these different constructs together in a developmental perspective, an integrative approach to the study of autism is possible. For example, although each construct was studied independently, it was shown that developmentally, communicative intent, communicative comprehension, and social engagement all involve integrating linguistic information from various sources in order to derive the communicative functions and pragmatic force of messages communicated. In situations in which typically developing children show communicative intent, young children with autism fail to attend to speech or to show the same attentional preferences as other children.

There is evidence that people with autism show atypical sequences of development and other developmental discontinuities. Although the majority of persons with autism function within the range of mental retardation, even in high functioning people with autism, disassociations in specific domains are evident at every stage of development, and while some difficulties fade, others persist throughout life. Conversely, development sometimes appears typical at young ages when simple understanding is required, but appears deficient at later stages when more complex behavior is required. Thus, it is clear that abilities undergo changes with age. For example, research has demonstrated that imitation skills—vocal and gestural—are related to the development of language. The ability to form a friendship is linked with various developmental variables, such as receptive language level, mental age, representational abilities, and affective expressiveness. The interplay of the development of language and social skills has not always been a major area of research in autism, as researchers seemed inclined to investigate singular deficits as possible core deficits from which the other impairments stemmed. By grouping all these different constructs together in a developmental perspective, an integrative approach to the study of autism may be possible.

THE BIOLOGICAL APPROACH IN AUTISM

The biology of autism and its neurology, neurochemistry, and genetics have been ongoing areas of intensive research ever since the late 1960s, when it became apparent that the etiology of autism lay in the biological function of the brain, rather than in the psychological aspects of child rearing. Research in the biological aspects of autism has made great strides over the past several decades. Early evidence of the biological basis of autism came from clinical observations and empirical findings that the prevalence of seizures in adolescents and adults with autism is significantly higher than in the general population, and from the observed association of genetic and infectious neurological disorders, with autistic behaviors. For example, the finding of hyperserotonemia in 30% to 50% of individuals with autism led to further research in the neurochemistry of autism. The study of the developmental trajectory of a known genetic disorder, such as fragile X syndrome, which is associated with a high incidence of autism, is also helpful in genetic research of autism. Employing multiple measures of assessment and identifying environmental factors and assessing developmental outcomes could yield a more valid and richer understanding of risk factors and resilience. These techniques may help explain why some individuals with fragile X syndrome have autism, some have a subset of autistic features, and others have no autistic features. Such knowledge would not only help the fragile X population, but would also contribute to a further understanding of autism itself.

The results presented in the studies reported in this book point to increasing evidence for genetic etiological heterogeneity in autism and suggest that the liability for autism may cause milder difficulties that resemble the characteristics of autism. Family studies have played an important role both in clarifying the genetic etiology of autism and in characterizing the broader phenotype or lesser variant of autism. Such research may assist in early identification of developmental difficulties and in implementing appropriate interventions for siblings, who, in addition to facing possible genetic liability, also experience difficulties associated with living with a sibling with autism. Although the results from the studies presented in the book were mixed, they imply that demonstrating an association between known genetic polymorphisms and the autistic phenotype may provide biological markers for different etiological and phenotypical forms of autism. This would further enhance a more accurate biological classification of the phenomenological syndrome of autism, which would result in a more rational approach to diagnosis, management, therapeutic interventions, and genetic counseling.

INTERVENTIONS BASED ON RESEARCH RESULTS

As suggested in the preceding discussion, although autism is seen as a disorder that continues throughout life, its expression changes as the individual develops and learns new adaptive skills. Since appropriate intervention is based on the individual's profile of abilities and disabilities, the first step is establishing a correct diagnosis for the individual. Diagnosing a young child with autism is particularly difficult and requires a thorough understanding of the disorder across differing levels of severity as well as an understanding of differences that are related to chronological age. The purpose of diagnosing "as early as possible" is to clarify the nature of the child's developmental problems, obtain appropriate intervention services, and provide parents with helpful information and support that will assist them in coping with their child's disability. The trend toward very early diagnosis has been fueled by increased knowledge of typical and atypical developmental patterns. With better understanding of significant developmental markers for autism (e.g., joint attention, eye gaze, and other aspects of nonverbal communication), the chances of correct early diagnosis will increase. There is little doubt that providing education and treatment for very young children with autism should target core areas of dysfunction in autism and can have a very positive effect on their development. It is important to emphasize that intervention must combine a thorough understanding of the nature of autism with an individualized program that is based on a comprehensive assessment of the child's abilities and difficulties. Clarifying meaningful information for the child, providing an organized schedule of activities, and generalizing skills across settings and people are some of the intervention strategies that are most helpful to young children with autism. The teaching should be individualized, providing visual support when necessary. Likewise, programs should be based on strengths and interests of the child with autism to help with weak areas of development. Curriculum in all preschool programs should emphasize attention and compliance, imitation, language, and social skills and should be implemented in a highly structured teaching environment, which can address the child's need for predictability and routine. Family involvement should be encouraged as much as possible.

Since the intervention needs of individuals with autism change as they reach different developmental levels, learning and rehabilitation are lifelong activities. Adults with autism continue to require treatment to enhance the quality of their lives and their ability to function as independently as possible in the community. The goals include the acquisition of and the independent use of adaptive skills and the reduction of inappropriate behaviors. The living environment should incorporate aspects of both a home and a learning environment. A positive, proactive environment that takes into account the unique needs of people with autism and their family should be created.

THE MULTIDISCIPLINARY APPROACH IN AUTISM

Employing a multidisciplinary approach toward scientific inquiry and clinical applications should be taken into consideration in the field of autism. For example, it has been clinically established that the autistic phenotype is associated with inherited impairments in stress responses, and researchers investigating stress have suggested that the long arm of chromosome 7 may be the site for candidate loci of genes responsible for the autistic phenotype. As a result of this line of thought, it was suggested that the recently discovered polymorphism in the extended promoter of chromosome 7 gene (*ACHE*), which is persistently up-regulated under stress, should be surveyed in families with and without members with autism to establish the frequency of this particular polymorphism and its association with autism. Although this association has not been confirmed, this type of multidisciplinary research contributes toward the possible localization of the specific genes involved in the etiology of the autistic phenotype.

Intervention programs for individuals with autism should also adapt a multidimensional framework, involving people working in different disciplines, to germinate new ideas from complementary professions. Our understanding of autism should be based on an ecological concept of the disorder, and intervention strategies should include parents, teachers, peers, and other professionals. Although much is currently known about autism, there still is no one method of treatment for autistic children and it is essential to form an integral and holistic approach for treatment. For example, interventions may be most effective if they incorporate real experiences in which the individual with autism can practice and learn skills in actual ongoing situations. Since the individual's environment plays a significant role in helping establish and maintain skills, there should be a close collaboration among all agents—peers, parents, teachers, and therapists—who operate in a shared environment and are thus interrelated. The professional community is obliged not only to investigate, develop, and provide the best practices available, but also to do so as a partnership between researchers, practitioners, and parents.

THE CULTURAL APPROACH IN AUTISM

In addition to cooperation, shared efforts, and open communication between school and home, we should remember the importance of belief and faith. We should be aware of the cultural, psychological, and emotional realms of individuals whose lives are affected by autism, whether they are parents, professionals, or the autistic persons themselves. It is in the mutual interest of both parents and professionals to bridge the gaps mentioned between scientifically proven methods and nonscientific methods.

Every disorder is perceived differently by society. Cultural and societal values affect the way in which individuals deal with disorders and influence coping mechanisms and interventions that society adopts regarding the disorder. Different cultures may define and relate to a given disorder, and the definition of a particular disorder may influence specific interventions and reflect societal beliefs and values. An example of this can be seen in the manner in which the Jewish ultraorthodox community in Israel adopted facilitated communication (FC) techniques. Although this community generally relates to mental disorders as a form of social deviance, individuals with autism have been used by them to strengthen their core values and belief system. The person with autism, whose messages are interpreted through FC, is believed to serve as evidence of the innate human spirituality and of the unity of the Jewish people. This can be seen as an especially cogent example of how a system of local knowledge within a particular community can substantially alter the manner in which autism is viewed by its members.

One recurrent theme throughout this book is our obligation to try to learn as much as possible about the nature of autism, by conducting more research to determine the uniqueness of the disorder. As always, the more we investigate and the more we further our knowledge, the more questions arise. Our goal should be not only to look for answers but also to perfect the way we ask questions. Are we looking at developmental discontinuities along the same spectrum or are we looking at disparate and separate syndromes? Should we focus on subclassifying individuals with autism into smaller and more homogeneous groupings? If so, according to what criteria? Possible systems for classifying children with autism into subgroups based on their profiles may help develop understanding, and can be invaluable in planning more appropriate interventions in order to better service individuals with autism and their families.

Although we have not devoted a separate chapter to families, the centrality of the family in both research and intervention is addressed in each individual chapter. Etiological, biological, molecular-genetic, and familial research addresses both the genotype and phenotype of autism. In addition to the scientific study of families, there are emotional and practical issues that continually confront parents of children with autism and extended family members. Involving professionals and parents together in the continual challenge of treating and living with autism requires perseverance and collaboration.

As our understanding of the disorder improves, so will the strategies for intervention. Interventions should be based on an in-depth understanding of the nature of the impairment, and should follow a careful assessment of the autistic individual in different areas of functioning. It is immensely important to take into consideration the person's family and cultural surroundings. All attempts at planning interventions and treatments should involve a close working relationship between the professional and the family, always keeping in mind the need to bridge the gap between science, beliefs, culture, and the individual needs of children and their families. It is our hope that as our understanding of autism improves, it will enhance our ability to identify and meet the needs of individuals with autism.

Index